R. Hetzer

J. S. Rankin

C. A. Yankah (Eds.)

Mitral Valve Repair

R. Hetzer
J. S. Rankin
C. A. Yankah (Eds.)

Mitral Valve Repair

With 384 Figures and 31 Tables

Springer

Roland Hetzer, MD, PhD
Chairman
Professor of Surgery
Charité Medical University Berlin
Deutsches Herzzentrum Berlin
Augustenburger Platz 1, 13353 Berlin
Germany

Charles A. Yankah, MD, PhD
Professor of Surgery
Charité Medical University Berlin
Consultant Cardiothoracic & Vascular Surgeon
Deutsches Herzzentrum Berlin
Augustenburger Platz 1, 13353 Berlin
Germany

J. Scott Rankin, MD
Associate Clinical Professor of Surgery
Department of Cardiac Surgery
Vanderbilt University Medical Center
320 Lynnwood Blvd.
Nashville, TN 37205
USA

ISBN 978-3-7985-1972-5 Springer-Verlag Berlin Heidelberg New York

Bibliographic information Deutsche Bibliothek
The Deutsche Bibliothek lists this publication in Deutsche Nationalbibliographie;
detailed bibliographic data is available in the internet at <http://dnb.ddb.de>.

SpringerMedizin
Springer-Verlag GmbH
ein Unternehmen von Springer Science+Business
springer.de

Softcover re-print of the Hardcover 1st edition 2011

Planning: Renate Scheddin, Heidelberg
Project management: Ulrike Dächert, Heidelberg
Copy-Editing: Dr. Mary Gossen, Dietzenbach
Cover design: WMX Design GmbH, Heidelberg
Typesetting: TypoStudio Tobias Schaedla, Heidelberg, Germany

SPIN 12589470 18/5141 – 5 4 3 2 1 0

Preface: A success story in medicine

»There can be no more fascinating problem in surgery than the relief of pathological conditions of the valves of the heart.« ***Sir Henry Souttar, 1925***

Cardiac valve surgery was first proposed a century ago by Dr. Harvey Cushing at the Johns Hopkins Hospital, which is ironic since Cushing is generally considered the father of neurosurgery. However, it was Cushing's influence on his most illustrious student and successor in the Surgical Chairmanship at the Peter Bent Brigham hospital, Dr. Elliot Cutler, that led to the first heart valve operation – a mitral »valvotomy« for rheumatic mitral stenosis in 1923. But Cutler's concept of incising the anterior mitral leaflet led to worsening heart failure, and the operation was eventually abandoned.

Sir Henry Souttar at the London Hospital then performed a transatrial »commissurotomy« in 1925. The operation was successful, but was met with overwhelming criticism by the medical physician-in-charge, Sir James MacKenzie, who taught that heart failure in rheumatic disease was due primarily to myocarditis. So Sir Henry was referred no more patients for potential valve operations. In 1948, Dr. Charles Bailey performed the first successful modern mitral commissurotomy, amid clouds of controversy due to multiple previous fatal attempts. At that point, »closed mitral commissurotomy« and, more importantly, the surgical treatment of cardiac valve disease, attained general acceptance and, in appropriately selected patients, this first method of mitral repair was carried to high levels of efficacy by Brock, Dubost, Edwards, Logan, Smithy, Harken, and others.

With the advent of prosthetic mitral valves in the early 1960s, valve replacement for mitral disease became the primary therapy. However, through the late 1960s and the 1970s, mitral valve replacement was associated with operative mortality rates that were among the highest of any heart surgery, approximating 20-30% in many centers. Several individuals continued to work on mitral repair, most notably Ellis, McGoon, Kay, Gerbode, Frater, Wooler, Paneth, and Carpentier. Frater's statement published in 1962 was prophetic: *»The patient with a mitral prosthesis is a patient for life«* (The Lancet, 1962). By 1980, Carpentier had combined leaflet resection, ring annuloplasty, and chordal procedures into a unified approach, and his 1983 lecture before the American Association for Thoracic Surgery launched mitral repair as a routine clinical procedure. Subsequent work has shown better outcomes in virtually every mitral disease category with valve repair versus replacement and, a steadily widening spectrum of mitral repair is becoming the dominant procedure in mitral valve surgery. Currently, mitral repair is associated with less than a 1% operative mortality in many centers, and late results continue to improve to unprecedented levels. It is clear that the development of effective autologous reparative procedures for the treatment of mitral valve disease is one of the all-time ***success stories in medicine***.

Most cases of mitral valve disease can be successfully approached by repair in the developed countries, where mitral incompetence of degenerative and ischemic origin now prevail. Rheumatic valve disease is almost eradicated in this part of the world; however, it is still pertinent in areas which are still developing modern standards of medicine. Repair in rheumatic valve disease has been performed either by commissurotomy in pure stenosis or by newer complex techniques with autologous pericardial leaflet augmentation and chordal replacement. Still, in this disease a certain proportion of chronic cases with calcification may require valve replacement. Similarly, in active infective endocarditis, at least in cases with advanced destruction of the valve apparatus, repair may be unsuccessful. It may, however, be attempted even with some residual incompetence, well accepting that re-operation may become necessary at a time when the infection has been cured. Likewise mitral repair is the concept of choice in infancy and childhood, even with less than perfect immediate results, with planned re-operation when the child has thrived and grown, and even then repeat repair may be accomplished. Ischemic mitral incompetence, with its spectrum of pathomechanisms and degrees of severity of left ventricular function impairment, is steadily growing in terms of numbers of patients and will be an important mitral disease of the future. Indications for mitral operation and appropriate repair techniques for this setting are still under debate. There is now great enthusiasm for »minimally invasive« approaches to the mitral valve, either by small chest incisions and peripheral cannulation or even with the use of robotic techniques. Many patients are attracted by the cosmetic results and the rapid postoperative recovery after such procedures. However, a somewhat larger sub-mammary chest incision may add to safety and flexibility during the procedure and still be cosmetically acceptable.

The Berlin Mitral Valve Repair Symposium held at the joint meeting of the Society for Heart Valve Disease and the Heart Valve Society of America in June 2009 and this volume of proceedings were conceived to showcase current techniques and outcomes for mitral valve repair by many of the experts in the field. A variety of approaches have been described to give the reader a reference for critical assessment of multiple different surgical philosophies. It was felt that the presentation of several diverse approaches was a healthy concept to allow the reader to review options for future practice improvement. The individual authors have done an excellent work in presenting their information, and it is hoped that the surgical readership will appreciate and enjoy this book. Most importantly, it is our wish that patients worldwide will benefit from its contents.

R. Hetzer, A., J. S. Rankin, C. A. Yankah

Table of Contents

List of Authors

David H. Adams, MD
Professor and Chairman
Department of Cardiothoracic Surgery
The Mount Sinai Medical Center
New York, NY 10029
USA

Adanna Akujuo, MD
Department of Cardiothoracic Surgery
Mount Sinai School of Medicine
1190 Fifth Avenue
New York, NY 10029
USA

Ottavio Alfieri, MD
Professor and Chairman of Cardiac Surgery
Cardiac Surgery Department
San Raffaele University Hospital
20132 Milan
Italy

Aref Amiri, MD
Deutsches Herzzentrum Berlin
Department of Cardiothoracic and Vascular Surgery
Augustenburger Platz 1
13353 Berlin
Germany

Anelechi C Anyanwu, MD
Associate Professor
Department of Cardiothoracic Surgery
The Mount Sinai Medical Center
New York, NY 10029
USA

Robert S. Binford, MD
Attending Surgeon
Centennial Medical Center
Nashville, TN 37203
USA

Calvin A. Burrichter, MD
Attending Anesthesiologist
Centennial Medical Center
Nashville, TN 37203
USA

Louis A. Brunsting III, MD
Attending Surgeon
Centennial Medical Center
Nashville, TN 37203
USA

Javier G. Castillo, MD
Resident Physician
Department of Cardiothoracic Surgery
The Mount Sinai Medical Center
New York, NY
USA

Elena Cavarretta, MD
Cardiac Surgeon
Department of Molecular Medicine
»Sapienza« University of Rome
Viale Regina Margherita, 324
00161 Rome
Italy

Joanna Chikwe, MD
Department of Cardiothoracic Surgery
Mount Sinai School of Medicine
1190 Fifth Avenue
New York, NY 10029
USA

W. Randolph Chitwood, Jr., MD, FACS, FRCS (Eng.)
Professor and Chairman
Department of Cardiovascular Sciences
East Carolina Heart Institute
East Carolina University
Greenville, NC 27834
USA

Mani A. Daneshmand, MD
Fellow in Cardiothoracic Surgery
Duke University Medical Center
Durham, NC 27710
USA

Michele De Bonis, MD
Staff Cardiac Surgeon
Cardiac Surgery Department
San Raffaele University Hospital
20132 Milan
Italy

Eva Maria B. Delmo Walter, MD, MSc, PhD
Department of Cardiothoracic and Vascular Surgery
Deutsches Herzzentrum Berlin
Augustenburger Platz 1
13353 Berlin
Germany

Dr. Robert W.M. Frater, MBChB, MS(Surg), FRCS, FACS
Emeritus Professor of Cardiothoracic Surgery
Albert Einstein College of Medicine and
Montefiore Medical Center
24 Prescott Ave
Bronxville, NY 10708
USA

Jeffrey G. Gaca, MD
Assistant Professor of Surgery
Duke University Medical Center
Durham, NC 27710
USA

Donald D. Glower, MD
Professor of Surgery
Duke University Medical Center
Durham, NC 27710
USA

Andrew B. Goldstone, MD
Department of Cardiothoracic Surgery
Mount Sinai School of Medicine
1190 Fifth Avenue
New York, NY 10029
USA

Roland Hetzer, MD, PhD
Chairman
Professor of Surgery
Charité Medical University Berlin
Deutsches Herzzentrum Berlin
Augustenburger Platz 1
13353 Berlin
Germany

Michael Hübler, MD
Deutsches Herzzentrum Berlin
Dept. of Cardiothoracic and Vascular Surgery
Augustenburger Platz 1
13353 Berlin
Germany

Afksendiyos Kalangos, MD, PhD, FETCS, DSci (Hon)
Professor and Chairman
Division of Cardiovascular Surgery
University Hospitals of Geneva
Rue Gabrielle-Perret-Gentil 4
1211 Geneva 14
Switzerland

Carmelo A. Milano, MD
Professor of Surgery
Duke University Medical Center
Durham, NC 27710
USA

Friedrich Wilhelm Mohr, MD, PhD
Professor and Chairman
Leipzig Heart Center
Leipzig University
Struempellstrasse 39
04289 Leipzig
Germany

Michele Musci, MD, PhD
Cardiac Surgeon
Deutsches Herzzentrum Berlin
Department of Cardiothoracic and Vascular Surgery
Augustenburger Platz 1
13353 Berlin
Germany

Nicole Nagdyman, MD, PhD
Pediatric Cardiologist
Deutsches Herzzentrum Berlin
Department of Cardiothoracic and
Vascular Surgery
Augustenburger Platz 1
13353 Berlin
Germany

Boris A. Nasseri, MD
Attending Cardiac Surgeon
Deutsches Herzzentrum Berlin
Augustenburger Platz 1
13353 Berlin
Germany

Miralem Pasic, MD, PhD
Professor of Surgery
Deutsches Herzzentrum Berlin
Department of Cardiothoracic and
Vascular Surgery
Augustenburger Platz 1
13353 Berlin
Germany

J. Scott Rankin, MD
Associate Clinical Professor of
Surgery
Department of Cardiac Surgery
Vanderbilt University Medical Center
320 Lynnwood Blvd.
Nashville, TN 37205
USA

Evelio Rodriguez, MD, FACS
Department of Cardiovascular Sciences
East Carolina Heart Institute
East Carolina University
Greenville, NC 27834
USA

Loris Salvador, MD, FECTS
Head of the Cardiac Surgery Division
San Bortolo Hospital
Viale Rodolfi, 37
36100 Vicenza
Italy

Joerg Seeburger, MD
Leipzig Heart Center
Leipzig University
Struempellstrasse 39
04289 Leipzig
Germany

Henryk Siniawski, MD, PhD
Charité Medical University Berlin
Deutsches Herzzentrum Berlin
Augustenburger Platz 1
13353 Berlin
Germany

Peter K. Smith, MD
Professor of Surgery and Chief Cardiothoracic
Surgery
Duke University Medical Center
Durham, NC 27710
USA

Christof Stamm, MD, PhD
Attending Cardiac Surgeon
Professor
Deutsches Herzzentrum Berlin
Augustenburger Platz 1
13353 Berlin
Germany

Carlo Valfrè, MD
Head of Cardiovascular Department
Treviso Regional Hospital
piazza Ospedale, 1
31100 Treviso
Italy

Walter G. Wolfe, MD
Professor of Surgery
Duke University Medical Center
Durham, NC 27710
USA

Yuguo Weng, MD
Deutsches Herzzentrum Berlin
Dept. of Cardiothoracic and Vascular Surgery
Augustenburger Platz 1
13353 Berlin
Germany

Charles A. Yankah, MD, PhD
Professor of Surgery
Charité Medical University Berlin
Consultant Cardiothoracic & Vascular Surgeon
Deutsches Herzzentrum Berlin
Augustenburger Platz 1
13353 Berlin
Germany

I Imaging of the mitral valve

Perioperative echocardiographic imaging of mitral valve incompetence

H. Siniawski, M. Hübler, A. Amiri, C.A. Yankah, R. Hetzer

1.1 Introduction

The concept of using the echocardiography machine in the operating room fulfills the need for intraoperative diagnosis. Immediately after the completion of a surgical intervention the outcome can be verified and, if the initial results are not optimal, surgical correction may be performed. Examination by stethoscope in the operating room is not sufficient and it was discovered that patients were doing poorly after closed commissurotomy if a systolic murmur was present, whereas those without a systolic murmur did not suffer from hemodynamic problems and had satisfactory outcomes. Persistent mitral regurgitation after commissurotomy was recognized as a significant clinical problem that needs to be avoided. This fact probably triggered the surgeons' desire for a precise intraoperative diagnostic method, and the requirements of such a method caused them to fix on echocardiography as the ideal tool for this function.

Perioperative echocardiography means that echocardiographic investigation is undertaken for assessment in the preoperative period, usually to establish the indication for surgery, in many cases with the consequence of follow-up in the operating room and, in the majority of patients, in the postoperative period for follow-up investigation after surgery.

Preoperative and intraoperative investigation challenges the echocardiographer to take on at least partial responsibility for the outcome of surgery, rather than his or her role being limited to establishing the indication for surgery. As a consequence, in many surgical cases, incluing reconstruction operations and even routine operations, more pharmacological intervention is possible, and this helps a better quality of treatment to be reached. Mitral valve reconstruction surgery is a procedure in which intraoperative investigation is obligatory.

1.2 Historical development of perioperative echocardiography

Before color Doppler was invented by the Japanese surgeon Riso Omoto (ALOKA, Japan), the investigation was based on black-and-white two-dimensional (2D) open chest (epicardial) echocardiography. In general, mitral regurgitation assessment was based on a single window of pulsed Doppler requiring »mapping« of the left atrium (LA). The term mapping indicates the time-consuming procedure of searching for a regurgitant jet in the LA by measuring the blood flow velocity in different directions in the atrium (jet area). The problem of this time-consuming assessment of mitral regurgitation was later avoided by intraoperative use of a simple contrast agent, which helped to identify the regurgitant area in the LA [1, 2].

The introduction of the echocardiography machine with color Doppler by ALOKA Japan in 2001 revolutionized intraoperative investigation. Color Doppler or multipulsed coded Doppler gives details of flow characteristics and the distribution of jets inside the chamber in real time and real motion. In other words, visualization of intracardiac flow gives us the opportunity not only to view but also to measure flow phenomena, including a regurgitant jet, immediately after the surgical procedure is completed. Color Doppler has also significantly shortened the time required for quantitative mitral regurgitation assessment after mitral valve reconstruction and after basic recovery of the circulation after cardiopulmonary bypass is stopped [3, 4].

Open chest echocardiography allowed us to use a high frequency echocardiographic probe to achieve high resolution images without artifacts. The transducer was covered in a plastic sleeve to maintain a sterile operating field. It was necessary to place ultrasonic gel inside the sleeve to obliterate the air space between the face of the transducer and the sleeve.

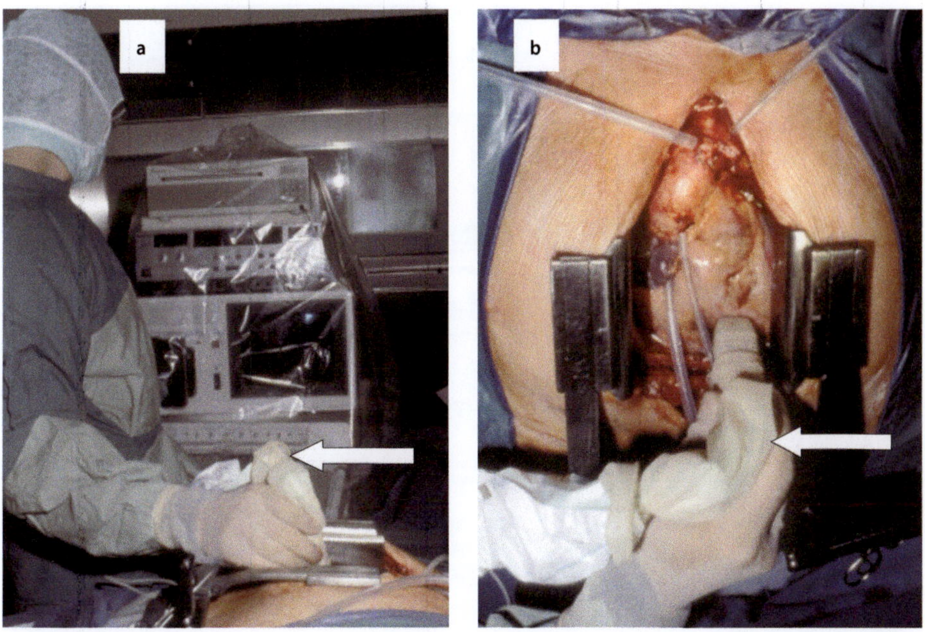

Fig. 1.1. Photographs taken in an operating room at the end of the 1980s during open chest color Doppler echocardiography. **a** Note the preparations made by the echocardiographer. At that time industry was not always able to supply sterile plastic sleeves of adequate size. Instead sterile surgical gloves (white arrow) filled with sterile physiological saline were used to cover the echocardiographic probe (5.0 MHz). **b** Open chest and opened pericardium during echocardiographic investigation

The covered transducer was positioned directly on the heart to view the heart structures and function, as in transthoracic echocardiographic examination (Fig. 1.1a, b).

Epicardial investigation interfered with surgical activity; nevertheless the investigation remained in use, especially in reconstructive surgery, until the end of the 1980s and in some cases is still a time honored investigation. The high quality 2D and color Doppler images satisfied operating teams (Fig. 1.2). What was most important in this means of investigation was that the number of heart sections was not limited by the anatomical position of the heart inside the chest, as is the case when using the transthoracic or even transesophageal approach. All heart structures could be visualized, including the papillary muscle and chordae, and the artifacts produced by chest structures did not interfere with or obscure the echocardiographic views. Some surgeons even preferred to use the echocardiographic transducer themselves to complete the diagnostic work, believing that first hand images are better than the second hand information from the cardiologist.

Nevertheless, the invention of transesophageal investigations (TEE) revolutionized intraoperative echocardiographic activity and opened up new possibilities. The idea of using a flexible gastroscope armed with an ultrasound transducer came from Europe but the technical development was performed in Japan. Dr. Feigenbaum from Minneapolis (MN) was the first to use a prototype of the transesophageal transducer around 1970. It was suggested that he undertake development of the TEE technology but he declined to explore this tool and several years later explained, »I could not imagine that the patient would swallow such a probe for the sake of diagnosis« [5]. The first prototype was not as small as the models used today, but numerous

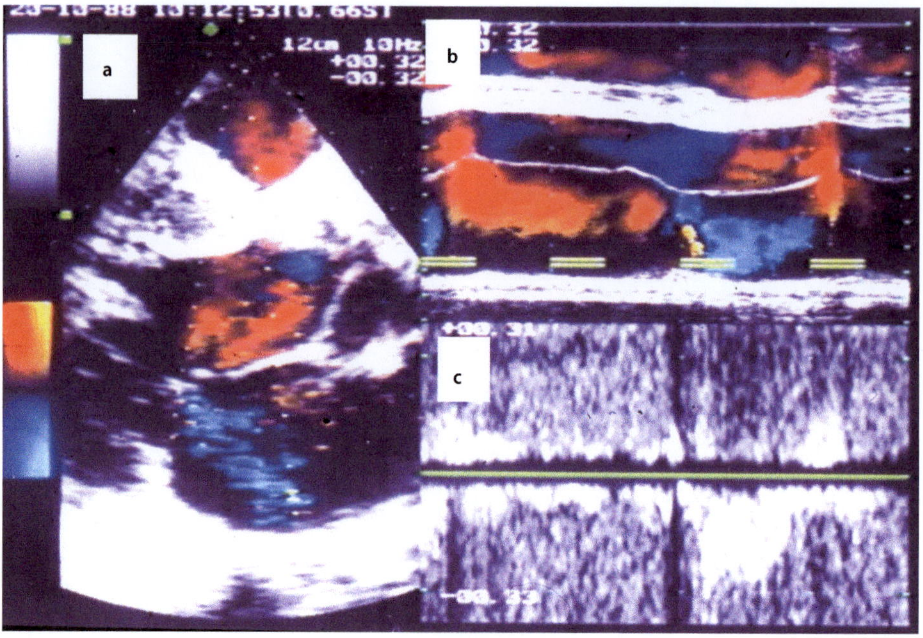

Fig. 1.2. Open chest mode of investigation (1988); images of the heart recorded in real time/real motion mode simultaneously by the following echocardiographic techniques: long-axis 2D color Doppler (**a**), M-mode color picture of left atrium (**b**), pulsed Doppler placed on the mitral regurgitation jet area (**c**)

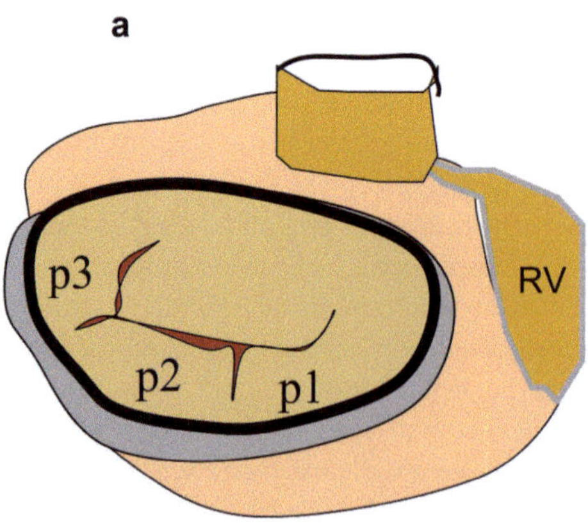

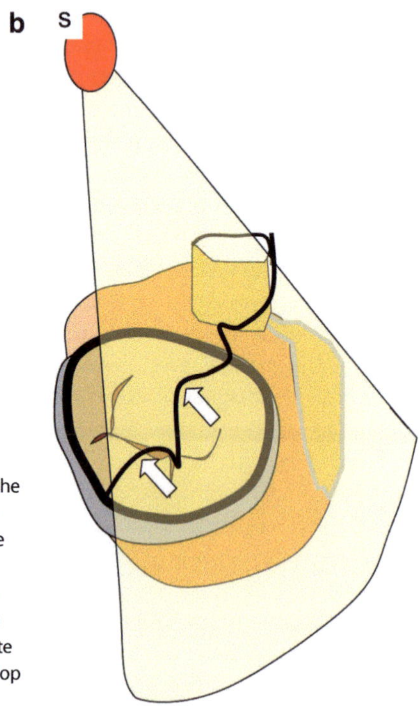

Fig. 1.3. a Schematic drawing of mitral valve, viewed from the esophagus after left atrium excision. Posterior mitral leaflet in normal patients demonstrates visible scallops (*P1* to *P3*), while the anterior mitral leaflet does not show functional scallops if the disease is not severely extended. **b** Section of TEE taken from upper part of esophagus (*s* echocardiographic probe) to demonstrate the 5-chamber view which is able to demonstrate only the central part of anterior mitral leaflet and middle scallop of posterior mitral leaflet (*P2*) (*arrows*). *RV* right ventricle

technical developments led to optimized resolution and a decrease in size, making the device applicable for investigation using the transesophageal approach. This new equipment not only heralded new possibilities in cardiology; it was also very useful in the operating room.

The images were similar in quality to those received using the epicardial approach and it was not necessary to interrupt the surgeons. However there are some limitations of heart structure visualization. The location of some anatomical structures of the mitral valve and its mitral apparatus means that visualization is not always easy and in some situations, for example hypovolemia, special maneuvers are necessary (◘ Figs. 1.3–1.5). Visualization of all scallops of the mitral valve requires multisectional visualization (◘ Figs. 1.3–1.7) and a lower view known as the »gastric« view is usually necessary to complete the investigation (◘ Fig. 1.7). In

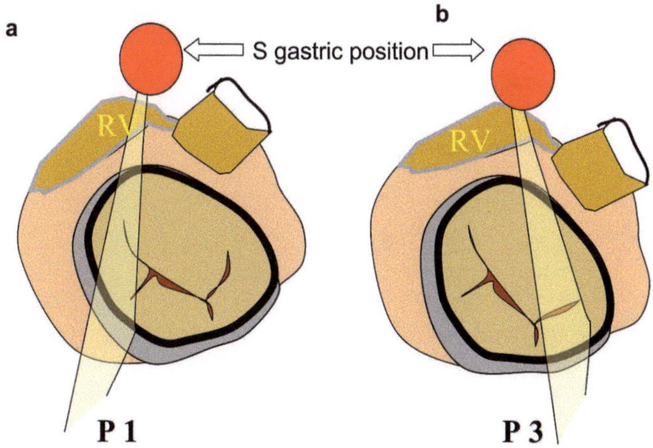

◘ **Fig. 1.4.** Section of TEE taken from gastric view (gastric position of echocardiograph probe »*s*«) for visualization of P1 (**a**) and P2 (**b**). *RV* right ventricle

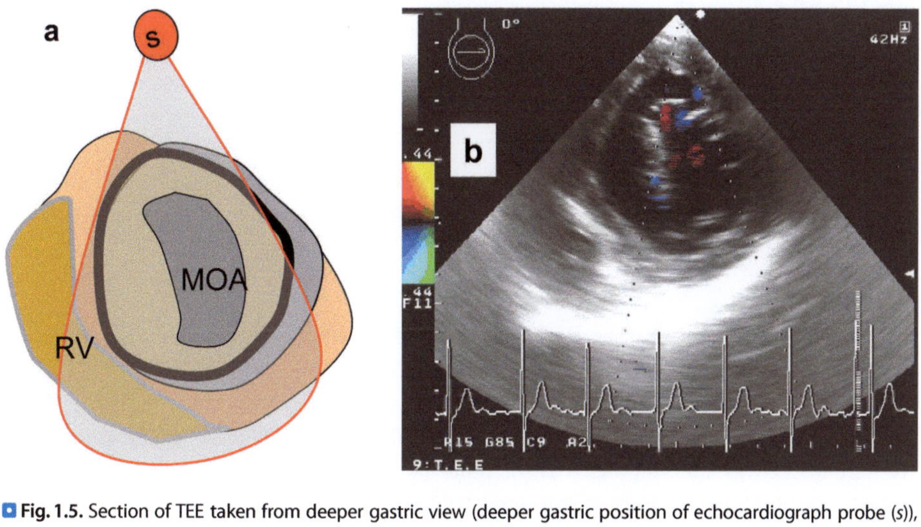

◘ **Fig. 1.5.** Section of TEE taken from deeper gastric view (deeper gastric position of echocardiograph probe (*s*)), **a** for visualization of the opening area of the mitral valve (*MOA*). **b** Echocardiographic image of the section presented schematically in **a**. *RV* right ventricle

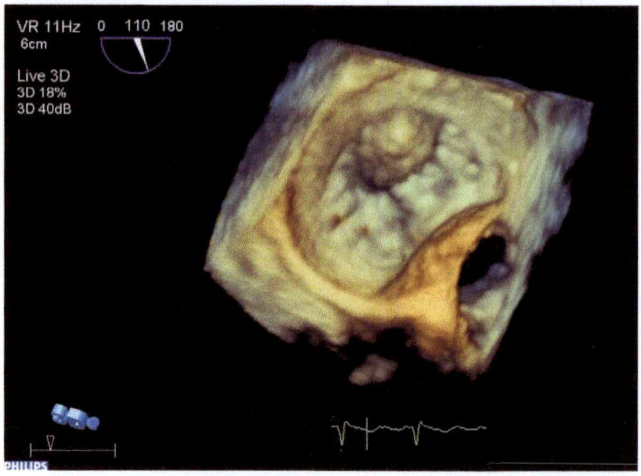

Fig. 1.6. Three-dimensional TEE image of mitral valve disease. (We thank Michael Gräfe MD, PhD for providing this image.)

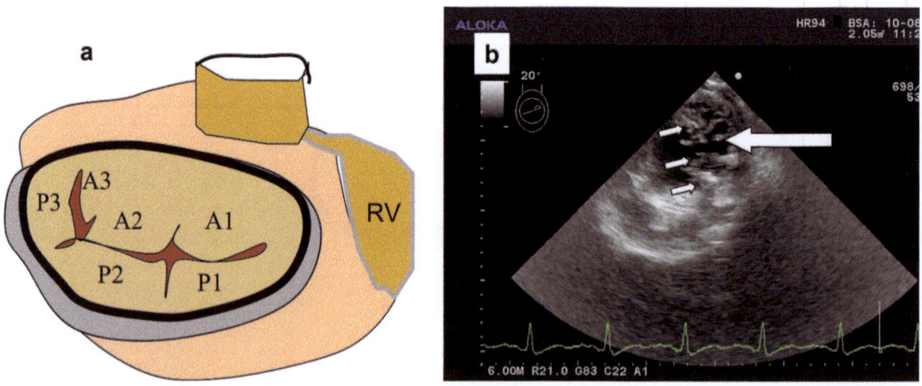

Fig. 1.7. a Schematic presentation of marfanoid (Barlow's) mitral valve in the short-axis view. The anterior mitral valve is composed of structures like scallops (*small arrows*) which are not formed in a regular way as the posterior mitral leaflet (ruptured PML, *large arrows*) but indicates presence of excessive tissue. The accessory scallops can also be present in the PML. Large opening area and mitral annulus dilatation are also present. *RV* right ventricle

addition, three-dimensional (3D) images of the mitral valve are not always precise enough to make intraoperative decisions based on the 3D images alone; however, the images are very helpful in understanding the anatomic topography of the pathology (Fig. 1.6).

1.3 Perioperative echocardiography at the Deutsches Herzzentrum Berlin

Since the Deutsches Herzzentrum Berlin (DHZB) was founded in 1986, the initiative of Professor Roland Hetzer was to establish well-functioning perioperative echocardiography. We were facing the same problems as the other pioneers at that time. The most important problem was the quantification of mitral regurgitation when focusing on mitral reconstruction. Angiography–at that time–was generally recognized as the gold standard for regurgitation quantification so the challenge was to try to find correlations between color Doppler

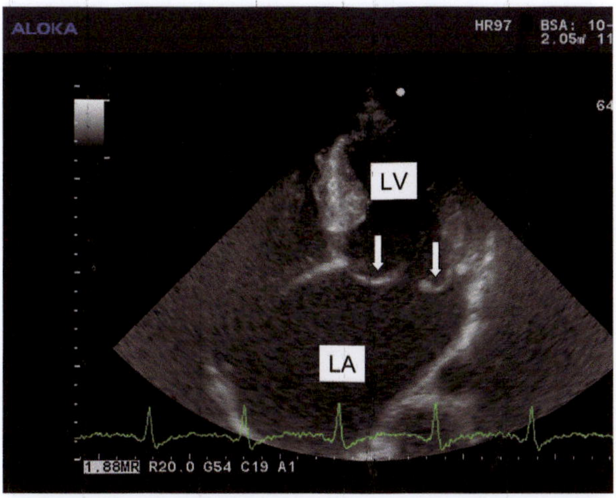

Fig. 1.8. Closed chest (TTE) 4-chamber view of »marfanoid« (Barlow's) valve. Thickened mitral valve and prolapsed AML and PML indicate pathology (*arrows*). *LV* left ventricle, *LA* left atrium

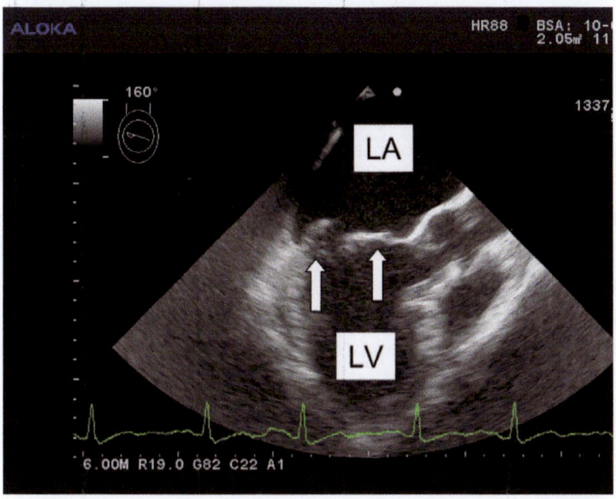

Fig. 1.9. TEE of marfanoid (Barlow's) valve. Prolapsing thickened valve is indicated by *arrows* (PML and AML). *LV* left ventricle, *LA* left atrium

phenomena and intraoperative angiography. Mitral reconstruction and angiography were performed by Professor Hetzer after cardiopulmonary bypass weaning intraoperatively and the angiographic assessment was correlated with epicardially assessed color flow phenomena. After completing investigations in ten reconstructive procedures, we established that early postoperative angiography in the operating room does not help to define the mitral reconstruction procedure and that echocardiographic assessment as a monitoring option represents a stable method of investigation, although the criteria were not optimal. Special attention was paid to preoperative assessment of the disease.

The introduction of echocardiographic examination into the operating room in the DHZB was based on the epicardial mode of investigation (Fig. 1.1). Intraoperative assessment of valvular lesions was able to add vital information to the diagnosis established preoperatively (Fig. 1.8–1.10).

Before the cardiopulmonary bypass machine is running or any surgical or interventional repair [6] is started, basic measurements should be undertaken and the results should be

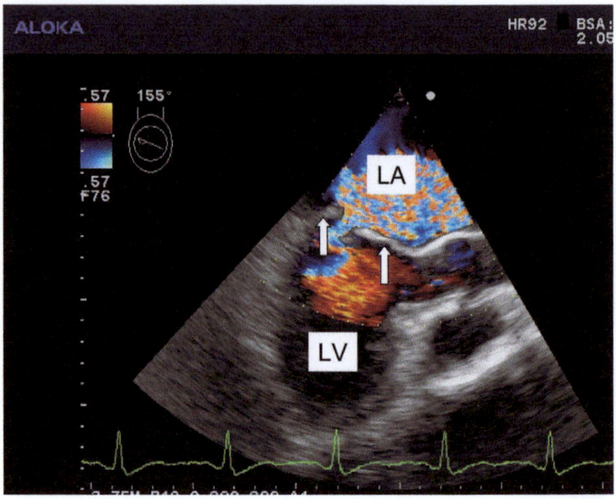

Fig. 1.10. Color Doppler TEE of the same patient as in Fig. 1.9. The prolapsing valve is marked by *arrows*. A large regurgitation jet filling the left atrium is visible. *LV* left ventricle, *LA* left atrium

compared to those found preoperatively. Anesthesia and other medication [7] can strongly influence the preoperative results, mainly by reducing afterload and preload and lowering the grade of the valve incompetence. Ischemic mitral incompetence–especially if it is purely functional (not dependent on scar but on ischemic myocardium)–can be significantly reduced, but only temporarily. The intraoperative investigation should include measurement of the mitral valve opening area and assessment of mitral regurgitation and wall motion disturbances, right ventricle (RV) and left ventricle (LV) global function and volume, and valvular and subvalvular apparatus function. In the great majority of cases, valve function assessment after reconstruction does not identify any remaining problems, if the surgeon is skilled and mitral repair is optimal. The reconstructed valve is usually competent or only slightly incompetent and a small jet means only slight regurgitation. Quantification of regurgitation is very seldom of use. If it emerges that regurgitation is present postoperatively, the preoperative investigation is very helpful as a guide for the evaluation of the jet and of valve function in general. Basic hemodynamic stabilization has to be maintained after the repair procedure is finished to make Doppler recording possible. Before hemodynamics are stabilized, the morphology of the reconstructed valve can be assessed and hemodynamic valve function can be evaluated by spontaneous contrast observation, as reported elsewhere [8].

1.4 Mitral annulus

In our cohort, mitral annulus pathology was not the main causative factor for regurgitation; however, the function of this structure plays a secondary but still important role in almost all forms of mitral valve disease. This is in agreement with the findings of other publications dealing with the function of the mitral ring [9]. This statement does not contradict findings that the function of the mitral ring cannot be neglected after mitral reconstruction surgery. The size of the mitral annulus has been measured in the past in autopsy and during surgical investigations [10], and more recent investigative methods (including MRI) have clarified the functional importance of this 3D structure [11]. Mitral valve reconstruction surgery should not use artificial fabric materials to avoid the risk of endocarditis, also in nonendocarditic mitral valve disease. This is the official policy of the DHZB and the pericardium is used as a source for reinforcement of the mitral annulus plasty (Gerbode–Hetzer) to keep the reconstructed ring flexible [12]. Since 2002, the pericardial strip has been used in all cases for this purpose. Our echocardiographic studies revealed good results (mitral regurgitation of <grade 1 and mitral opening area >2.7 cm²) of reconstruction procedures in 97% of patients suffering from nonischemic mitral valve disease early after operation and in long-term studies. The good results of mitral reconstruction surgery prompt early correction of mitral regurgitation in symptomatic as well as asymptomatic patients, instead of a »watch and wait« strategy.

1.5 Importance of the subvalvular apparatus

The importance of the subvalvular apparatus is well documented [13, 14, 15]. Our study comparing the long-term outcome of mitral reconstruction and mitral replacement with complete subvalvular apparatus reconstruction in patients suffering from ischemic mitral incompetence also proved the importance of integration of the subvalvular apparatus after mitral surgery (◘ Figs. 1.11 and 1.12). Surgical correction of mitral valve disease is still based on mitral replacement. The technique of replacement with full preservation of the subvalvular apparatus published by Hetzer et al. in 1983 [16] opened the way for the Rushmer [17] and later the Lillehei [18] concept to restore heart function postoperatively in patients suffering from mitral valve disease. The preservation of the subvalvular apparatus in ischemic and nonischemic mitral surgery became a fundamental achievement in developing optimal surgical results [19]. The preserved papillary muscles provide systolic–diastolic elastic support similar to the two »hands« in ◘ Fig. 1.12. Nevertheless, perfectly performed mitral valve reconstruction offers better early and long-term results [20] and is the first choice for mitral surgery [21].

1.6 Echocardiographic assessment of mitral regurgitation

There are several problems to be avoided in measuring mitral regurgitation quantitatively but, if important principles are adhered to, and in experienced hands, echocardiography can be a very accurate method [22, 23]. Historically, the severity of mitral regurgitation was assessed qualitatively by measuring the area of regurgitation jet propagation by pulse Doppler [24] and, later, by color flow imaging [25, 26]. The regurgitation can be semi-quantified–as in angiography–on a scale of 1/4 to 4/4 [27]. This method has not lost its value today. The principle »a large jet indicates great regurgitation and a small jet small regurgitation« continues to be valid. Quantification of mitral regurgitation can be undertaken using Doppler echocardiography (if the hemodynamics allow it) by measurement of the differences between mitral stroke and aortic stroke volume [28, 29]. The phenomenon of proximal isovelocity flow area, which corresponds to anatomic leakage, is used to measure the regurgitant volume known as proximal flow convergence [30]. All modern echocardiography machines possess a program for easy measurement of the regurgitation volume based on these principles. Regurgitation volume <30 ml indicates mild regurgitation, 30–59 ml moderate, and >60 ml severe regurgitation [31]. Speaking generally the proximal isovelocity area and distal jet area, which are both measures of the leakage area of the mitral valve in Doppler, virtually define regurgitation. In other words, both methods are trying to describe the same thing (exemplified in the sketch by an animal) or, so to speak, the animal based on either the proximal area (head) or from

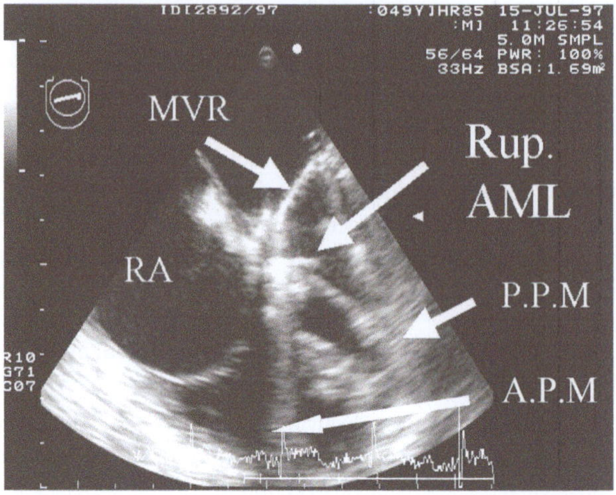

Fig. 1.11. Transesophageal 4-chamber view of the heart after mitral valve replacement (St. Jude Medical prosthesis) with totally preserved subvalvular apparatus. *MVR* mitral valve replacement, *P.P.M* posterior papillary muscle, *A.P.M* anterior papillary muscle, *Rup.* small chordae rupture after subvalvular apparatus reconstruction without clinical significance, *RA* right atrium

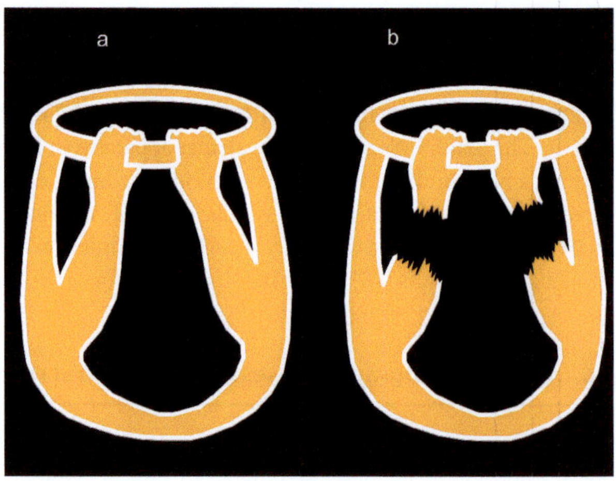

Fig. 1.12. Schematic illustration of the importance of the subvalvular apparatus, with subvalvular papillary muscle preservation (**a**) and without preservation (**b**)

behind (the body) or from the neck only (vena contracta) (Fig. 1.13) [32]. In some ways, the three methods should be complementary to each other. However, certain factors of flow mechanics can influence all phenomena. One of these is asymmetric jet or asymmetric area of proximal isovelocity area produced by the nonregular morphology of the valve. In such cases, the problem of energy being absorbed by the atrial wall diminishes the color Doppler area and falsely indicates a negative regurgitant grade.

1.7 Importance of intraoperative investigation: can the durability of reconstruction surgery be predicted?

In the literature, it is well documented that the spectrum of valve dysfunction is generally well defined on the basis of 2D and Doppler echocardiography [33, 34, 35]; both preoperatively [36] and intraoperatively, these investigations become important in directing surgical activ-

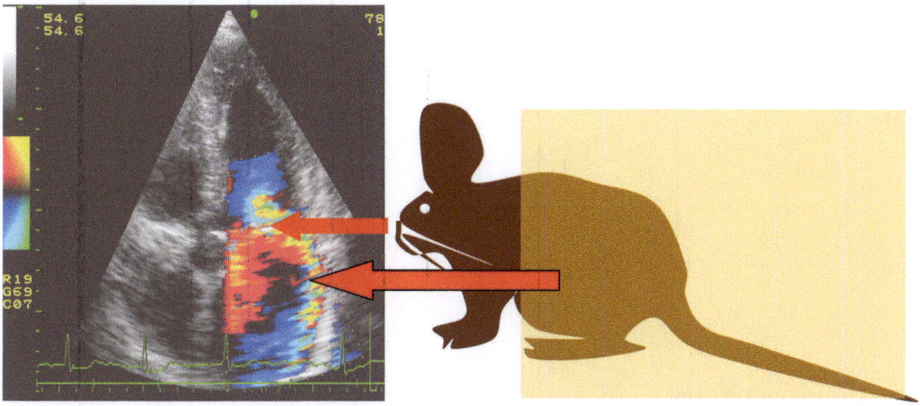

Fig. 1.13. Schematic giving an impression of two different regurgitation assessments based on color Doppler TTE; proximal to the anatomic location of leakage isovelocity area (convergence) indicated as the head of the animal and the colored area in the image representing jet regurgitation located behind anatomical leakage indicated by the corpus of animal

ity (Figs.1.14 –1.18) [37, 38]. This is probably one of the most important factors helping surgeons not only to reach the title of »experienced valve surgeon« but also to gain the title »reference valve surgeon« [39].

Our study [42] revealed the importance of intraoperative transthoracic echocardiography (TEE) investigation for surgical ischemic mitral reconstruction in improving long-term outcome. The excellent surgical results deemed to show no or only small (<grade I) regurgitation resulted in significantly better long-term outcome than in the group of patients whose surgical results were assessed intraoperatively as »acceptable« (<grade II regurgitation). This study also revealed that only reconstruction with excellent results offers better long-term outcome (7 years) than mitral valve replacement with complete subvalvular apparatus preservation [40]. The significance of intraoperative investigation depends not only on the echocardiographer's experience but also on the surgical technique, which is presumably why some other researchers found an absence of a correlation between the intraoperative echocardiographically assessed surgical quality and durability of the mitral reconstruction in the long term [41].

1.8 Degenerative mitral valve disease

Degenerative mitral valve disease is a frequent valve disorder and is continually the subject of error in terms of its clinical importance and mode of treatment. The basic information regarding this mitral lesion may be traced to the early 1800s. In 1831, J. Hope recognized the relationship between auscultatory phenomena and mitral regurgitation [42] and C.J.B. Williams established the association between systolic murmur and postmortem diagnosed rupture of the mitral chordae [43].

The concept of the importance of mitral valve disease and the relation of the disease to connective tissue disorder was rediscovered in the 1960s and 1970s, among others by Read et al. [44], McKay and Yacoub [45], but Barlow's research is probably the most recognized in this respect. There is a broad spectrum of degenerative mitral valve disease, ranging from

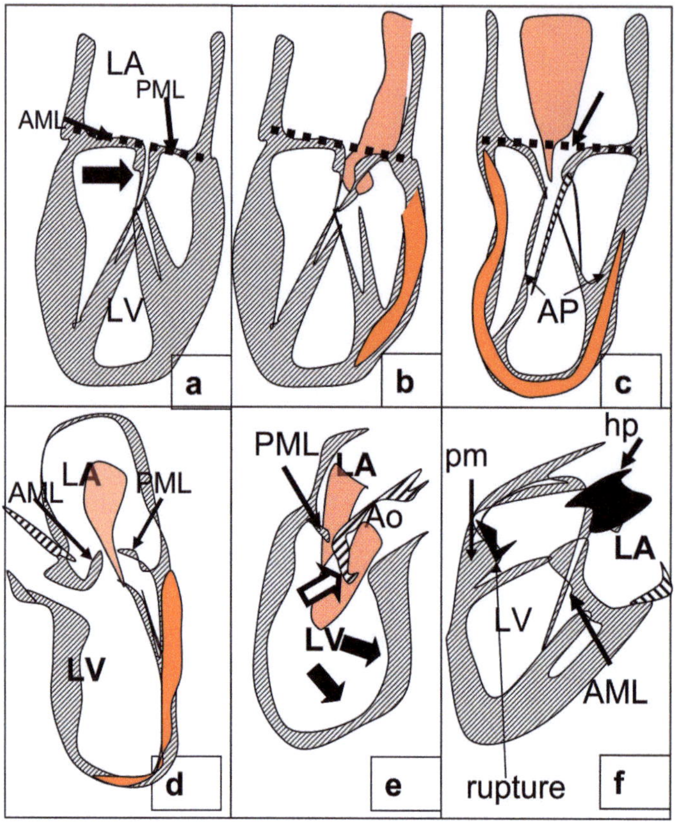

Fig. 1.14. Spectrum of mitral incompetence of ischemic origin: **a–c** show drawings similar to TEE 4-chamber view; **d, e** TEE modified 5-chamber view; **f** modified 2-chamber view from transesophageal image. Scar of the myocardium after myocardial infarction is shown in *orange*. Regurgitation jet in the left atrium (*LA*) is *red*. **a** Normally functioning left ventricle (*LV*) chamber, mitral valve, and subvalvular apparatus. *Dashed line* indicates mitral ring position with preserved mitral valve function by restoration of physiological position of the anterior mitral leaflet (*AML*) and posterior mitral leaflet (*PML*) tips visible as sufficient coaptation (*black arrow*). **b** Asymmetrical restriction of the mitral valve in patients after myocardial infarction localized at the lateral wall. In this case the posterior leaflet is more restricted than the AML. This constellation (the position of the AML and PML) also produces an asymmetrical mitral regurgitation jet steered toward the lateral wall of the atrium. In such cases, it is important to not underestimate the severity of the mitral regurgitation because the Conanda effect (absorption of the jet's energy by the atrial wall) is responsible for energy loss of the jet. **c** Anterolateral scar responsible for the same grade of anterior and posterior wall dysfunction and producing AML and PML symmetrical restriction indicated by central regurgitation jet in left atrium. **d, e** TEE 5-chamber view. Note **D** is drawn with classical localization of the aorta on the left side, while **e** is the mirror image of **d** (aorta at the right side). **d** This sketch represents rather seldom occurring constellation of mitral valve prolapse probably caused by scar formation extended to the posterior papillary muscle with consequent significant dilatation of the subvalvular apparatus (posterior part) leading to prolapse of the AML and PML. This situation is possible when patients are suffering from a prolapsing mitral valve primarily with development of infarction. **e** Intraoperative development of de novo systolic anterior movement (SAM) phenomenon after urgent surgical revascularization of patients suffering from enzyme positive instable angina and mitral repair of coexisting degenerative mitral valve disease (P2 rupture). Note the color flow pattern configured in TEE as »Y« steering with high velocity from the left chamber into the aorta (*Ao*) and left atrium at the same time. The cause of SAM (*white arrow*) is provoked by anterior wall dyskinesia and posterior wall hyperkinesia (two *black arrows*). **f** Rupture of the head of posterior papillary muscle in a case with isolated circumflex occlusion. The »flail« posterior muscle hanging on the anterior and posterior leaflet in systole is visible in the left atrium (*black object*). *AP* anterior/posterior, pm papillary muscle, *hp* ruptured papillary muscle

the simple form to severe degenerative pathomorphological lesions [46] usually known as Barlow's mitral valve.

Barlow's mitral valve is known for deformation of the valve and enlarged opening area, in some individuals up to 12.5 cm^2, with excessive enlargement of the leaflet tissue leading to prolapse and anatomical rupture of multiple scallops. In such cases, it is possible to distinguish the presence of scallops on the anterior mitral leaflet (AML) (◘ Figs. 1.7–1.9). At the DHZB, the frequently encountered degenerative form of mitral valve disease was traditionally called »marfanoid mitral valve«, which corresponds with Barlow's valve, and was found in 15% of our preoperatively studied cohort of patients (◘ Figs. 1.8–1.10).

1.9 Ischemic mitral incompetence

Ischemic mitral incompetence is a subdivision of functional mitral incompetence and is a complication of ischemic heart disease leading to congestive heart failure [47] and doubling

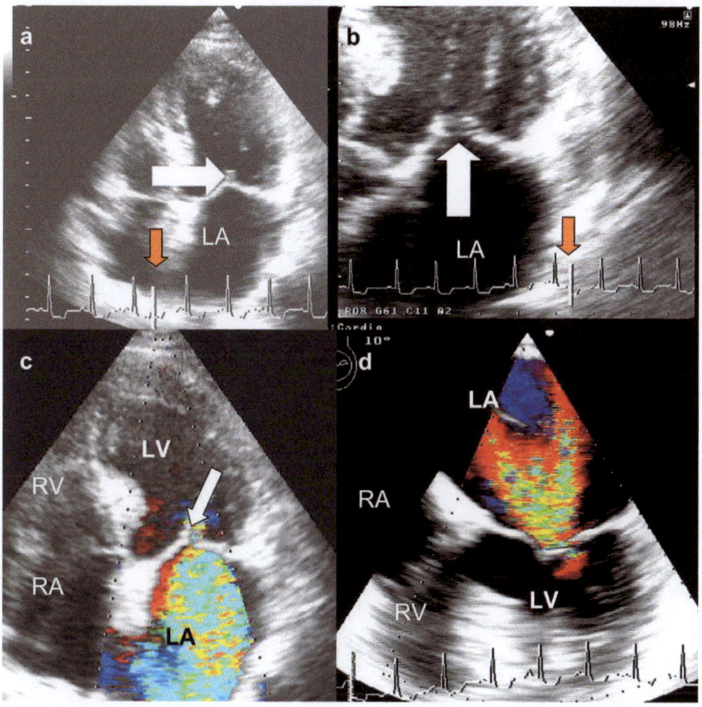

◘ **Fig. 1.15a–d.** Echocardiographic images taken during midejection (*red arrows* indicate on echocardiography (ECG) the time the image was taken) from the some patient suffering from ischemic mitral incompetence. Only **d** is taken using the transesophageal approach during the same period as **a**. **a** The 4-chamber view demonstrating a symmetric type of restrictive pattern of the mitral valve. Coaptation seems to be preserved (*white arrow*) because the section is through the preserved part of the mitral valve (to aid understanding see ◘ Fig. 1.4). **b** Echocardiographic image showing modification of the previously taken section. In this view, a gap between the AML and PML is clearly visible (*white arrow*). This middle part of the mitral valve is severely restrictive and causes severe mitral incompetence as shown in **c** and **d**. *LV* left ventricle, *LA* left atrium, *RV* right ventricle, *RA* right atrium

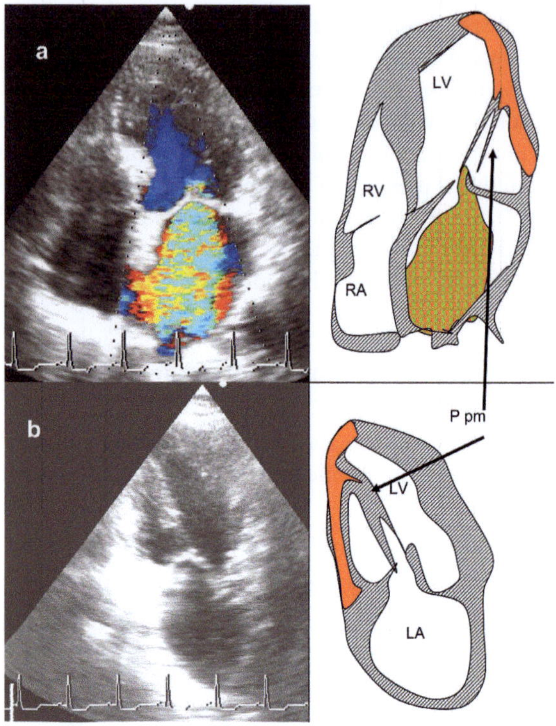

Fig. 1.16. Mitral valve prolapse coexists with ischemic heart disease (persistent myocardial infarction scar area in *orange*). **a** Beginning of systole with pronounced mitral valve prolapse; **b** late systole with profound mitral prolapse causing severe mitral regurgitation (not presented in color Doppler). *LV* left ventricle, *LA* left atrium, *RV* right ventricle, *RA* right atrium, *P pm* posterior papillary muscle

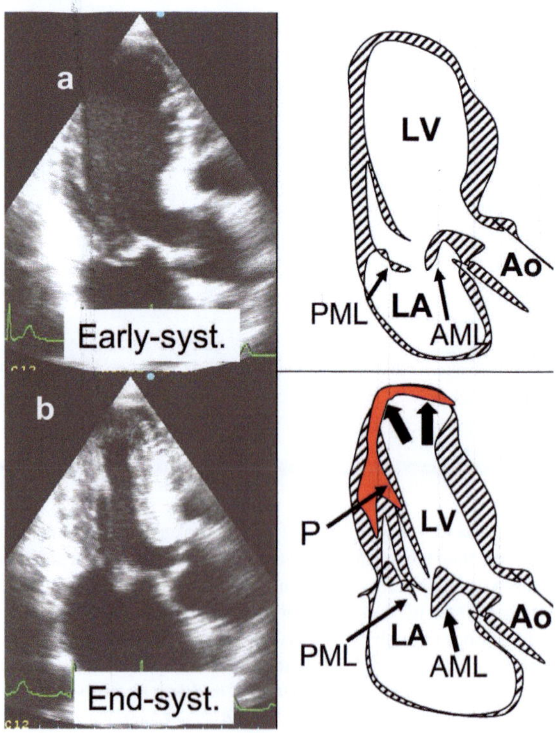

Fig. 1.17. Echocardiographic examinations in **a** and **b** belongs to the same patient as in Fig. 1.15. The images demonstrates localization of scar (*orange area*) on the posterior and lateral wall and scarification of posterior papillary muscle (*P pm*; *arrows* in **a** and **b**). This posterior papillary muscle is connected to both the anterior mitral leaflets (*AML*) and the posterior mitral leaflet (*PML*). Elongation of muscle is present but not sufficient to maintain correct coaptation. Both leaflets remain in restrictive position, producing significant restrictive mitral regurgitation. *LA* left atrium, *Ao* aorta, *P* posterior infarction, *LV* left ventricle

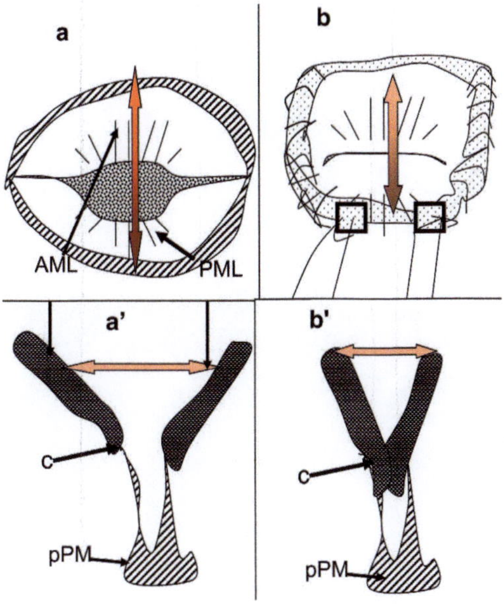

Fig. 1.18. Schematic presentation of Paneth plasty modified by Hetzer. **a** Drawing of the mitral valve in systole demonstrates leakage of the mitral valve produced by tethering of the subvalvular apparatus (**a'**). **b** After successfully performed annulus plasty with reconstruction of the coaptation of the mitral valve (**b'**). *AML* anterior mitral leaflet, *PML* posterior mitral leaflet, *pPM* posterior papillary muscle, *c* coaptation

the risk of late death [48,49]. The mechanism of ischemic incompetence is produced by motion of the leaflet towards the apex [50] in systole not allowing leaflets to achieve adequate coaptation (Figs. 1.14b, c, 1.15, 1.16). Incomplete closure of the leaflet produced by tethering of the subvalvular apparatus is the most frequent mechanism of ischemic incompetence; however, prolapse of the mitral valve can be demonstrated in some cases (Figs. 1.14c and 1.17).

The aim of surgical treatment is to restore myocardial perfusion and at the same time correct mitral dysfunction. Generally speaking, coronary artery disease leads to ischemia and/or scar formation affecting the regional function of the heart muscle and can influence the function of the subvalvular apparatus. The great majority of the experts dealing with this pathophysiology in recent times agree that ischemic incompetence of the mitral valve is produced by wall motion disturbances [51, 52, 53, 54] rather than by papillary muscle dysfunction alone [55, 56, 57, 58]. Most often the constellation appears in which posterior wall or apex dyskinesia is produced by the coronary heart disease, affecting the subvalvular apparatus and causing mitral valve dysfunction. There are also acutely developing forms of ischemic valve dysfunction that occur in the course of myocardial infarction or ischemic mitral valve incompetence as a complication of chronic ischemic heart disease. These two conditions are also different in terms of outcome.

There are several surgical proposals on how best to repair the dysfunctional valve and the subvalvular apparatus, including use of devices to stabilize the subvalvular and valvular apparatus [59, 60]. The classical reconstruction surgery offers good outcome and better results than replacement [61]. Rankin reported significantly better 2-year survival rate after valve reconstruction compared to replacement (80% vs. 58%) [62]. The repair technique should be perfect to ensure good long-term results, as published previously; significant mitral incompetence after reconstruction leads to poor prognosis in our long-term observations [40].

To aid understanding of echocardiography images, a schematic presentation of different forms of ischemic mitral incompetence is given in Fig. 1.14. The classical restrictive form (usually known as type IIIa of the Carpentier functional classification) [63] is demonstrated

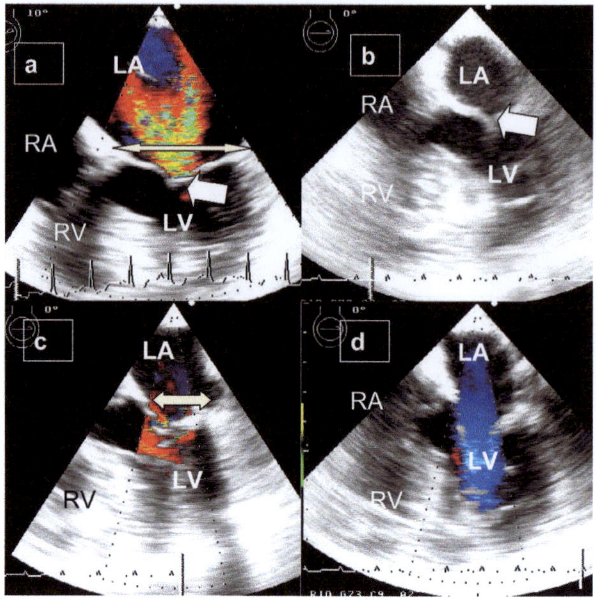

Fig. 1.19. Intraoperative TEE sequences of the same patient as in Fig. 1.16. **a** Intraoperative TEE section with arrow indicating mitral ring dimension before mitral reconstruction was performed. **b–d** Images taken early after cardiopulmonary bypass cessation. **b** Systolic TEE section demonstrating restored coaptation visible in the 2D image (*white arrow*). **c** TEE postoperative color Doppler taken in systole. The pictures have the same grade of magnification. Note that a significant reduction of mitral ring dimension (*white arrow*) was achieved (see **a**). The valve is competent and the opening area is preserved, ranging from 3.1–3.2 cm^2, as visible in **d** in diastole. *LV* left ventricle, *LA* left atrium, *RV* right ventricle, *RA* right atrium

in Figs. 1.15 and 1.16. The reconstruction procedure of the ischemic mitral valve Paneth plasty with Hetzer modification [64] is schematically presented in Fig. 1.18 and the next intraoperative images (Figs. 1.19b–d and 1.20) demonstrate good results of the reconstruction procedure (see figure legends).

In patients suffering from ischemic mitral regurgitation, the constellation of wall motion dysfunction and type of mitral pathology can be extended to a mixed form (any kind of mitral valve disease may coexist with ischemic heart disease) but classical forms are presented in Fig. 1.14b–d and f. In general, mitral leaflets are tethered towards the apex (coaptation is shifted below the dotted line) resulting in a deficit of coaptation as presented in Fig. 1.14b. The insufficient coaptation can be produced by the asymmetrically tethered posterior leaflet producing a regurgitation jet toward the atrial wall (Fig. 1.14b) or by symmetrical tethering toward the apex of both mitral leaflets producing a centrally blowing regurgitation jet in the left atrium (Fig. 1.14c). It is important to remember that in the wall jet (eccentrically blowing jet steering to the wall of the left atrium) the color Doppler phenomenon representing regurgitation usually underestimates the grade of regurgitation. This phenomenon is produced by atrial surface adherence (Coanda effect) which reduces jet size and color encoding, causing smaller color Doppler jet areas [65].

1.10 Inflammatory valve disease

Active infective endocarditis (AIE) is a malignant disease seldom heralded by a recognizable event or even if such an event is present it is usually obscured by noncharacteristic »infectious« symptoms that delay diagnosis [66]. The scarcity of characteristic symptoms in patients suffering from destructive forms of endocarditis makes echocardiographic investigation very important [67]. Echocardiography with the transesophageal mode of insertion can visualize the extent of the abscess and valve regurgitation, the main factors influencing morbidity and mortality [68] and, thus, aids the decision-making process preoperatively and intraoperatively [69]. It should be stated that only serial preoperative investigations can lead to precise assessment and prediction of destructive forms of endocarditis. The timing for surgery is defined by classical indications for surgery as described by Hetzer et al. [70] (severe valve dysfunction, paravalvular abscess formation, septic shock, septic emboli, and persistent sepsis despite adequate antibiotic therapy, leading to kidney failure or congestive heart failure) including lack of clinical improvement termed »no go endocarditis« [71]. The factors that make surgery difficult are detectable and can be precisely assessed by perioperative echocardiography. The value of echocardiography in the assessment of these endocarditic lesions and unusual complications, such as secondary mitral valve involvement as an extension of pathological processes primarily localized elsewhere (aortic root), is well established in the literature [72]. In patients suffering from destructive mitral valve endocarditis, reconstructive surgery should be given the highest priority to reach a good outcome [73]. To achieve this aim, the surgery should be performed early so that there is still a »pool« of nondiseased tissue to make mitral valve repair possible [74], but also late enough to treat peripheral sources of pathognomic microorganisms to lower the risk of extracardial reinfection after surgical treatment.

1.11 Systolic anterior motion (SAM)

Systolic anterior motion movement of the AML and subvalvular apparatus produces a lack of mitral valve coaptation such that various degrees of mitral regurgitation occur (◘ Fig. 1.14e; ◘ Figs. 2.17–2.20 in the chapter »Perioperative echocardiographic imaging after mitral valve repair for ischemic, inflammatory, and degenerative incompetence« in this book). New onset of SAM implies that this pathology was not present preoperatively. The severity of mitral regurgitation (grades 0–4) can be assessed according to standard color Doppler criteria [75]. Continuous wave Doppler signals can be recorded during transthoracic echocardiography (TTE) from the 5-chamber view or during transesophageal echocardiography (TEE) from the transgastric view to demonstrate the presence of high gradients in the left ventricular outflow tract (LVOT). The »dagger«-shaped Doppler spectrum can help to distinguish between aortic valve pathology (if mitral reconstruction coexists with aortic pathology) and identified new-onset SAM.

Few hypotheses can be put forward to explain new-onset SAM in patients following MVR. From the technical-surgical viewpoint, the complication of SAM after mitral valve surgery can be caused by »overreconstruction« [76]. After tight annulus plasty, the posterior leaflet can be significantly reduced and the posterior part of the mitral annulus can be shifted toward the outflow tract of the left ventricle. In this situation, there may be two causes of systolic motion of part of the mitral valve and its subvalvular apparatus. First, the AML is relatively longer than the posterior leaflet and in systole can be pushed toward the LVOT. This mechanism was postulated by Schwammenthal et al. [77] as the cause of SAM in hypertrophic cardiomyopathy (HOCM). Second, the inflow tract overlaps with the outflow tract as a consequence of posterior mitral ring reduction–the »overreconstruction« effect. The other cause can be a postoperative mismatch between (inadequate) volume supplementation (»empty left chamber«) and catecholamine administration (increase vascular resistance to keep vascular tonus). This is the »hypovolemic state« of the heart early after cardiopulmonary

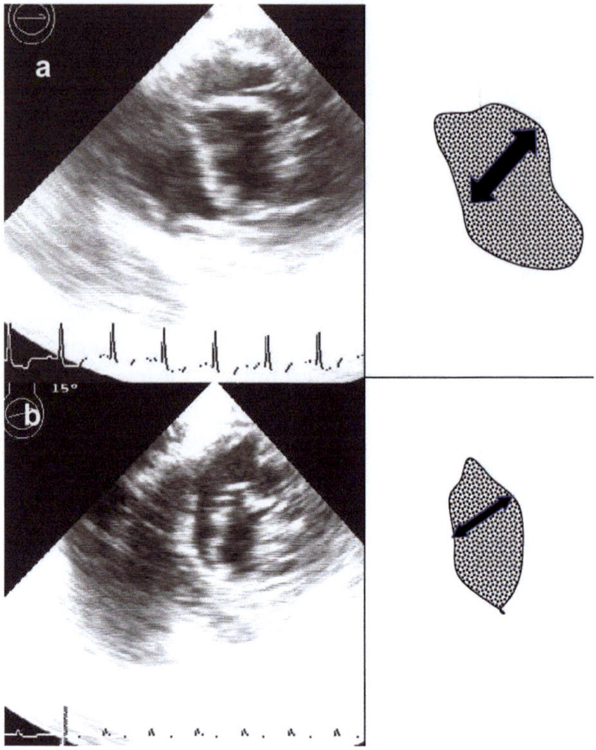

Fig. 1.20. Opening area in a patient after successful Paneth plasty with Hetzer modification: **a** before starting cardiopulmonary bypass (CPB) and **b** after weaning from CPB

bypass which can be compensated hemodynamically with an »overdose« of catecholamines (epinephrine). Prolongation of such a situation may produce a hyperkinetic left ventricle in a dyssynchronic manner where the posterior wall is hyperkinetic and the LVOT is obstructed due to shrinkage of the chamber cavity and shifting of the subvalvular apparatus of the mitral valve into the LVOT (see Figs. 2.17–2.20 in the chapter »Perioperative echocardiographic imaging after mitral valve repair for ischemic, inflammatory, and degenerative incompetence« in this book). In some patients, the presence of concomitant coronary artery disease provoking anterior wall dyskinesis can produce SAM, especially if concomitant mitral repair was performed. An explanation of this state may lie in ischemic wall motion disturbance injury, which is the subject of controversial discussion. Increased stiffness [78] of the myocardium, seen as a consequence of ischemia, could produce a hemodynamic state similar to that found in patients suffering from HOCM. Septum hypertrophy is not a condition sine qua non for the development of SAM [79].

1.12 Conclusion

There are several questions waiting to be answered. Among others, the problem of optimal timing of surgery in patients suffering from regurgitation is constantly the subject of controversy. We believe that adequate echocardiographic monitoring of patients suffering from valve diseases will help to solve this problem in the near future.

Acknowledgments

We thank Anne M. Gale, Editor in the Life Sciences, for editorial assistance.

References

1. Goldman ME, Mindich BP, Teichholz LE, Burgess N, Staville K, Fuster V (1984) Intraoperative contrast echocardiography to evaluate mitral valve operations. J Am Coll Cardiol 4:1035–1040
2. Eguaras MG, Pasalodos J, Gonzalez V, Montero A, Garcia MA, Moriones I, Granados J, Valles F, Concha M (1985) Intraoperative contrast two-dimensional echocardiography: Evaluation of the presence and severity of aortic and mitral regurgitation during cardiac operations. J Thorac Cardiovasc Surg 89:573–579
3. Czer LS, Maurer G, Bolger AF, DeRobertis M, Resser KJ, Kass RM, Lee ME, Blauche C, Chaux A, Gray RJ, Matloff JM (1987) Intraoperative evaluation of mitral regurgitation by Doppler color flow mapping. Circulation 76(Suppl III):III-108–116
4. Maurer G, Czer LSC, Chaux A, Bolger AF, DeRobertis M, Resser K, Kass RM, Lee ME, Matloff JM (1987) Intraoperative Doppler color flow mapping for assessment of valve repair for mitral regurgitation. Am J Cardiol 60:333–337
5. Feigenbaum H (1989) Personal communication, Indianapolis, Spring 1989
6. St. Goar FG, Fann JI, Komtebedde J, Foster E, Oz MC, Fogarty TJ, Feldman T, Block PC (2003) Endovascular edge-to-edge mitral valve repair: short-term results in a porcine model. Circulation 108:1990–1993
7. Levine HJ, Gaacsh WH (1996) Vasoactive drugs in chronic regurgitant lesions of the mitral and aortic valves J Am Coll Cardiol 28:1083–1091
8. Siniawski H, Weng Y, Hetzer R (1991) Decision-making aspects in the surgical treatment of ischemic mitral incompetence. In: Vetter HO, Hetzer R, Schmutzler H (eds) Ischemic mitral incompetence. Steinkopff, Darmstadt, pp 137–147.
9. Bulkley BH, Roberts WC (1975) Dilatation of the mitral annulus. A rare cause of mitral regurgitation. Am J Med 59: 457–463
10. Davies MJ, Moore BP, Baimbridge MV (1978) The floppy mitral valve: study of incidence, pathology and complications in surgical, necropsy and forensic material. Br Heart J 40:468–481
11. Komoda T, Hetzer R, Uyama C, Siniawski H, Maeta H, Rosendahl UP, Ozaki K (1994) Mitral annular function assessed by 3D imaging for mitral valve surgery. J Heart Valve Dis 3:483–490
12. Komoda T, Hetzer R, Oellinger J, Siniawski H, Hofmeister J, Hübler M, Felix R, Uyama C, Maeta H (1997) Mitral annular flexibility. J Card Surg 12(2):102–109
13. David TE, Uden DE, Strauss HD (1986) The importance of the mitral apparatus in left ventricular function after correction of mitral regurgitation. Circulation 74:116–120
14. Horstkotte D, Schulte HD, Birks W, Strauer BE (1993) The effect of chordal preservation on late outcome after mitral valve replacement: a randomized study. J Heart Valve Dis 2:150–158
15. Komeda M, Tirone ED, Rao V, Sun Z, Weisel RD, Burns RJ (1994) Late hemodynamic effects of the preserved papillary muscles during mitral valve replacement. Circulation 90(Suppl II):II190–II194
16. Hetzer R, Bougioukas G, Franz M, Borst HG (1983) Mitral valve replacement with preservation of papillary muscles and chordae tendineae. Revival of a seemingly forgotten concept. I. Preliminary clinical report. Thorac Cardiovasc Surg 31:291–296
17. Rushmer RF (1956) Initial phase of ventricular systole: asynchronous contraction. Am J Physiol 184:188–194
18. Lillehei CW, Levy MJ, Bonnabeau RC (1964) Mitral valve replacement with preservation of papillary ,muscles and chordae tendinae. J Thorac Cardiovasc 47: 532–543
19. Siniawski H, Warnecke H, Weng Y, Drews T, Hetzer R (1991) Perioperative echocardiographic assessment of the heart function in the patients treated by mitral reconstruction or replacement with complete papillary-annular continuity. Circulation 84(Suppl 2):II-577
20. David TE (2007) Outcomes of mitral valve repair for mitral regurgitation due to degenerative disease. Semin Thorac Cardiovasc Surg 19:116–120
21. Bonow RO, Carabello BA, Chatterjee K, et al. (2006) ACC/AHA 2006 guidelines for the management of patients with valvular heart disease: a report of the American College of Cardiology/American Heart Association Task Force on Practice Guidelines (Writing Committee to revise the 1998guidelines for the management of patients with valvular heart disease) developed in collaboration with the Society of Cardiovascular Anesthesiologists endorsed by the Society for Cardiovascular Angiography and Interventions and the Society of Thoracic Surgeons. J Am Coll Cardiol 48:e1–148

22. Enriquez-Sarano M, Avierinos JF, Messika-Zeitoun D, Detaint, Capps M, Nkomo v,Scott C, Schaff HV, Tajik AJ (2009) Quantitative determinants of the outcome of asymptomatic mitral regurgitation. N Engl J Med 352:875–883
23. Grayburn PA (2008) How to measure severity of mitral regurgitation. Heart 94(3):376–383
24. Omoto R, Yokote Y, Takamoto S, Kyo S, Ueda K, Asano H, Namekawa K, Kasai C, Kondo Y, Koyano A (1984) The development of real-time two-dimensional Doppler echocardiography and its clinical significance in acquired valvular diseases: with special references to the evaluation of valvular regurgitation. Jpn Heart J 25:325–340
25. Miyatake K, Izumi S, Okamoto M, Kinoshita N, Asonuma H, Nakagawa H, Yamamoto K, Takamiya M, Sakakibara H, Nimura Y (1986) Semiquantitative grading of severity of mitral regurgitation by real-time two-dimensional Doppler flow imaging technique. J Am Coll Cardiol 7:82–88
26. Spain MG, Smith MD, Grayburn PA, Harlamert EA, DeMaria AN (1989) Quantitative assessment of mitral regurgitation by Doppler color flow imaging: angiographic and hemodynamic correlations. J Am Coll Cardiol 13:585–590
27. F Helmcke, NC Nanda, MC Hsiung, B Soto, CK Adey, RG Goyal, RP Gatewood, Jr (1987) Color Doppler assessment of mitral regurgitation with orthogonal planes. Circulation 75:175–183
28. Rokey R, Sterling LL, Zoghbi WA, et al. (1986) Determination of regurgitant fraction in isolated mitral or aortic regurgitation by pulsed Doppler two-dimensional echocardiography. J Am Coll Cardiol 7:1273–1278
29. Enriquez-Sarano M, Seward JB, Bailey KR, Tajik AJ (1994) Effective regurgitant orifice area: a noninvasive Doppler development of an old hemodynamic concept. J Am Coll Cardiol 23:443–451
30. Vandervoort PM, Rivera JM, Mele D, et al. (1993) Application of color Doppler flow mapping to calculate effective regurgitant orifice area: an in vitro study and initial clinical observations. Circulation 88:1150–1156
31. Dujardin KS, Enriquez-Sarano M, Bailey KR, Nishimura RA, Seward JB, Tajik AJ (1997) Grading of mitral regurgitation by quantitative Doppler echocardiography: calibration by left ventricular angiography in routine clinical practice. Circulation 96:3409–3415
32. Hall SA, Brickner ME, Willett DL, Irani WN, Afridi I, Grayburn PA (1997) Assessment of mitral regurgitation severity by Doppler color flow mapping of the vena contracta. Circulation 95:636–642
33. Zoghbi WA, Enriquez-Sarano M, Foster E, et al. (2003) Recommendations for evaluation of the severity of native valvular regurgitation with two-dimensional and Doppler echocardiography. J Am Soc Echocardiogr 16:777–802
34. Irvine T, Li XK, Sahn DJ, Kenny A (2002) Assessment of mitral regurgitation. Heart 88(Suppl 4):iv11–iv19
35. Dujardin KS, Enriquez-Sarano M, Bailey KR, Nishimura RA, Seward JB, Tajik AJ (1997) Grading of mitral regurgitation by quantitative Doppler echocardiography: calibration by left ventricular angiography in routine clinical practice. Circulation 96:3409–3415
36. Enriquez-Sarano M, Tajik A, Schaff H, Orszulak T, Bailey K, Frye R (1994) Echocardiographic prediction of survival after surgical correction of organic mitral regurgitation. Circulation 90:830–837
37. Bech-Hanssen O, Ryden T, Schersten H, Oden A, Nilsson F, Jeppsson A (2003) Mortality after mitral regurgitation surgery: importance of clinical and echocardiographic variables. Eur J Cardiothorac Surg 24:723–730
38. Anyanwu AC, Adams DH (2009) Why do mitral valve repairs fail? J Am Soc Echocardiogr 22:1265–1268
39. Adams DH, Rosenhek R, Falk V (2010) Degenerative mitral valve regurgitation: best practice revolution. Eur Heart Journal 31:1958–1967
40. Hausmann H, Siniawski H, Hotz H, Hofmeister J, Chavez T, Schmidt G, Hetzer R (1997) Mitral valve reconstruction and mitral valve replacement for ischemic mitral insufficiency. J Card Surg 12:8–14
41. Bouchard D, Demers P, Coutu M, Pellerin M, Carrier M, Perrault LP, Cartier R, Pegé P, Cossete P, Basmadijan AJ (2006) Is a good perioperative echocardiographic result predictive of durability in ischemic mitral incompetence? J Thorac Cardiovasc Surg 131:565–573
42. Keele KD (1973) The application of the physics and sounds to 19th century cardiology: with the particular reference to the part played by CJB Williams and James Hope. Clio Med 8:191–221
43. Vander Veer JB (1958) Mitral insufficiency. Historical and clinical aspects. Am J Cardiol 2:1–6
44. Read RC, Thal AP, Wendt VE (1965) Symptomatic valvular myxomatous transformation (the floppy valve syndrome). A possible forme fruste of the Marfan syndrome. Circulation 897–910
45. McKay R, Yacoub MH (1973) Clinical and pathological finding in patients with »floppy« valve treated surgically. Circulation 47(Suppl):63–73
46. Demaria AN, King JF, Bogren HG,Lies JE, Mason DT (1974) The variable spectrum of echocardiographic manifestations of the mitral valve prolapse syndrome. Circulation 50:33–41
47. Grigioni F, Detaint D, Avirinos JF (2005) Contribution of ischemic mitral regurgitation to congestive heart failure after myocardial infarction. J Am Coll Cardiol 45:260–267
48. Rankin JS, Hickey MSJ, Smith LR, et al. (1989) Ischemic mitral regurgitation. Circulation 79(Suppl I):I-116–I-121

49. Frater RWM, Cornelissen P, Sisto D (1991) Mechanisms of ischemic mitral insufficiency and their surgical correction. In: Vetter HO, Hetzer R, Schmutzler H (eds) Ischemic Mitral Incompetence. Springer, New York, NY, pp 117–130
50. Hider CF, Taylor DEM, Wade JD (1965) The effect of papillary muscle damage on atrioventricular valve function in the left heart. Q J Exp Physiol 50:15–22
51. Tsakiris AG, Rastelli GC, Amorim D, et al. (1970) Effect of experimental papillary muscle damage on mitral valve closure in intact anesthetized dogs. Mayo Clin Proc 45:275–285
52. Mittal AK, Langston M Jr, Cohn KE, et al. (1971) Combined papillary muscle and left ventricular wall dysfunction as a cause of mitral regurgitation: an experimental study. Circulation 44:174–180
53. Kaul S, Spotnitz WD, Glasheen WP, et al. (1991) Mechanism of ischemic mitral regurgitation: an experimental evaluation. Circulation 84:2167–2180
54. Burch GE, De Pasquale NP, Phillips JH (1963) Clinical manifestations of papillary muscle dysfunction. Arch Intern Med 59:508–520
55. Phillips JH, Burch GE, De Pasquale NP (1963) The syndrome of papillary muscle dysfunction. Ann Intern Med 59:508–520
56. Godley RW, Wann LS, Rogers EW, et al. (1981) Incomplete mitral leaflet closure in patients with papillary muscle dysfunction. Circulation 63:565–571
57. Kisanuki A, Otsuji Y, Kuroiwa R, et al. (1993) Two-dimensional echocardiographic assessment of papillary muscle contractility in patients with prior myocardial infarction. J Am Coll Cardiol 21:932–938
58. Inoue M, McCarthy P, Popovic Z (2004) The Coapsys device to treat functional mitral regurgitation: in vivo long-term canine study. J Thorac Cardiovasc Surg 127:1068 –1077
59. Langer F, Kunihara T, Hell K, Schramm R, Schmidt KI, Aicher D, Kindermann M, Schäfers HJ (2009) RING+STRING: successful repair technique for ischemic mitral regurgitation with severe leaflet tethering. Circulation 120:S85–S91
60. Miller DC (2001) Ischemic mitral regurgitation redux–to repair or to replace? J Thorac Cardiovasc Surg 122:1059–1062
61. Rankin JS, Feneley MP, Hickey MSTJ, et al (1988) A clinical comparison of mitral valve repair versus valve replacement in ischemic mitral regurgitation. J Thorac Cardiovasc Surg 95:166–177
62. Rankin JS, Hickey MSTJ, Smith LR, et al (1991) Current concepts in the pathogenesis and treatment of ischemic mitral regurgitation. In: Vetter HO, Hetzer R, Schmutzler H (eds) Ischemic Mitral incompetence. Spinger Verlag, New York, NY, pp 157–178
63. Fischer GW, Anyanwu AC, Adams DH (2009) Intraoperative classification of mitral valve dysfunction: the role of the anesthesiologist in mitral valve reconstruction. J CardiothoracVasc Anesth 23:531–543
64. Siniawski H, Weng Y, Hetzer R, et al (1991) Decision making aspects in the surgical treatment of ischemic mitral incompetence. In: Vetter HO, Hetzer R, Schmutzler H (eds) Ischemic Mitral Incompetence. Springer Verlag, New York, pp 137–147
65. Chao K, Moises VA, Shandas R, Elkadi T, Sahn DJ, Weintraub R (1992) Influence of the Coanda effect on color Doppler jet area and color encoding in vitro studies using color Doppler flow mapping. Circulation –341
66. Saners PJ, Neubuerger KT, Ravin A (1957) Rupture of papillary muscles: occurrence of rupture of the posterior muscle in posterior myocardial infarction. Dis Chest 36:166–177
67. Stevenson RR, Tunrer WJ (1935) Rupture of a papillary muscle in the heart as a cause of sudden death. Bull John Hopkins Hosp 57:235.95
68. Gula G, Yacoub MH (1981) Surgical correction of complete rupture of the anterior papillary muscle. Ann Thorac Surg 32:88–91
69. Stewart JA, Silimperi D, Harris P, Wise NK, Fraker TD Jr, Kisslo JA (1980) Echocardiographic documentation of vegetative lesions in infective endocarditis: clinical implications. Circulation 61:374–380
70. Hetzer R, Deyerling W, Borst HG (1984) Herzklappenchirurgie bei aktiver infektiöser Endokarditis. In: Gahl K (ed) Infektiöse Endokarditis. Klinik, Diagnostik, Therapie. Steinkopff, Darmstadt, pp 148–176
71. Oakley CM, Hall RJC (2001) Endocarditis: problems of patients being treated for endocarditis and not doing well. Heart 85:470–474
72. Braimbridge MV (1969) Cardiac surgery and bacterial endocarditis. Lancet 1:1307–1309
73. Zegdi R, Debièche M, Latrémouille C et al. (2005) Long-term results of mitral valve repair in active endocarditis. Circulation 111:2532–2536
74. Hetzer R, Dalichau H, Borst HG (1975) Herzklappenchirurgie bei bakterieller Endocarditis. Thoraxchirurgie 23:427–430
75. Helmcke F, Nanda NC, Hsiung MC et al. (1987) Color Doppler assessment of mitral regurgitation with orthogonal planes. Circulation 74:175–183

76. Personal communication from Professor Hetzer. Berlin 1989
77. Schwammenthal E, Nakatani S, He S, Hopmeyer J, Sagie A, Weyman AE, Lever H M, Yoganathan PA, Thomas JD, Levine RA (1998) Mechanism of mitral regurgitation in hypertrophic cardiomyopathy: mismatch of posterior to anterior leaflet length and mobility. Circulation 98:856–865
78. Siniawski H, Lehmkuhl H, Weng Y, Hetzer R (2004) High pressure gradients in left ventricular outflow tract after aortic valve replacement. Acta Cardiologica 59(2):235–236
79. GS Mintz, MN Kotler, BL Segal, WR Parry (1967) Systolic anterior motion of the mitral valve in the absence of asymmetric septal hypertrophy. Circulation 57:256–263

Perioperative echocardiographic imaging after mitral valve repair for ischemic, inflammatory, and degenerative incompetence

H. Siniawski, M. Hübler, A. Amiri, C.A. Yankah, R. Hetzer

2.1 Introduction

Perioperative echocardiographic imaging has become an indispensable component of contemporary mitral valve repair. Mitral valve reconstruction surgery was popularized by the French surgeon Alain Carpentier and has continuously gained popularity over prosthetic valve replacement. At our institution, the Deutsches Herzzentrum Berlin (DHZB), Roland Hetzer modified the Gerbode and the Paneth techniques of mitral valve reconstruction effectively without using fabric material.

Between January 1988 and December 2009, a total of 2409 mitral valve reconstructions were performed at the DHZB. Over the past 5 years (1 January 2005 to 31 May 2010), 44.9% of all patients who received mitral surgery were treated using reconstruction procedures. Our study revealed that, of patients classified as having nonischemic mitral valve disease (MVD), 65% had the degenerative form, 15% endocarditic, 12% rheumatic, and 8% miscellaneous forms (◘ Fig. 2.1). The most frequent findings in our studies based on 609 preoperative patients suffering from degenerative MVD classified for mitral reconstruction were as follows: rupture of the posterior mitral leaflet (PML; posterior chordal) 78%, rupture of the anterior mitral leaflet (AML; anterior chordal) in 3%, and both AML and PML rupture in 4%. Annular dilatation and elongation of the chordae were recognized as being responsible for the mitral pathology in 15% of cases (◘ Fig. 2.2). In a population suffering from posterior chordae rupture, in the great majority of the cases rupture was localized to the middle scallop (P2, 92%), while the anterior or posterior scallop (P1 and P3) was affected in 3% and 5% of cases, respectively (◘ Fig. 2.3). Ruptured scallop is also called »flail mitral leaflet« and lack of central coaptation of the mitral valve causes significant mitral regurgitation, as demonstrated in color Doppler transesophageal echocardiography (TEE) investigations (◘ Fig. 2.4). The possible coexistence of another pathology, e.g., persistent foramen ovale, requires TEE examination preoperatively to exclude or confirm a concomitant pathology.

2.2 Degenerative mitral valve disease

Mitral reconstruction: Gerbode with Hetzer modification

Echocardiographic investigation of patients during or after mitral reconstruction requires knowledge of the basic concept of technical aspects of reconstruction (surgical or interventional repair) to be able to correctly interpret the results. At the DHZB, the technique most commonly used for the treatment of patients suffering from degenerative mitral valve disease is based on the Gerbode technique and the Hetzer modification performed using classical or minimally invasive access.

The risk of error during the assessment of valve function may not be neglected during intraoperative investigation or early postoperatively in the intensive care unit. In both situations, the patients are not always adequately supplied with volume, and sinus rhythm has often not been restored. The influence of vascular resistance modified by vasoactive pharmacological agents should not be ignored. It should be kept in mind that all these factors influencing the pulmonary wedge »v« wave limit its diagnostic value in regurgitation assessment early after reconstruction [1].

The first echocardiographic assessment can be undertaken very early after weaning from cardiopulmonary bypass has begun. The first action of the heart, although not adequately

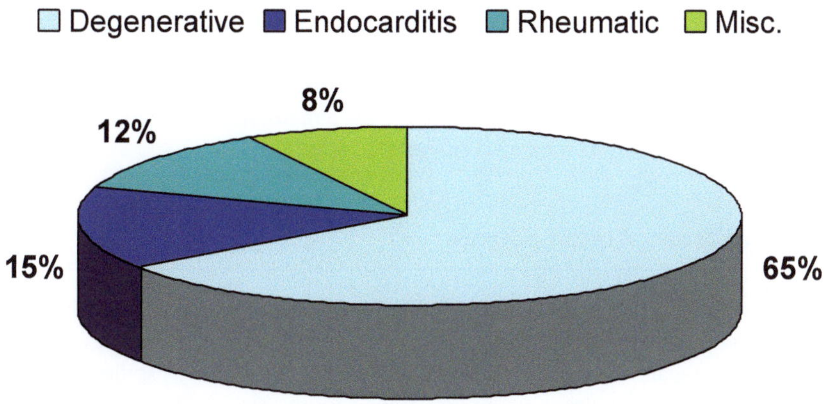

Fig. 2.1. Etiology of surgical nonischemic mitral valve regurgitation as established by echocardiography in 609 patients treated by mitral valve reconstruction at the Deutsches Herzzentrum Berlin

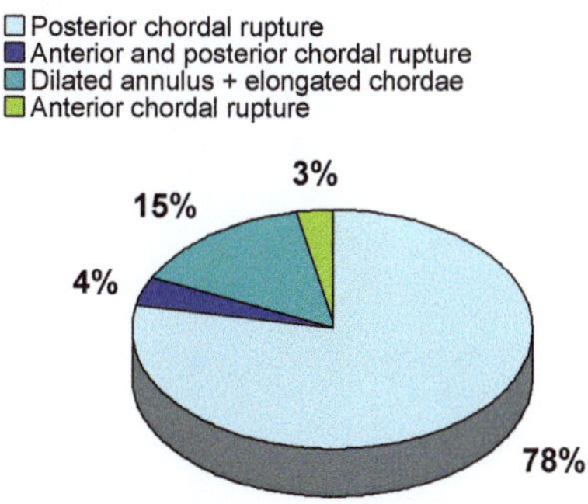

Fig. 2.2. Anatomic characteristics of degenerative mitral valve disease as identified by echocardiography in 521 patients treated by mitral valve reconstruction at the Deutsches Herzzentrum Berlin. *Ant* anterior, *post* posterior, *ch* chordae

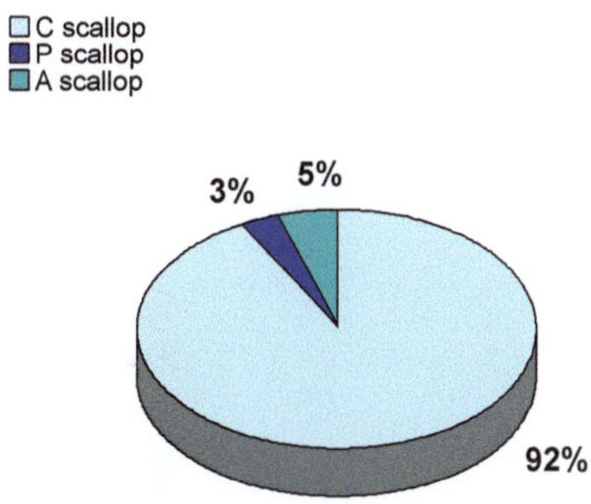

Fig. 2.3. Incidence of scallop rupture of the posterior mitral leaflet (*PML*) in 246 patients with degenerative mitral valve regurgitation treated by mitral valve reconstruction at the Deutsches Herzzentrum Berlin. *A* anterior (P1), *C* middle (P2), *P* posterior (P3)

filled, produces spontaneous diffusion of the contrast medium to the left atrium, making initial valve function assessment possible (Fig. 2.5), as has been published elsewhere [2]. There is also the possibility of testing the reconstruction procedure when the heart surgeon is removing the air bubbles from the left chamber by massaging the heart (Fig. 2.6). These tests are the earliest, even before color Doppler assessment can be used.

In addition, during the intraoperative monitoring of patients after mitral reconstruction, echocardiographic examination can be accomplished and should include Doppler flow and the two-dimensional (2D) opening area of the mitral valve measurements. In our series, the success rate of mitral reconstruction in patients suffering from different stages of degenerative mitral valve disease was 97% with good results in long-term follow-up [3].

Echocardiographic follow-up of patients after Gerbode–Hetzer plasty (Fig. 2.7) in the parasternal short-axis and 4-chamber view demonstrates excellent coaptation and opening area, and no regurgitation of the mitral valve as documented in 2D and Doppler measurements (Figs. 2.8 and 2.9). Normalization of the LV dimension and function after valve reconstruction can be observed soon after surgery (Fig. 2.10).

2.3 Ischemic mitral incompetence

Surgery after an acute coronary infarction (during the acute phase) is generally associated with a high risk of death but, if carcinogenic shock is produced by acute severe mitral incompetence, surgical repair can save the patient's life. Acute rupture of the papillary muscle leads to such a complication, requiring urgent life-saving surgery (Fig. 2.11).

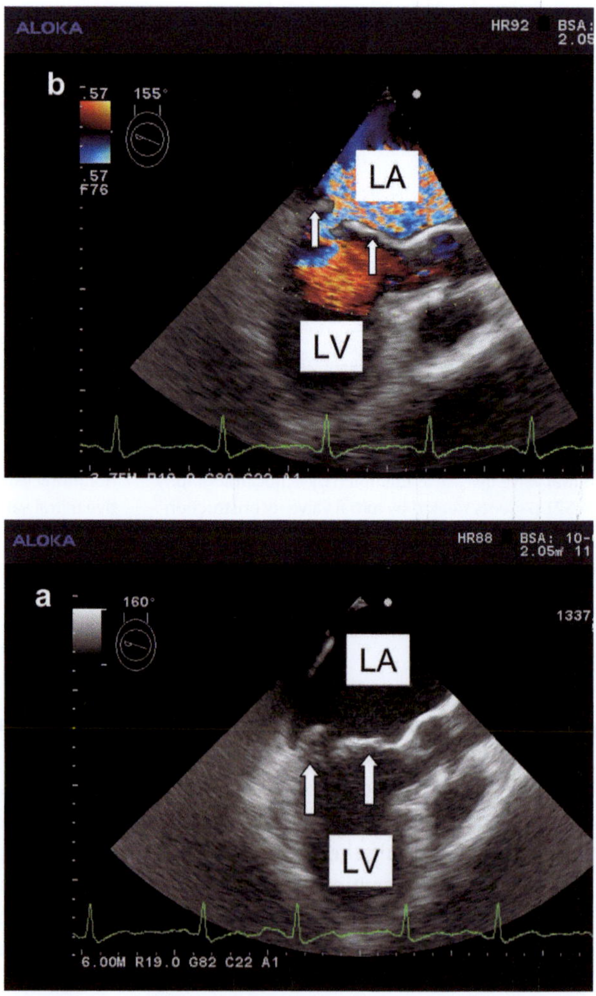

Fig. 2.4. Color Doppler TEE of the same patient as in Fig. 2.9. **a** Two-dimensional 4-chamber view. **b** A large regurgitation jet filling the left atrium is visible. *Arrows* indicate prolapsing anterior mitral leaflet. *LA* left atrium, *LV* left ventricle

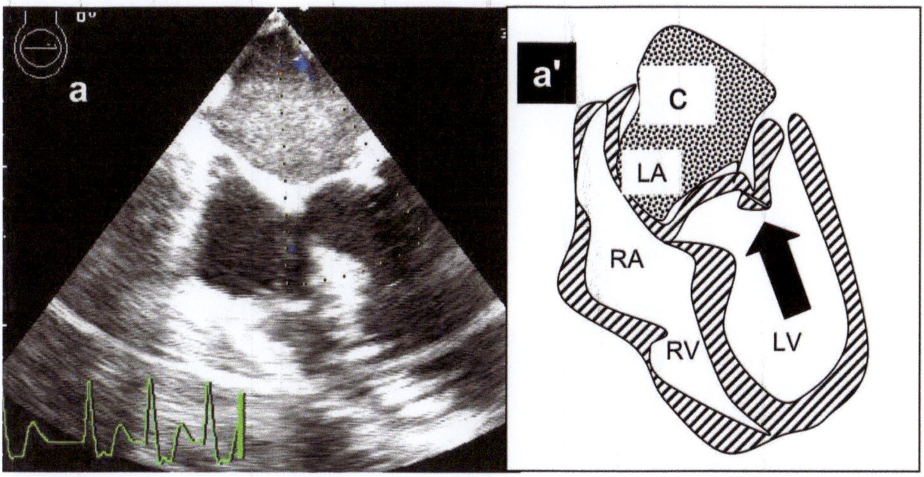

Fig. 2.5. Spontaneous contrasting period of left atrium (*c*) at the time of cardiopulmonary bypass weaning in a patient after mitral valve reconstruction; patient suffered from destruction of the mitral valve by endocarditis. The flow in the left ventricle (*LV*) vanishes during spontaneous contrasting and if the mitral valve is incompetent it will produce a visible jet in the left atrium (*LA*) at the time of spontaneous contrasting. Lack of such a jet indicates a competent mitral valve. Color Doppler is useless because hemodynamics are not restored. Thus, there is sufficient coaptation of the reconstructed valve. *RA* right atrium, *RV* right ventricle

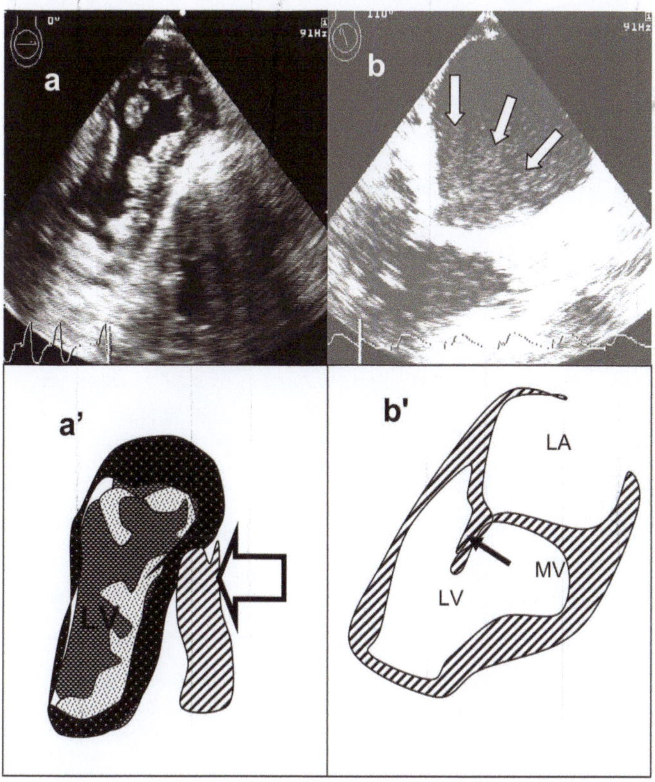

Fig. 2.6. Intraoperative TEE images taken during cardiopulmonary bypass at the time when the surgeon is removing air bubbles by massaging the heart. The surgeon's finger is visible, located on the lateral wall of the heart (**a**). At the same time, movement of the mitral valve (*MV*) and spontaneous contrasting of left atrium (*LA*) demonstrating good coaptation of the valve (*arrows*) and no regurgitation during the passively produced stroke can be observed (**b**)

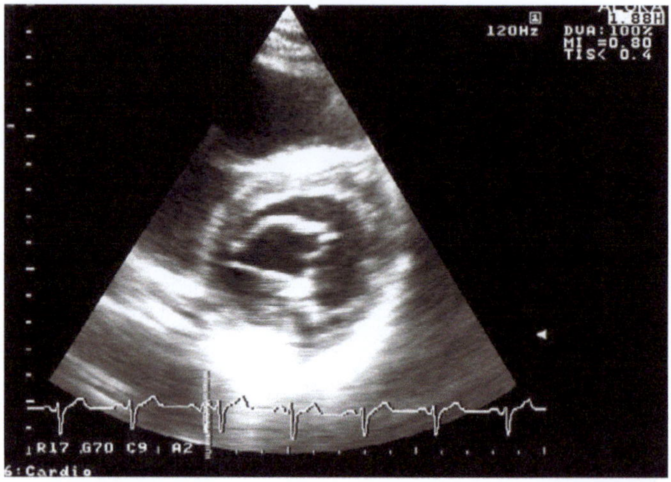

Fig. 2.7. Gerbode–Hetzer mitral reconstruction. Short-axis view in postoperative TTE visualizes mitral opening area

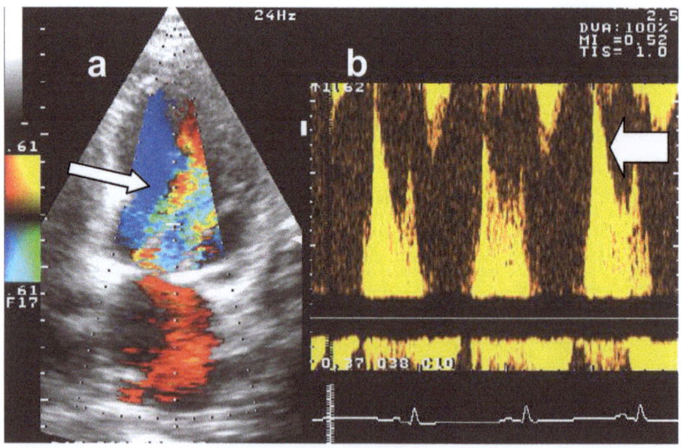

Fig. 2.8. The postoperative TTE Doppler and phonocardiogram investigation reveals no stenosis (normal Doppler early wave E slope – ***white line***) and no regurgitation. There is no flow in diastole

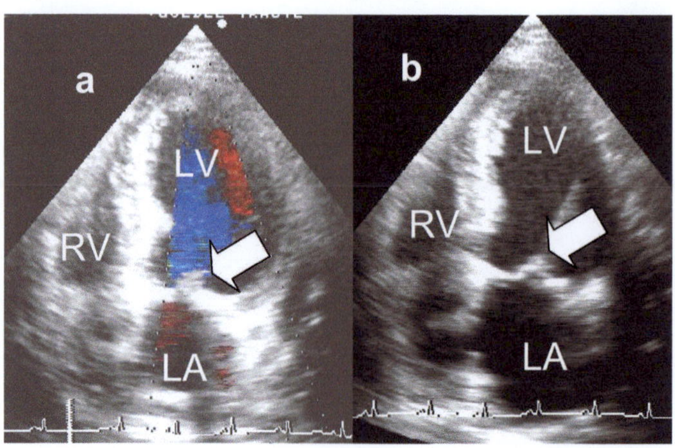

Fig. 2.9. A further case after Gerbode–Hetzer mitral reconstruction. **a** The 4-chamber view with color Doppler mitral early flow (early wave E – *arrow*) in diastole. **b** Doppler profile indicating adequate mitral opening area (*arrow*)

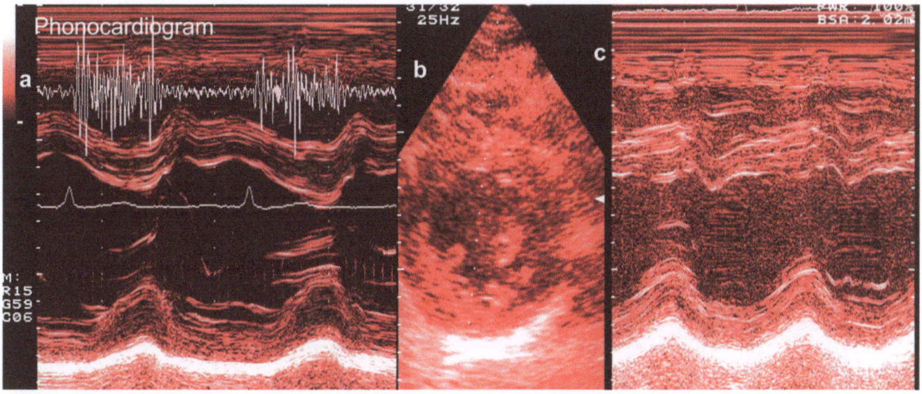

Fig. 2.10. M-mode TTE of a patient suffering from Barlow syndrome. **a** Preoperative M-mode of the left ventricle (LV) showing dilatation of the LV (63 mm) with preserved LV function (Fs=31%). Phonocardiogram of this patient (*top*) indicates nonejection click and systolic murmur. Two-dimensional TEE (**b**) and M-mode TEE (**c**) of the same patient taken intraoperatively after mitral valve reconstruction. The patient is without inotropic stimulation. LV is immediately significantly smaller (48 mm) and LV function is preserved (28%) but slightly reduced compared to the preoperative value

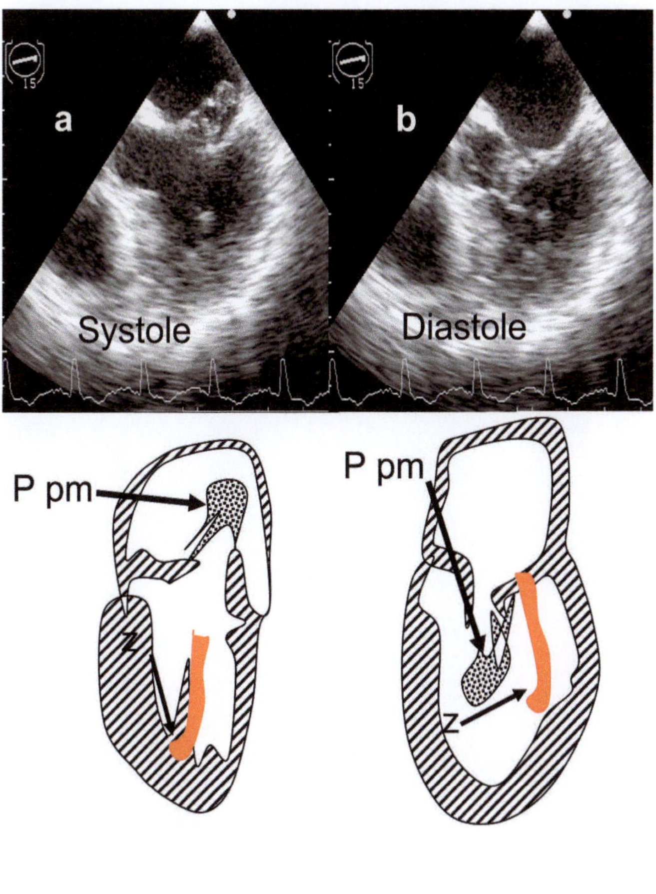

Fig. 2.11. Case with a ruptured posterior papillary muscle in the clinical course of acute myocardial infarction caused by severe single artery stenosis (circumflex). **a** Visible flail of the anterior mitral leaflet (AML) and posterior mitral leaflet (PML) with the head of the posterior papillary muscle (*P pm*). **b** In diastole, the subvalvular apparatus is moving into the inflow tract of the LV. *Z* intact part of the posterior papillary muscle

Rupture of the papillary muscle during myocardial infarction can be caused by a relatively small infarction in the posterior wall and because of severe acute mitral regurgitation this usually leads to shock and death [4] if surgery is not performed urgently. However, patients with rupture of the anterior papillary muscle have reached the operating room as reported by cardiac surgeons [5]. Early diagnosis is the key so that the patient may undergo emergency life-saving surgery. The standard treatment is mitral valve replacement as it has been for three decades [6], since suturing torn papillary muscles transmurally has not been proven to be successful [7, 8].

2.4 Inflammatory valve disease

Severe destruction of the annular and periannular structures of the aortic, mitral, and tricuspid valve due to infection can produce technical problems that can be managed only in each situation individually, giving surgeons satisfaction when success is reached [9, 10, 11]. Double

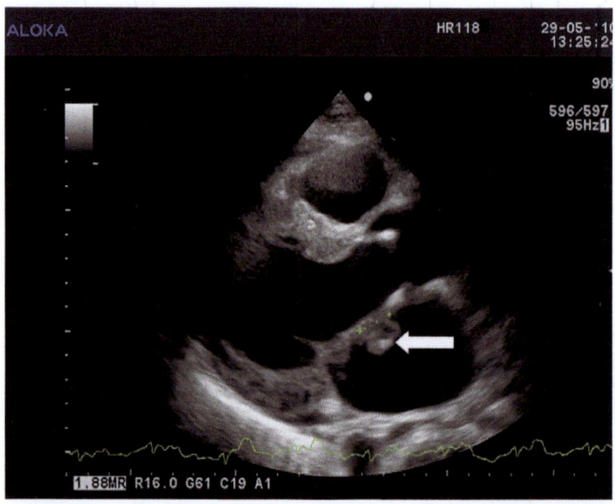

Fig. 2.12. Active infective endocarditis. Parasternal long-axis view (TTE) of a patient suffering from severe aortic insufficiency and a jet lesion at the base of the mitral valve

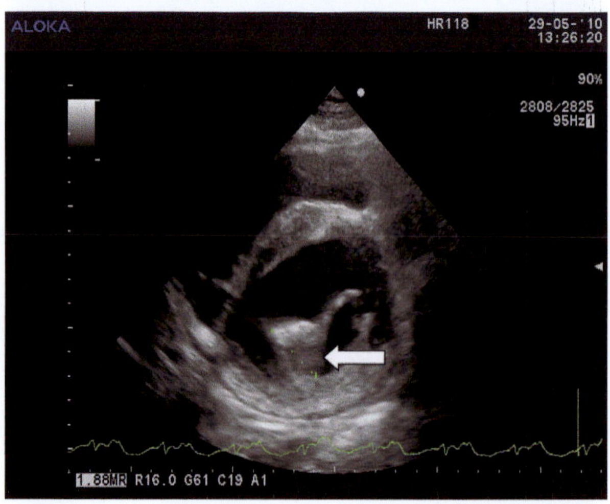

Fig. 2.13. TTE short-axis view allows localization of the jet lesion ulceration to be identified

valve disease where mitral ulceration with perforation was caused by an aortic jet lesion is shown in ◘ Figs. 2.12 and 2.13. Early identification of this lesion made mitral valve reconstruction possible [12].

2.5 Echocardiographic features of complications after mitral valve repair

Unfortunately, in a very small number of cases, complications may arise after surgery such as new development of the SAM (systolic anterior motion) phenomenon [13], new onset of myocardial ischemia producing wall motion dysfunction, or other surgical complications. Investigators should be aware of the possibility of the appearance of such complications and should be able to give advice to the surgeon and the anesthesiologist on overcoming the problem. The intraoperative decision-making process needs to be unerring and prompt in order to avoid the risk of final surgical treatment failure.

De novo obstructions of the left ventricular outflow tract (LVOT) in the early postoperative period can be attributed not only to anatomical but also to purely functional origin, as has been published by many institutions, including our own [8, 14].

2.6 Posterior wall ischemia

Ischemia of the posterior wall after mitral ring plasty is a rare complication that also arises in nonischemic mitral reconstructive surgery (◘ Figs. 2.14 and 2.15). If this complication occurs, it should be recognized early, allowing surgical intervention to be performed. Altogether in our institution, this complication was diagnosed intraoperatively in a few cases on the basis of ECG, hemodynamic condition, and echocardiography. The reason for it is that the posterior

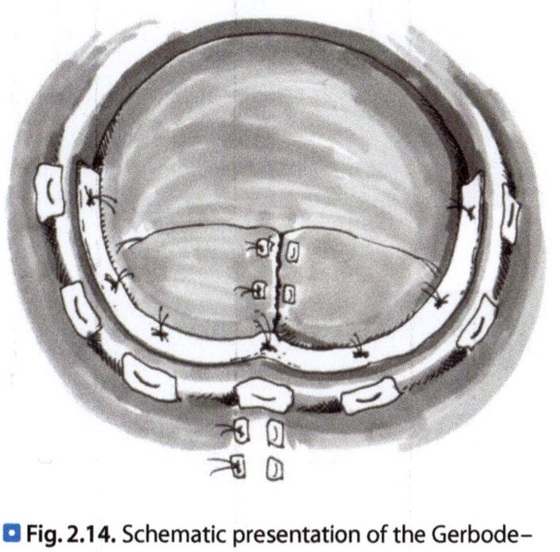

◘ **Fig. 2.14.** Schematic presentation of the Gerbode–Hetzer mitral valve reconstruction

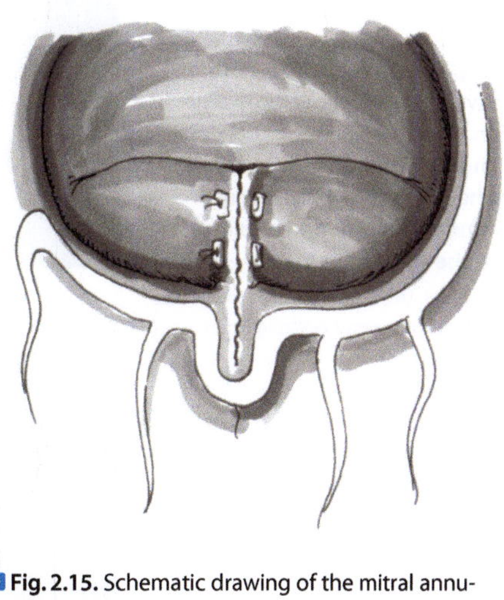

◘ **Fig. 2.15.** Schematic drawing of the mitral annuloplasty when the posterior ring plasty is too tight, which produces the risk of coronary artery deformation resulting in posterior wall ischemia

2

2.8 Mismatch of the prosthetic ring

There are several kinds of prosthetic ring on the market that are used for mitral reconstruction or for reinforcement of mitral repair [15, 16]. It should be noted that the natural dynamics and force distribution of the MV annulus are not physiological to the devices and the optimal design has still not been determined. The development of new optimal rings and surgical techniques is a continuous challenge to the technician and the surgeon [17, 18, 19]. Reconstruction based on a mitral ring is better standardized and easier to perform than mitral ring plasty. Perioperative echocardiographic investigation should be concentrated on leaflet movement and the relation of the prosthetic ring to the mitral annulus. Mismatch of the prosthetic ring to the native ring can produce restriction of the valve and severe mitral incompetence (Fig. 2.21) or late rupture of the mitral ring sutures with paravalvular leakage development. The suspicion of ring–ring mismatch requires close follow-up during the initial period after ring implantation to avoid the complication of native ring rupture over the long term.

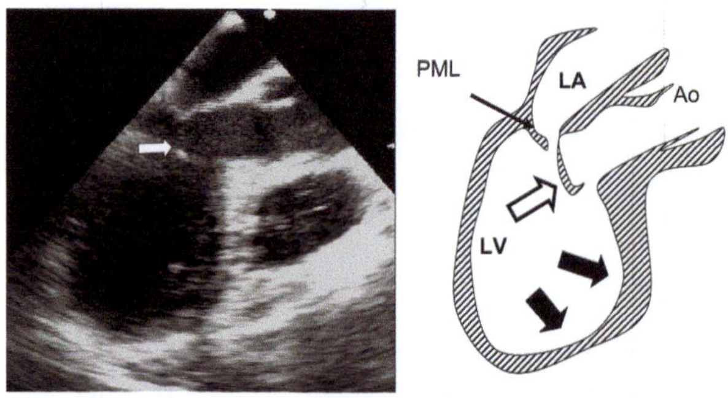

Fig. 2.20. The systolic anterior motion (SAM; *white arrows*) in this case was caused by anterior wall dyskinesia (*black arrows*) and posterior wall hyperkinesia after bypass surgery. *LA* left atrium, *LV* left ventricle, *Ao* aorta, *PML* posterior mitral leaflet

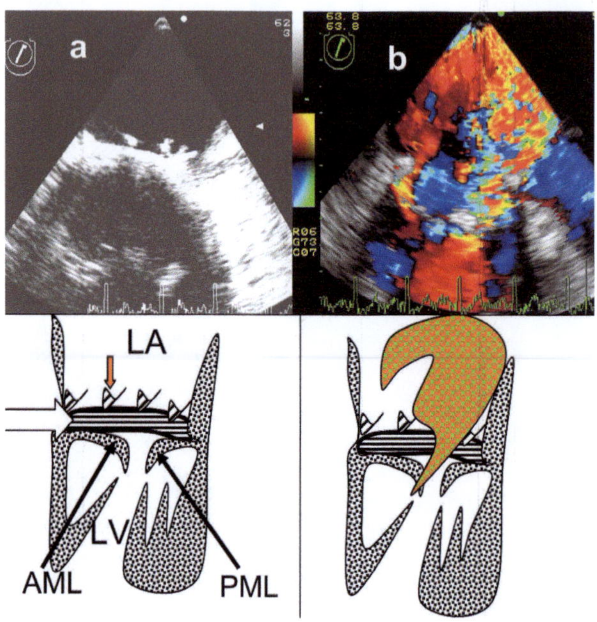

Fig. 2.21. Mitral repair using an elastic mitral ring (**a**) (surgical sutures are visible (*orange arrow*)). Note restriction of subvalvular apparatus which causes severe mitral regurgitation in color Doppler (**b**). *LA* left atrium, *LV* left ventricle, *AML* anterior mitral leaflet, *PML* posterior mitral leaflet

2.9 Conclusions

Although preoperative diagnosis is based on a spectrum of invasive and noninvasive non-echocardiographic tools, perioperative echocardiography plays a very important role in contemporary mitral valve repair. Reconstructive mitral valve surgery requires thorough preparation of the patients for the planned procedure. Echocardiography in experienced hands provides excellent information on cardiac morphology and function and can compete with other techniques, including magnetic resonance imaging and computed tomography. What is most important is that echocardiographic investigation, being a real time/real motion technique of visualization, can be undertaken at almost »any time and any place« to evaluate the results of mitral valve repair.

Acknowledgment

We would like to thank Anne M. Gale, Editor in the Life Sciences, for editorial assistance

References

1. Fuchs RM, Heuser RR, Yin FCP, Brinker JA (1982) Limitations of pulmonary wedge V-waves in diagnosing mitral regurgitation. Am J Cardiol 49:849–854
2. Siniawski H, Weng Y, Hetzer R (1991) Decision-making aspects in the surgical treatment of ischemic mitral incompetence. In: Vetter HO, Hetzer R, Schmutzler H (eds) Ischemic mitral incompetence. Steinkopff, Darmstadt, pp 137–147
3. Siniawski H, Warnecke H, Weng Y, Drews T, Hetzer R (1991) Perioperative echocardiographic assessment of the heart function in the patients treated by mitral reconstruction or replacement with complete papillary-annular continuity. Abstract. Circulation 84(Suppl 2):II577
4. Stevenson RR, Tunrer WJ (1935) Rupture of a papillary muscle in the heart as a cause of sudden death. Bull John Hopkins Hosp 57:235–242
5. Grula G, Yacoub MH (1981) Surgical correction of complete rupture of the anterior papillary muscle. Ann Thorac Surg 32:88–95
6. Gerbode FLA, Hetzer R, Krebber HJ (1978) Surgical management of papillary muscle rupture due to myocardial infarction. World J Surg 2:751–795
7. DiSesa VJ, Cohn JH, Collins JJ, et al. (1982) Determinants of operative survival following combined mitral valve replacement and coronary revascularization. Ann Thorac Surg 34:482–486
8. Carpentier A, Didier L, Deloche A (1987) Surgical anatomy and management of ischemic mitral valve incompetence. Circuation 76(Suppl. 111):111–446
9. Hetzer R (1981) Prosthetic valve endocarditis. In: Boerhave (ed) Causes of Infectious Endocarditis. Leiden
10. Easaw J, El-Omar M, Ramsey M (2000) Perivalvar abscess of the mitral valve annulus with perforation owing to infective endocarditis. Heart 83:261
11. Braimbridge MV (1969) Cardiac surgery and bacterial endocarditis. Lancet 1:1307–1309
12. Siniawski H, Grauhan O, Hofmann M, Pasic M, Weng Y, Yankah C, Lehmkuhl H, Hetzer R (2004) Heart Surg Forum 7(5):E405–410
13. Jebara VA, Mihaileanu S, Acar C, Brizard C, Grare P, Latremouille C, Chauvaud S, Fabiani JN, Deloche A, Carpentier A (1993) Left ventricular outflow tract obstruction after mitral valve repair. Results of the sliding leaflet technique. Circulation 88:II30–34
14. Siniawski H, Lehmkuhl H, Weng Y, Hetzer R (2004) High pressure gradients in left ventricular outflow tract after aortic valve replacement. Acta Cardiologica 59(2):235–236
15. Kunzelman KS, Reimink MS, Cochran RP (1998) Flexible versus rigid ring annuloplasty for mitral valve annular dilatation: a finite element model. J Heart Valve Dis 7:108 –116
16. Arita M, Kasegawa H, Umezu M (2004) Static analysis of annuloplasty rings sutured on an annulus model of the mitral valve: comparison between the Duran ring and the Carpentier Classic ring. J Artif Organs 7:30 –36

17. Salgo IS, Gorman JH, III, Gorman RC, Jackson BM, Bowen FW, Plappert T, St John Sutton MG, Edmunds LH Jr (2002) Effect of annular shape on leaflet curvature in reducing mitral leaflet stress. Circulation 106:711–717
18. Jimenez JH, Soerensen DD, He Z, He S, Yoganathan AP (2003) Effects of a saddle shaped annulus on mitral valve function and chordal force distribution: an in vitro study. Ann Biomed Eng 31:1171–1181
19. Jensen MO, Jensen H, Smerup M, Levine RA, Yoganathan AP, Nygaard HJ, Hasenkam M, Nielsen SL (2008) Saddle-shaped mitral valve annuloplasty rings experience lower forces compared with flat rings. Circulation 118: S250– S255

II Congenital mitral and tricuspid disease

Mitral valve repair in children

E.M. Delmo Walter, R. Hetzer

3

3.1 Introduction

Surgical management of mitral valve disease in infants and children has been a major therapeutic challenge for many years. It poses special surgical difficulties because of the wide spectrum of morphological abnormalities requiring meticulous modifications of the valve repair techniques [1, 2, 3], a high incidence of associated cardiac anomalies [4, 5], and relatively limited experience in each surgical center. At our institution, mitral valve (MV) reconstruction is the preferred technique for any kind of MV disease in infants, children, and adolescents. This avoids the need for valve replacement with all its drawbacks, particularly in infants and small children, in the face of the complete lack of prostheses suitable for this age group. Even when the primary repair result is not optimal, time is gained for repeated repair until an appropriate adult-size prosthesis can be implanted. We believe that reconstruction allows for valve growth without the need of anticoagulation. This is best achieved by using a spectrum of repair techniques applied individually and avoiding any prosthetic material. We have reviewed our 20-year experience with surgical reconstruction of the MV in pediatric age groups to assess our techniques and determine early and long-term survival and freedom from reoperation and valve replacement.

3.2 Patient population

Between June 1987 and December 2007, we surgically treated 437 pediatric patients (age <18 years) with MV diseases, 173 (39.6%) of whom underwent mitral valve surgery for either congenital or acquired MV diseases. Excluded from this study were 62 patients with type II mitral insufficiency, in whom the severely dysplastic annulus, leaflets, and deformed subvalvular apparatus were initially repaired but intraoperative echocardiography showed persistent severe mitral insufficiency; hence, after several reconstructive attempts, the decision to replace the MV was made during the same surgical procedure. Likewise, patients with left-sided atrioventricular valve anomalies associated with septal defects and those with Marfan's syndrome and other degenerative diseases were excluded (*n*=264). Thus, data were available for 111 (25.5%) children who had MV reconstruction using various surgical techniques. Demographic data, surgical techniques used, postoperative course, and follow-up data provided by the Departments of Pediatric Cardiology and of Clinical Studies, Deutsches Herzzentrum Berlin as well as by the referring physicians were reviewed.

3.3 Demographic data

The series comprised 67 boys and 44 girls whose mean age was 7.5±5.9 years (range 1 day–17.8 years). The children were divided into three age groups: <3 months old (*n*=6), >3 months –2 years old (*n*=28), and 2–18 years old (*n*=77). At the time of surgery, 32 (27.9%) patients were in NYHA class II, 45 (40.5%) in class III, and 34 (30.6%) in class IV. Degree of MV lesions, left ventricular function, and associated anomalies were assessed by echocardiography or cardiac catheterization, or by a combination of the two techniques.

3.4 Classification of mitral valve lesions

As several anomalies may coexist, the predominant anomaly was used to classify the lesion according to Carpentier's functional classification [3]. The distribution of children according to this classification is shown in Table 3.1. Grading of mitral valve insufficiency (MI) was based on echocardiographic measurements of regurgitant fraction (RF) (none=no RF; mild=RF <20%, moderate=RF 20–40%; moderate to severe= RF 40–60%; severe=RF >60%).

In a total of 22 (19.8 %) children, mitral valve stenosis (MS) was associated with Shone's anomaly in 8 patients (all with parachute valves), isolated parachute valve in 4 patients, presence of supramitral membrane in 2 patients, and anomalies of the subvalvular apparatus (e.g., papillary muscle fibrosis, shortened papillary muscles, chordal agenesis, chordal thickening, and chordal fusion) in 8 patients. Severity was evaluated based on echocardiographic measurements of the mitral valve orifice area (cm^2), i.e., none=4–6 cm^2; mild=2–4 cm^2; moderate=1–2 cm^2; severe$\leq$1 cm^2.

Table 3.1. Classification of the mitral valve lesions according to Carpentier functional approach

	<3 months (*n*=9)	>3 months–2 years (*n*=29)	>2–18 years (*n*=73)
Type I: normal leaflet motion			
Annular dilatation	[5][a]	[11][a]	[15][a]
Mitral cleft		4	10
Leaflet defect/perforation		1	8
Type II: leaflet prolapse			
Leaflet prolapse	3	6	15
Chordal elongation/rupture		2	8
Papillary muscle elongation/rupture	1	5	6
Absence of chordae	1		
Type III: restricted leaflet motion			
Normal papillary muscles			
Commissural fusion	2	2	13
Leaflet thickening	1	3	5
Short chordae/chordal fusion/thickening	1	1	5
Abnormal papillary muscle			
Parachute mitral valve		3	1
Hammock mitral valve		1	1
Papillary muscle hypoplasia		1	1

[a] Coexisted with other valve lesions; hence, numbers do not coincide with total number of patients

3.5 Associated lesions

Mitral valve lesions were associated with other congenital defects in 107 (96.3%) patients, while 28 (25.2%) had previous operations: 8 patients with Shone's anomaly, 6 had undergone repair of coarctation of the aorta, 2 of whom had additional aortic valve balloon dilatation, while another 2 had had aortic valve reconstruction and previous aortic valve balloon dilatation, 1 of whom had previous mitral commissurotomy and aortic valve balloon dilatation. Previous operations were also recorded for 17 patients with mitral insufficiency (MI) and 3 patients with mitral stenosis (MS), either on the mitral or aortic valve or for other cardiac anomalies.

Concomitant repair of associated lesions was performed in 74 (66.7%) patients and included repair of complex cardiac anomalies in 47 (63.5%) patients, while the other 27 (36.5%) had concurrent repair of the aortic, tricuspid, and/or pulmonary valve.

3.6 Mitral valve reconstruction

All mitral valve reconstructions were performed through a median sternotomy under cardiopulmonary bypass and moderate systemic hypothermia (rectal temperature 28–32 °C). Antegrade intermittent cold crystalloid cardioplegia with topical hypothermia was used for myocardial protection. Through a left atriotomy along the interatrial groove, annulus, leaflets, chordae tendineae, and papillary muscles were exposed and meticulously inspected to determine the precise nature of the lesion and plan the procedure. Particular attention was given to the leaflet motion and position of the papillary muscles. The concept followed in our institution is preservation of the native valves and avoidance of any prosthetic materials, except for suture materials, whenever possible.

Depending on the underlying valve pathology, various reconstruction techniques were used. Because malformation usually implies several anomalies, several repair steps may have to be used in the same patient. Sutures used for repair in children were 5-0 to 7-0 polypropylene, according to age. Whenever necessary, pledgets and annular reinforcement strips from untreated autologous pericardium were used.

Intravalvular saline injection and intraoperative transesophageal echocardiography (TEE) were routinely performed to assess the adequacy of repair. Postoperative transthoracic echocardiography (TTE) was carried out annually, or if clinically indicated on the basis of symptoms. Regardless of the underlying pathology and techniques used, no patient was discharged from hospital with more than mild MI.

Modified Kay-Wooler annuloplasty was most frequently used in small infants with annular dilatation, performed by shortening the segments of the posterior annulus next to both trigones by polypropylene sutures pledgeted with untreated autologous pericardium (◘ Fig. 3.1a, b) [6].

Modified Paneth annuloplasty was used mostly in children and adolescents with severely dilated annulus of any origin, performed by shortening the posterior annulus with polypropylene sutures anchored to both trigones with pledgets of untreated autologous pericardium (◘ Fig. 3.2a) [6]. The degree and extent of shortening are chosen to effect good leaflet coaptation, according to the calculated weight-related valve size. The shortened posterior annulus is stabilized with a strip of untreated autologous pericardium (◘ Fig. 3.2b, c) [6].

Modified Gerbode plication plasty was used for ruptured chordae of the central scallop of the posterior leaflet (◘ Fig. 3.3a) [6].The flail leaflet segment is plicated towards the ventricle

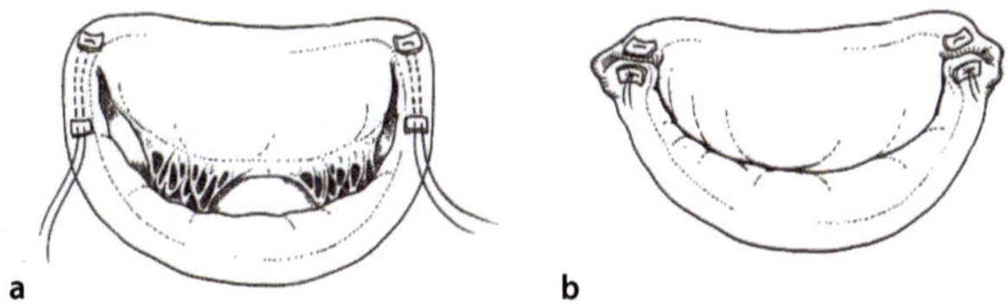

Fig. 3.1. a Modified Kay–Wooler annuloplasty, **b** completed repair

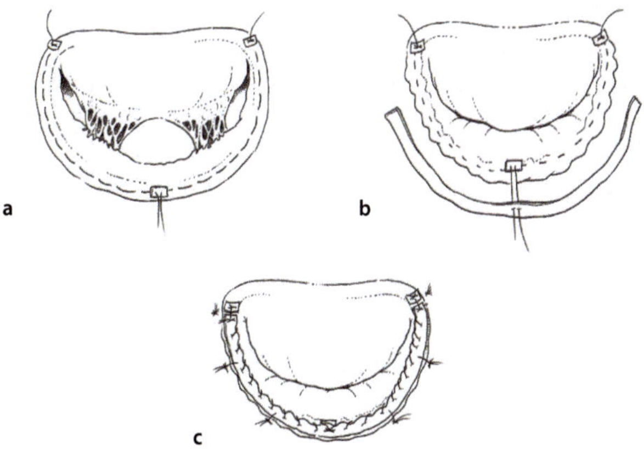

Fig. 3.2. a Modified Paneth posterior annulus shortening plasty, **b** reinforcement with autologous pericardial strip (Hetzer's technique), **c** completed repair

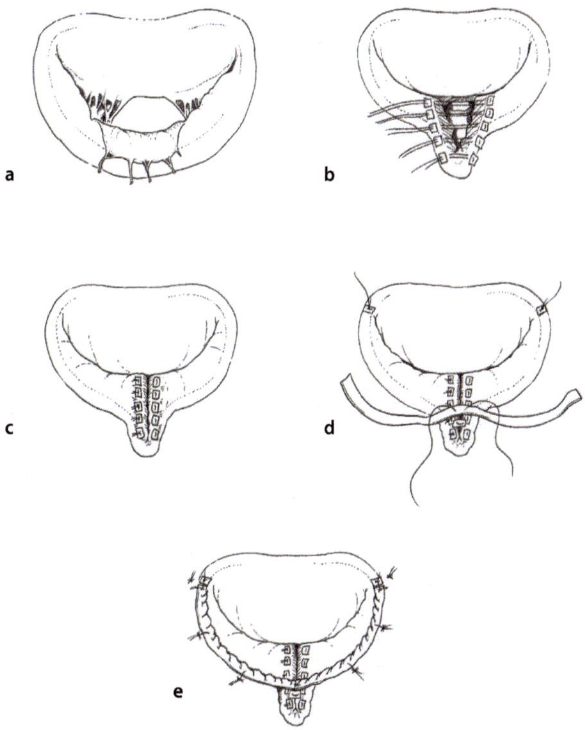

Fig. 3.3. Modified Gerbode plication plasty: **a** ruptured chordae of posterior leaflet, **b** Gerbode plication plasty, **c** completed Gerbode plication plasty, **d** reinforcement with untreated autologous pericardial strip (Hetzer's technique), **e** completed repair

by a V-shaped suture line of polypropylene mattress sutures pledgeted with untreated autologous pericardium (◘ Fig. 3.3b, c) [6]. When valve competence is assured, the posterior annulus is stabilized with a strip of untreated autologous pericardium anchored to both trigones with separate pledgeted mattress sutures (◘ Fig. 3.3d, e) [6].

Anterior leaflet retention plasty (ALRP) was employed for the treatment of hypertrophic obstructive cardiomyopathy (HOCM) and prevention of systolic anterior motion (SAM). In these patients, no distinct abnormalities of the chordae tendineae and papillary muscles were apparent. Repair was guided by TEE with careful assessment of the septal anatomy and thickness, MV function, and anatomy and mobility of the subvalvular apparatus. Segments of the anterior leaflet closest to the trigones were sutured to the corresponding posterior annulus with polypropylene mattress sutures pledgeted with untreated autologous pericardium. Sutures are passed through the coaptation line of the anterior leaflet and the corresponding posterior annulus (◘ Fig. 3.4a, b) [6]. Thus, the anterior MV leaflet becomes limited in its mobility in the segment near the trigones and is, therefore, unable to produce systemic anterior motion (SAM) and MI (◘ Fig. 3.4c, d) [6]. Intraoperative MV orifice measurement is facilitated by using a Hegar dilator based on an age-related minimal normal valve diameter to ensure that no MS is produced. ALRP has always been accompanied by a Morrow-type subaortic septal myectomy via a transaortic approach.

Direct intracardiac pressures were measured simultaneously in the left ventricle and aorta. If the left ventricular outflow tract (LVOT) gradient is low (<30 mmHg) because of anesthesia, isoproterenol is administered or premature ventricular contractions are induced to determine the maximal gradient. An oblique aortotomy is made, rightward down to the noncoronary sinus toward the aortic annulus. The aortic valve is inspected and the subvalvular region exposed. We make parallel incisions into the septum directly opposite the anterior mitral leaflet. Resection of long blocks of septal myocardium between the two incisions is started just below the aortic annulus of the right coronary sinus and the commissure between the right and the left coronary sinuses (◘ Fig. 3.4e) [6].The incision should be continued apically beyond the point of mitral–septal contact, which is usually marked by a fibrous band. This wide incision beneath the aortic valve improves exposure of the important area towards the apex. Intraoperative preseptal myectomy pressure gradient ranged from 40–105 (mean 60±25) mmHg and postseptal myectomy gradient ranged from 0–18 (mean 5±6) mmHg. After septal myectomy and ALRP, the aortic and mitral valves are inspected to ensure that they had not been injured. Pressures are remeasured in the left ventricle and aorta, and the TEE evaluation is repeated after weaning from cardiopulmonary bypass. If myectomy has been successful, there will be little or no residual gradient, and little or no systolic anterior motion of the mitral valve. Overall, postmyectomy mitral insufficiency was reduced to a regurgitant fraction of 0–10%. There was no early or late mortality, nor reoperation for repeat myectomy or repeat mitral valve repair or replacement. No instance of MS occurred.

Repair of hammock valve (◘ Fig. 3.5a) [6]. In the absence of any papillary muscle, a suitably thick part of the posterior left ventricular wall carrying the rudimentary chordae is carved off the wall (◘ Fig. 3.5b) [6]. Then it must be assured that both the remaining left ventricular wall and the »new papillary muscles« maintain sufficient muscle thickness to perform their function (◘ Fig. 3.5c) [6].

Repair of parachute valve. The most appropriate site for leaflet-splitting incisions is defined on both sides from the common papillary muscles towards the »assumed« trigones (com-

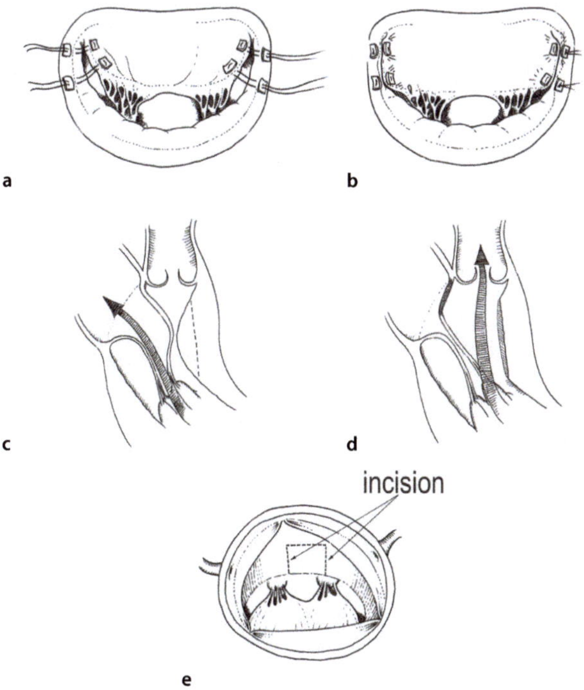

Fig. 3.4. a Anterior leaflet retention plasty (ALRP) for hypertrophic obstructive cardiomyopathy (HOCM) and systolic anterior motion (SAM) (Hetzer's technique). **b** Completed repair (atrial view). **c** Mitral insufficiency in HOCM and SAM before repair. **d** Redirection of mitral insufficiency following septal myectomy and ALRP. **e** Septal myectomy (aortic view) opposite anterior mitral valve leaflet (Hetzer's technique) (*dashed lines* indicate myocardial septal incisions)

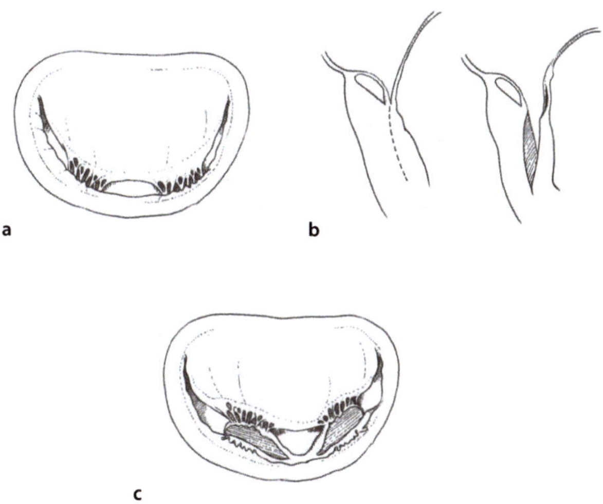

Fig. 3.5. Hammock valve: **a** pre-repair, **b** splitting off a papillary muscle from the posterior ventricular wall, **c** post-repair

misurotomy and fenestration, Fig. 3.6a, b) [6] These incisions are extended into the body of the papillary muscle which is split toward its base assuring sufficient thickness of both new »papillary muscle heads« (Fig. 3.6c–e) [6].

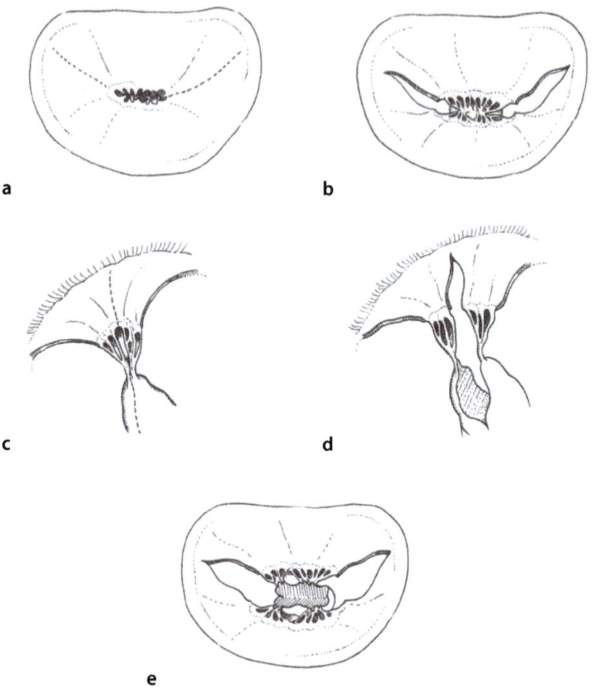

Fig. 3.6. Parachute valve: **a** pre-repair, **b** commissurotomy and fenestration, **c, d** commissurotomy and splitting of the papillary muscles, **e** completed repair

Repair in mitral valve endocarditis. Standard operative principles were adequate debridement of all infected tissues, meticulous washing of all affected areas with 7.5 g povidone containing 10% iodine solution regardless of the presence or absence of purulence or vegetations, meticulous removal of vegetations when present, and reconstruction using untreated autologous pericardial strips and pledgets for suture reinforcement. MV reconstruction was performed as follows: anterior commissuroplasty (Fig. 3.1a, b) [6] in 2 patients, posterior commissuroplasty with leaflet resection (Fig. 3.2a) in another 2 patients, posterior commissuroplasty with pericardial strip reinforcement (Fig. 3.2b, c) [6] in 3 patients, and chordal rupture repaired by chordal reimplantation in 1 patient.

Other repair strategies. Flexible ring annuloplasty was used in 4 (3.6%) patients in our early years. The mitral cleft in this series was restricted to the anterior leaflet. The posterior leaflet appeared normal in size. There was no accompanying annular dilatation or abnormal subvalvular apparatus or subaortic obstruction due to the chordal attachments of the cleft. The isolated anterior mitral leaflet cleft was corrected by a direct suture technique, either completely or partially closed, as necessary, based on a minimal acceptable age-dependent mitral valve diameter to avoid mitral stenosis. In 2 patients in our series, suture of the cleft was impossible because of retraction of both parts of the anterior mitral valve leaflet. Augmentation of the anterior leaflet with a pericardial patch was accomplished in 1 patient, whereas the other underwent an Alfieri procedure. Leaflet perforation was directly sutured or closed with a pericardial patch. The supramitral membrane, when found, was excised. All concomitant congenital heart anomalies were repaired accordingly.

3.7 Results

3.7.1 Early mortality

Early death occurred in 5 (4.5%) patients, 4 with MI and 1 with combined lesions. One was a case of rescue MV reconstruction due to iatrogenic leaflet injury from balloon dilatation of an aortic isthmus stenosis in an 11-day-old infant. A 1-month-old infant with ischemic MI caused by Bland–White–Garland syndrome and associated cardiac anomalies received extracorporeal membrane oxygen (ECMO) support after surgery but died on postoperative day 7. A 3-month-old infant with Shone's anomaly and hypoplastic left heart syndrome underwent urgent MV repair. Postoperatively, he had heart failure and capillary leak syndrome and died on postoperative day 18. Another 5-month-old infant with severe anterior leaflet prolapse, associated hypoplastic ascending aortic root, and pulmonary hypertension, in whom ECMO was instituted because of low output syndrome, died on postoperative day 2. A 16-year-old adolescent with a double inlet left ventricle, L-TGA and rudimentary right ventricle, and severe tricuspid insufficiency underwent the modified Paneth technique for MI with concomitant modified De Vega tricuspid annuloplasty and had intraoperative ECMO because of heart failure. He underwent heart transplantation on postoperative day 3 but unfortunately died on postoperative day 14.

3.7.2 Late mortality

There were 9 (8.1%) late deaths among the 106 patients who were discharged from the hospital. A 2-month-old infant with congenital MS who underwent MV replacement with a heterograft 4 months after the initial reconstruction did not survive the second procedure. A child aged 7 months at the time of initial operation with severe anterior mitral prolapse died of a noncardiac event 5 years postoperatively. A 1-year-old child who had myocardial infarction due to an anomalous coronary artery died 11 months later. A patient aged 2 years at the time of initial operation with isolated parachute valve underwent repeat MV reconstruction 5 years postoperatively and then MV replacement 2 years later but died 8 years postoperatively. One 8-year-old patient with Shone's anomaly died from a noncardiac event 13 years postoperatively. Two 10-year-old children, both with cardiomyopathy, died of heart failure 2 and 7 months after the operation, respectively. Another 13-year-old who had Shone's anomaly died of unknown causes 2 years postoperatively. A 17-year-old girl with multiple endocrinological abnormalities and severe MI from dysplastic posterior leaflet died from a noncardiac cause 6 years after successful initial MV reconstruction.

Actuarial survival was 95.5±2.6% at 30 days, 88.4±3.2% at 1 year, 85.5±3.7% at 5 years, and 77.4±5.1% at both 10 and 20 years (◘ Fig. 3.7a). Overall survival rates by age group over a 20-year period are shown in ◘ Fig. 3.7b.

3.7.3 Reoperation

Overall freedom from reoperation was 88.8± 3.1, 86.2± 3.5, 79.2± 5.1, and 73.5± 7.2 at 1, 5, 10, and both 15 and 20 follow-up years (◘ Fig. 3.7c). There were 7 patients who underwent repeat MV reconstruction at a mean of 3.9 (range 1–6) years postoperatively. Mean age at reoperation was 7.8±1.75 (range 0.12–20.4) years. Two patients, both with isolated parachute valves,

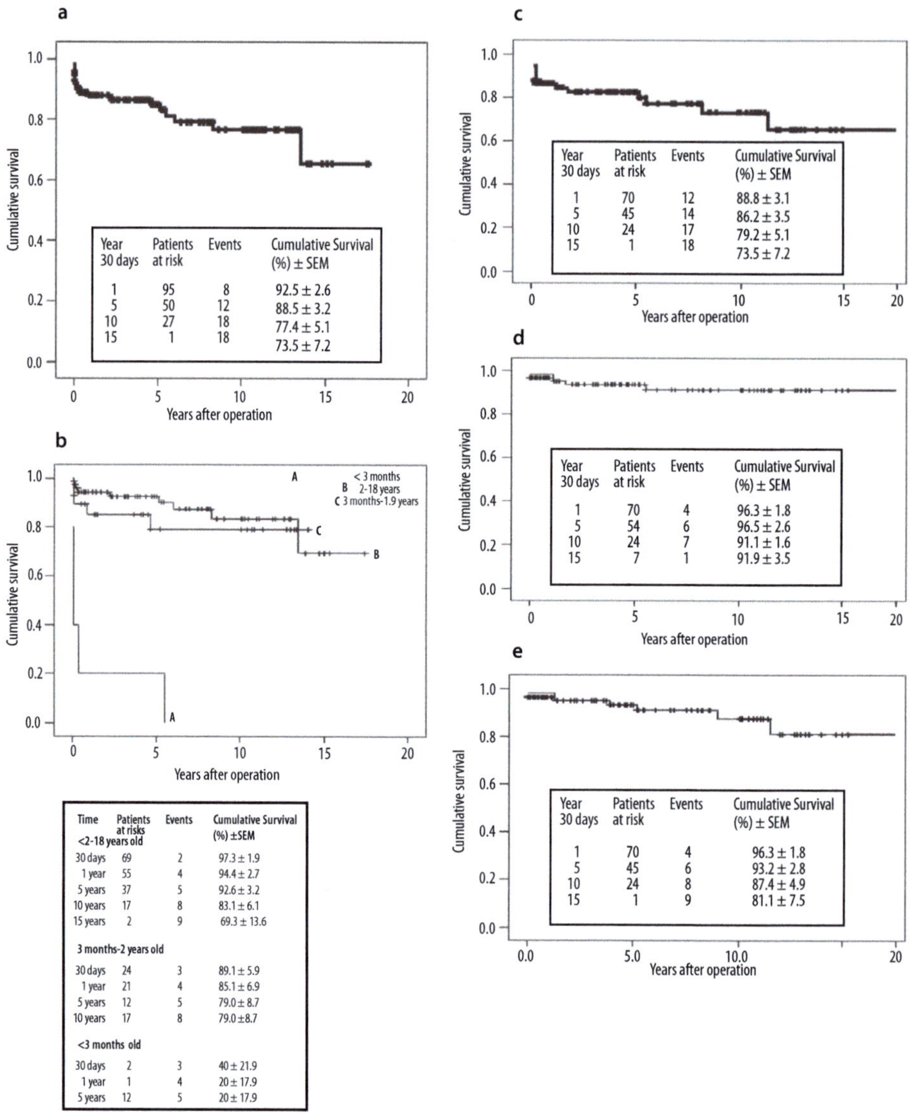

Fig. 3.7. Kaplan–Meier curves showing overall survival rate for a 20-year period (**a**), overall survival rates by age group over a 20-year period (**b**), overall freedom from reoperation over a 20-year period (**c**), freedom from repeat mitral valve reconstruction over a 20-year period (**d**), freedom from mitral valve replacement over a 20-year period (**e**)

were reoperated upon 2 and 5 years after the operation, respectively. One patient with papillary muscle fibrosis had repeat reconstruction 1 year later. A patient who had Shone's anomaly had another reconstruction 2 years postoperatively. Five years postoperatively, 2 patients, one with MV prolapse and another with combined mitral stenosis and insufficiency, underwent repeat MV reconstruction. One patient with mitral cleft had another reconstruction 6 years later. Freedom from repeat MV reconstruction was 96.3±1.8%, 96.5±2.6%, 91.1±1.5%, and 91.1±1.5% at 1, 5, 10 and 20 years, respectively (Fig. 3.7d).

Table 3.2. Multivariate Cox regression analysis of perioperative factors with regard to mortality and reoperation

	Odds ratio	95 % Confidence interval	p value
Gender	1.78	0.716–4.455	0.040
Age 2 vs.1[a]	0.07	0.02–0.26	<0.00
3 vs. 1[a]	0.05	0.01–0.14	< 0.001
Etiology: congenital vs. acquired	0.28	0.04–2.179	0.225
MI vs. MS	2.29	0.8–6.17	0.130
MS/MI vs. MI	2.90	0.79–10.63	0.108
Previous operation	1.42	0.97–1.43	0.098
Associated cardiac anomalies	1.87	0.67–1.29	0.23
Concomitant surgery	0.35	0.10–1.21	0.012
Urgent or emergency vs. elective	3.42	1.39–8.43	0.008
Bypass time	1.004	1.001–1.007	0.003
Ischemic time	1.10	0.99–1.02	0.003
Reperfusion time	1.006	1.002–1.009	0.004
Total operative time	1.004	1.001–1.006	0.004
Valve status on discharge	3.56	0.69–7.24	0.027

[a]1= ≤3 months old; 2= 3 months–2 years old; 3= >2–18 years old
MI mitral insufficiency, *MS* mitral stenosis

Eight patients eventually underwent MV replacement at a mean of 6.1 years (range 4 months–17 years) postoperatively. Overall freedom from MV replacement is 96.3±1.8%, 93.2±2.8%, 87.4±4.9%, and 81.1±7.5% at 1, 5, 10, and both 15 and 20 years, respectively (Fig. 3.7e).

Multivariate analysis revealed that age at operation, concomitant operations, urgency of operation, operative times, and valve status on discharge were risk factors for mortality and reoperation (Table 3.2).

3.7.4 Follow-up

Three patients from foreign countries were lost to follow-up at 4, 9, and 13 years. Follow-up of the remaining patients was complete and comprised 593 patient–years (mean 5.4±0.46 years). Improvements in degree of both insufficiency and stenosis after valve reconstruction were maintained until the last follow-up. An acceptable postoperative outcome was achieved in all 85 (76.6%) surviving patients. Mild stenosis was noted in 3 of the 13 patients who previously had severe MS. Among the 72 patients who had had MI as the predominant lesion, only 8 patients had mild to moderate insufficiency at their latest follow-up (Table 3.3).

Table 3.3. Most recent valve status among survivors (n=86[a])

Lesion	Follow-up	Current valve status				
Mitral valve insufficiency		0	I	II	III	IV
n (%)	Early term	61 (83.6%)	12 (16.4%)	–	–	–
	Mid-term	56 (76.7%)	17 (23.2%)	–	–	–
	Long-term	50 (68.4%)	15 (20.5%)	8 (10.9%)	–	–
Mitral valve stenosis		0	I	II	III	IV
n (%)	Early term	13 (100%)	–	–	–	–
	Mid-term	10 (77%)	3 (23%)	–	–	–
	Long-term	10 (77%)	3 (23%)	–	–	–

[a]Patients (n=8) who underwent eventual MV replacement are excluded. Echocardiographic grading of mitral valve insufficiency (based on regurgitant fraction) and mitral stenosis (based on mitral valve orifice area, cm^2 and mean resting end-diastolic gradient, mmHg)

Mitral insufficiency: *none* absence of regurgitant fraction; *mild* regurgitant fraction of <20%, *moderate* 20–40% regurgitant fraction; *moderate to severe* 40–60% regurgitant fraction; *severe* ≥60% regurgitant fraction

Mitral stenosis: *none* 4–6 cm^2, 0 mmHg; *mild* 2–4 cm^2, <5 mmHg; *moderate* 1–2 cm^2, 5–10 mmHg; *severe* ≤1 cm^2, >10 mmHg

0 none, *I* mild, *II* moderate, *III* moderate to severe, *IV* severe

3.7.5 Morbidity

Nonfatal complications affected 3 patients who returned to the operating room for management of postoperative bleeding. One patient required permanent pacemaker implantation for complete heart block and another had diaphragmatic plication to correct the paralysis, both performed within 30 days after the operation No patient had thrombotic problems.

3.8 Discussion

Although it is extremely challenging to reconstruct mitral valves in infants and children, not only because of their size, but also because of the immature and fragile leaflet tissues in infants and associated congenital cardiac abnormalities, we believe that this population gains optimally from reconstruction. Our results of repair in this group are encouraging, with actuarial survival rates of 77.4±5.1% at 20 years, comparable to or even higher than those reported in the literature [4, 7, 8], and actuarial freedom from repeat reconstruction and replacement comparable to that of reported series [9–12]. It is also important to note that 94% were in NYHA functional classes I and II with normal growth and development.

In addition, mitral valves significantly lacking in valve tissues, or severely dysplastic, with severe deformation of the subvalvular apparatus that rendered reconstruction impossible, as in 62 patients who were excluded from this study, were encountered. Attempts to reconstruct and preserve their valves proved futile, since satisfactory functional results could not be achieved; hence, their valves were replaced during the same surgical procedure. Based on this experience, we learned that the main goal of surgical repair should be to achieve satisfactory, if not ideal, MV function, rather than an ideal anatomical or morphological reconstruction.

We believe that the key to a satisfactory outcome is thorough preoperative evaluation and understanding of the valve abnormality with meticulous attention given to the anatomical and functional features of the MV apparatus and the precise mechanisms causing stenosis or insufficiency. Attempts to preserve the native mitral valve should be encouraged, especially in infants and young children since MV repair offers the advantages of avoiding thromboembolism, preserving chordal and subvalvular apparatus function, thus, making reoperation unnecessary [11].

In this population, annular dilatation and prolapsed leaflet were frequently present. We tried to avoid placement of a rigid ring prosthesis for stabilization or to correct annulus abnormalities because of concerns about anticoagulation, subsequent somatic growth problems and risk of a rigid prosthesis causing distortion of the heart cavities and/or contributing to left ventricular outflow tract obstruction [7]. Several studies consider ring annuloplasty for MV incompetence obligatory in children over 2 years of age [13–15]. This concept is supported by their experience of a 25% incidence rate of significant residual mitral regurgitation after repair without ring insertion [13]. Other groups demonstrated that other types of annuloplasty techniques can be employed successfully in children and that prosthetic rings are not indispensable for achieving favorable results [16, 17]. In most of our patients, commissure plication annuloplasty was employed to correct the annular dilatation, which was reported to yield adequate long-term functional results [18]. We found that annuloplasty using the techniques of Kay-Wooler, Paneth, and Gerbode with reinforcement by an autologous pericardial strip [19] proved to be highly satisfactory.

Hammock MV, dysplastic with shortened chordae directly inserted into a muscular mass of the posterior wall of the left ventricle, resulting in tethering of both leaflets, was one of the most challenging malformations to correct, as was also stated by other authors [5, 9, 16, 20, 21]. The key to a successful reconstruction was mobilization of these shortened chordae by splitting or incising them off the posterior muscular ventricular wall.

Surgical repair of congenital MS has been reported to be associated with greater postoperative mortality and morbidity [16, 20]. In this series, 12 of the 22 patients with MS had parachute MV. Leaflets and commissures were normal but the chordae tendineae were short and thickened, reducing leaflet motion. Reconstruction was a combination of splitting of the parachute, commissurotomy and fenestration. All patients did well.

In parachute and hammock valves, the degree and extent of incision or fenestration and commissurotomy are determined by measurement with a Hegar dilator, based on the minimal age-related acceptable MV diameter to avoid MS. Adequate reconstruction becomes a balance between residual stenosis and induced insufficiency, assessed intraoperatively with TEE.

Shone's anomaly requires an equally challenging surgical strategy. Understanding its mitral valve morphology is critical to determine the reconstructive approach. Parachute MV and supravalvular mitral ring are the most prevalent variants of mitral stenosis in this disease [22]. Supraannular fibrous ring, a characteristic feature, rarely occurs as an isolated lesion and is not usually severely obstructive. Resection of this ring should be straightforward [23]. Although recurrence has been described [23], our experience and that of others [23–25] show that it is rare. Even when the parachute is associated with significant subaortic stenosis, we believe that such lesions are amenable to repair, because the main obstructive mitral element is subvalvar. The majority of our patients presented initially in the neonatal period with coarctation of the aorta and some type of LVOT obstruction effectively treated by transaortic resection. Outcomes are related to the degree to which MS can be relieved. Satisfactory hemodynamic results have been achieved in this series by splitting the papillary muscle and releasing and separating the chordae tendineae to open the obliterated chordal spaces and increase the effective mitral orifice.

Surgery in children with HOCM was technically demanding because of the difficulty in exposing the smaller structures. Our 9 patients with HOCM had associated moderate-to-severe MI. Our reconstructive approach has been modified to avoid the potential development of SAM after septal myectomy and mitral leaflet repair. We addressed the prolapsing anterior leaflet by performing anterior leaflet retention plasty which we found to be excellent in restricting mitral valve motion, allowing more complete relief of subaortic obstruction and MI, and avoiding SAM. It is very important to evaluate the presence of abnormalities of the subvalvular apparatus in HOCM, since failure to recognize and treat them may be fatal or lead to incomplete relief of obstruction [26]. Symptomatic improvement of the 9 patients was gratifying and all remain improved by at least one functional class. There has been no incidence of MS following ALRP in this series.

In clefts with an otherwise normal MV, repair is accomplished by direct and complete suturing of the edges of the cleft in the majority, using the age-related minimal normal valve diameter as a guide to prevent valve stenosis.

Our study demonstrates that MV reconstruction can be safely performed in patients with MV lesions, e.g., complications of acute and chronic endocarditis, in agreement with the findings of Muehrcke and colleagues [27] who advocated early intervention and repair to prevent leaflet destruction and vegetation embolization, and to preserve left ventricular function. Likewise, Talwar and associates [28] found in their large series of 278 patients acceptable long-term results in repairing rheumatic valves. In our published report [29] of 8 children with infective endocarditis, all of them required an aggressive approach to valve preservation, and all did well postoperatively. The surgical approach we employed offered optimal ventricular remodeling owing to preservation of the valvular and subvalvular apparatus, absence of infection and, in general, absence of any anticoagulation therapy requirement.

No patients who underwent mitral valve reconstruction received anticoagulation, except for 2 patients who had undergone previous aortic valve replacement. There was no incidence of thromboembolism in this series. In contrast, Aharon et al. [4] reported that in their series they had 1 patient who had transient right-sided paralysis despite adequate anticoagulation after MV repair and aortic valve replacement.

Few reports on MV repair in children have identified predictors for poor outcome in this group of patients, probably because of the small numbers of patients in each report. We identified age <3 months, urgency of operation, concomitant procedures, operative times, and valve status on discharge as risk factors for mortality and reoperation.

Lack of durability of repair is a major setback of MV reconstruction in children. With meticulous intraoperative assessment of valve morphology and careful selection of the appropriate reconstruction strategy, repair can be long-lasting. Our actuarial freedom from reoperation at 10 and 20 years is encouraging, especially in this population where 30% of patients were less than 2 years of age. We have continued to modify our surgical techniques to optimize our results.

3.9 Conclusions

Mitral valve reconstruction is the surgical technique of choice for any kind of mitral disease in childhood. We believe that reconstruction allows continuous somatic and valve growth, delays or eliminates the need for future valve replacement and lifelong anticoagulation, and obviates the known complications of valve replacement which frequently requires subsequent reoperation to implant a larger prosthesis. It must be assumed that the majority of, if not all, valves repaired during childhood will eventually have to be replaced at some time in life. The concept of repair in childhood primarily aims to accommodate growth of the patient to an age when, if necessary, an adult size prosthesis can be implanted. Strong predictors for poor overall survival and freedom from reoperation are age less than 3 months, urgency of surgery, concomitant procedures, and long operative times.

Acknowledgment

We are grateful for the tremendous assistance of Anne Gale, Christine Detschades, Julia Stein, Astrid Benhennour, and Helge Haselbach in writing this chapter.

References

1. Murakami T, Yagihara T, Yamamoto F, Uemura H, Yamashita K, Ishizaka T (1998) Artificial chordae for mitral valve reconstruction inn children. Ann Thorac Surg 65:1377–1380
2. Aharon AS, Laks H, Drinkwater DC, Chugh R, Gates RN, Grant PW, Permut LC, Ardehali A, Rudis E (1994) Early and late results of mitral valve repair in children. J Thorac Cardiovasc Surg 107(5):1262–1270
3. Carpentier A (1994) Congenital malformation of the mitral valve. In: Stark, J, de Leval M (eds) Surgery for congenital heart defects. WB Saunders, Philadelphia pp 599–614
4. Lorier G, Kalil RA, Barcellos C, Teleo N, Hoppen GR, Netto AH, Prates PR, Vinholes SK, Prates PR, Sant Anna JRM, Nesralla LA (2001) Valve repair in children with congenital mitral lesions: late clinical results. Pediatr Cardiol 22:44–52
5. Naoki Yoshimura, Masahiro Yamaguchi, Yoshihiro Oshima, Shigeteru Oka, Yoshio Ootaki, Hiroshisa Murakami, Teruo Tei, Kyoichi Ogawa (1999) Surgery for mitral valve disease in the pediatric age group. J Thorac Cardiovasc Surg 118(1):99–106
6. Hetzer R, Delmo Walter EMB,Huebler M, Alexi-Meskishvili V, Weng Y, Nagdyman N, Berger F. (2008) Modified surgical techniques and long-term outcome of mitral valve reconstruction in 111 children. Ann Thorac Surg 86:604–613
7. Lessana A, Carbone C, Romano M, Palsky E, Quan YH, Escorsin M, Jegier B, Ruffenach A, Lutfalla G, Aime F, Guerin F (1990) Mitral valve repair: results and the decision-making process in reconstruction. Report of 275 cases. J Thorac Cardiovasc Surg 99(4):622–630
8. Kumar AS, Rao PN, Saxena A (1997) Mitral valve reconstruction: eight years' experience in 531 patients. J Heart Valve Dis 6 (6):591–593
9. McCarthy JF, Neligan MC, Wood AE. (1996) Ten years' experience of an aggressive reparative approach to congenital mitral valve anomalies. Eur. J. Cardio-thoracic Surg (7):534–539
10. Sousa UM, Gallenti L, Lacour-Gayet F, Piot D. Seraf A, Brumiax J, Comas J, roussin R, Touchot A, Binet JP, Planche C (1995) Surgery for congenital mitral valve disease in the first year of life. J Thorac Cardiovasc Surg 109(1):164–176
11. Stellin G, Padalino M, Milanesi O, Vida V, Favaro A, Rubino M, Bifafanti R, Casarotto D (2000) Repair of congenital mitral valve displasia in infants and children:is it always possible? Eur. J. Cardio-thoracic Surg 18 (1):74–82
12. Prifti E, Vanini V, Bonacchi M, Frati G, Bernabei M, Giunti G, et al. (2002) Repair of congenital malformations of the mitral valve: early and midterm results. Ann Thorac Surg 73:614–621
13. Chauvaud S, Fuzellier JF, Houel R, Berrebi A, Mihaileanu S, Carpentier A (1998) Reconstructive surgery in congenital mitral valve insufficiency (Carpentier's techniques): long-term results. J Thorac Cardiovasc Surg 115:84–93
14. Chauvaud SM, Mihaileanu SA, Gaer JAR, Carpentier A (1997) Surgical treatment of mitral valvar insufficiency. Cardiol Young 7:5–14
15. Wood AE, Healy DG, Nolke L, Duff D, Oslizlok P, Walsh K (2005) Mitral valve reconstruction in pediatric population: Late clinical results and predictors of long outcome. J Thorac Cardiovasc Surg 130(1):66–73
16. Zias EA, Mavroudis C, Backer CI, Kohr LM, Gotteiner NI, Rocchini AP (1998) Surgical repair of the congenitally malformed mitral valve in indfants and children. Ann Thorac Surg 66:1551–1559

17. Uva MS, Galletti L, Gayet FL, et al. (1995) Surgery for congenital mitral valve disease in the first year of life. J Thorac Cardiovasc Surg 109:164–176
18. Ohno H, Imai Y, Terada M, Hiramatsu T (1999) The long term results of commissure plication annuloplasty for congenital mitral insufficiency. Ann Thorac Surg 68(2):537–541
19. Komoda T, Hübler M, Siniawski H, Hetzer R (2000) Annular stabilization in mitral repair without a prosthetic ring. J Heart Valve Dis 9(6):776–782
20. Moran AM, Däbritz S, Keanne JF, Mayer JE (2000) Surgical management of mitral regurgitation after repair of endocardial cushion defects early and midterm results. Circulation 102:III160–165
21. Thieme C, Frescura C, Daliento L (1986) The pathology of the congenitally malformed mitral valve. In: Marcelletti C, Anderson RM, Becker AE, Corno A, Di Donato RM, Mazzera E (eds) Pediatric cardiology Churchhill-Livingstone New York, pp 225–239
22. Brown JW, Ruzmetov M, Palaniswamy V, Hoyer M, Girod D, Rodefeld D, Turrentine MW (2005) Operative results and outcomes in children with Shone's anomaly. Ann Thorac Surg 79:1358–1365
23. Tulloh RM, Bull C, Elliott MJ, Sullivan ID (1995) Supravalvar mitral stenosis: risk factors for recurrence or death after resection. Br Heart J 73:164–168
24. Serraf A, Zoghbi J, Belli E, et al. (2000) Congenital mitral stenosis with or without associated defects: an evolving surgical strategy. Circulation 102(Suppl III):166–171
25. Brown JW, Ruzmetov M, Vijay P, Rodefeld MD, Turrentine MW (2003) Surgery for aortic stenosis in children: a forty-year experience. Ann Thorac Surg 76:1398–1411
26. Minakata K, Dearani JA, Nishimura RA, Maron BJ, Danielson GK (2004) Extended septal myectomy for Hypertrophic obstructive cardiomyopathy with anomalous mitral papillary muscles or chordae. J Thorac Cardiovasc Surg 127(2):481–489
27. Muehrcke DD, Cosgrove DM 3rd, Lytle BW, Taylor PC, Burgar AM, Durnwald CP, Loop FD (1997) Is there an advantage to repairing infected mitral valve. Ann Thorac Surg 63(6):1718–1724
28. Talwar S, Rajesh MR, Subramanian A, Saxena A, Kumar S (2005) Mitral valve repair in children with rheumatic heart disease. J Thorac Cardiovasc Surg 129(4):875–879
29. Delmo Walter EM, Musci M, Nagdyman N, Huebler M, Berger F, Hetzer R (2007) Mitral valve repair for infective endocarditis in children. Ann Thorac Surg 84:2059–2065

Mitral valve repair using biodegradable annuloplasty rings

A. Kalangos

4.1 Evolution of the mitral and tricuspid annuloplasty concept using biodegradable suture materials and rings

The idea of developing a biodegradable ring is not a recent one. Already in 1983, Professor A. Carpentier predicted the potential use of biodegradable material for annuloplasty in his article entitled *Cardiac valve surgery–the French correction* by stating that the »reinforcement of the dysplastic annulus using a polyethyl-collagenol resorbable ring, which dissolves spontaneously in 12 months...« is »...replaced by strong connective tissue by a process of creeping substitution« [1].

In 1986, after this insight, Duran et al. [2] developed an absorbable flexible ring comprised of ox bovine fibrin and sewed it around the tricuspid annulus of dogs using a running 4-0 monofilament polypropylene suture. They noticed that the ring had completely disappeared by 1 to 2 months after its implantation in 9 of 10 dogs, and in all 10 dogs after 2 months. In dogs sacrificed between 2 and 4 weeks after implantation, histological analyses showed mild to moderate ring erosion and fibrous tissue covering the ring.

In 1990, Chachques et al. [3] described their experimental findings for a polydioxanone absorbable ring similar in shape to that of the rigid Carpentier–Edwards ring, covered with an extensible sewing sheath of high-porosity polyester, which they implanted onto the native mitral annulus as for a conventional ring. At 1 year, histological analyses showed only small residual particles of polydioxanone surrounded by collagen and elastic fibers, with fibroblasts in mitotic activity. No stenotic effect or other adverse affection of leaflet motion or pliability were demonstrated in growing animals, despite the presence of a fibrous reaction covering the ring within the first 2 weeks, increasing in thickness thereafter.

In 1992, Duran et al. [4] reported the histological results of a DeVega annuloplasty performed using a 2-0 polydioxanone suture in an experimental sheep model. The polydioxanone suture material remained practically intact during the first 3 months and its partial resorption at 5 months allowed the native tricuspid annulus to restore its initial dimensions. The authors concluded that temporary reinforcement of the tricuspid annulus was, hence, possible due to the gradual resorption of polydioxanone within 6 months. In 1993, Duran et al. [5] reported their clinical results for 73 patients with functional tricuspid regurgitation using a 2-0 polydioxanone suture. Based on the low rate of recurrent tricuspid insufficiency over the maximum follow-up of 2 years, they concluded that patients with functional tricuspid regurgitation and low pulmonary resistance could be adequately treated with the vanishing DeVega annuloplasty that stabilizes the tricuspid annulus for 4 months.

In 1994, Miyamura et al. [6] published their short- and midterm follow-up results for a clinical study carried out in children who underwent correction of their atrioventricular septal defect using a totally circular mitral annuloplasty with 4-0 poydioxanone or 4-0 polygalactin suture materials. Of these children, 77% maintained satisfactory valve function with gradual growth of the native mitral annulus over the follow-up period. There is no information in the literature with regard to the long-term fate or durability of mitral or tricuspid annuloplasty using such absorbable suture material. Indeed, the major disadvantages of polydioxanone and polygalactin sutures are the redilatation of the native annulus with the degradation process of the biodegradable material and the difficulties associated with precisely plicating the dilated posterior and the two commissural annulus segments according to the surface of the anterior mitral leaflet. For this reason, absorbable suture materials can sometimes result in residual valvular stenosis or insufficiency due to over- or undercorrection of annular dilatation.

Other potential disadvantages of such absorbable suture materials are their insufficient thickness with respect to pediatric needle sizes. A minimal thickness of suture material is required to generate an optimal intraannular fibrous reaction. Moreover, the lack of predesigned absorbable ring shapes in conformity with the shape of the entire or posterior part of the mitral orifice for mitral annuloplasty–and with that of the anteroposterior part of the tricuspid annulus for tricuspid annuloplasty–may hinder homogeneous fibrous remodeling of the mitral annulus and, hence, no longer respect the 3:4 relationship between the anteroposterior and lateral diameters of the mitral orifice, and thereby predispose the three-dimensional contractile geometry of the mitral annulus to subsequent deformity. In spite of all the above-mentioned disadvantages of such absorbable suture materials, we were encouraged by these annuloplasty techniques and especially the use of polydioxanone polymers in pediatric operations, and started developing a new biodegradable annuloplasty ring in 1994, which finally received CE (Conformity Marking Europe) approval in May 2005. It is currently undergoing clinical investigation by the FDA for the »humanitarian device exemption« procedure.

4.2 Characteristics of the biodegradable ring

The Kalangos® biodegradable ring has a curved »C« segment comprised of a poly-1,4-dioxanone polymer, located at the middle of a nondegradable suture material (2-0 polyvinyl monofilament for adult sizes and 3-0 for pediatric sizes) equipped with a stainless steel needle at each extremity (◘ Fig. 4.1). The suture material is in continuity over the entire central portion of the biodegradable ring in order to increase the resistance to tensile redilatory stretch of the dilated mitral and tricuspid annulus. The specific molecular weight of polydioxanone polymers, contrary to that of the biodegradable sutures, ensures structural memory against subsequent deformity, a key factor in initiating the generation of fibrous tissue leading to secondary annular remodeling; it also adds three-dimensional flexibility to the ring. The ring is available in various sizes (range 16–36) for both mitral and tricuspid annuloplasty; these sizes represent the intertrigonal distances for mitral annuloplasty. The ring has been designed to remodel the posterior and both commissural annulus segments in the mitral position and the anteroposterior part of the annulus in the tricuspid position, by inducing progressive fibrous tissue formation during its degradation by hydrolysis within

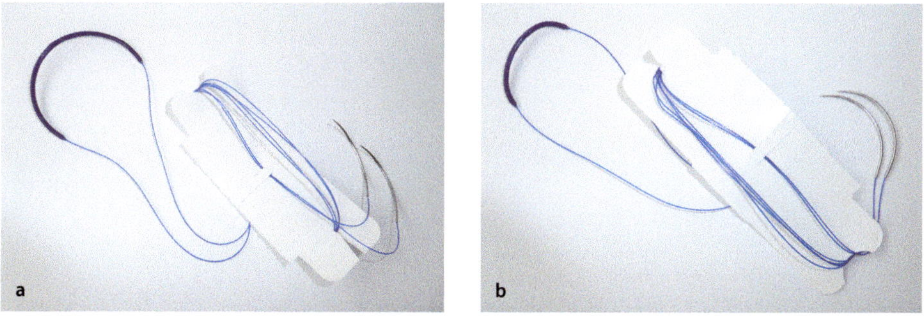

◘ Fig. 4.1. The biodegradable mitral (**a**) and tricuspid (**b**) rings

6 months after implantation. The gradual degradation of the ring within 6 months after implantation into the native annulus and the gradual increase in thickness of the fibrous tissue, which fills the space left by the degraded implant material and reaches the diameter of the implant at 12 months after implantation, is shown in ▣ Fig. 4.2 [7]. The degrading polymer stimulates inflammation that activates macrophages to secrete growth factors aimed at fibroblastic cell proliferation. The histological analysis of the conversion of the degradable ring into fibrous tissue at 1 month, 6 months, and at 1 year after implantation into the tricuspid annulus are shown in ▣ Fig. 4.3 [7].

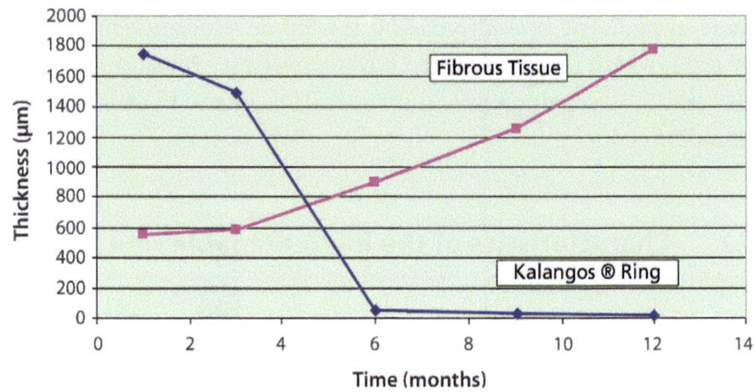

▣ **Fig. 4.2.** Ring degradation over time and the gradual induction of fibrous tissue ([7], © J Heart Valve Dis)

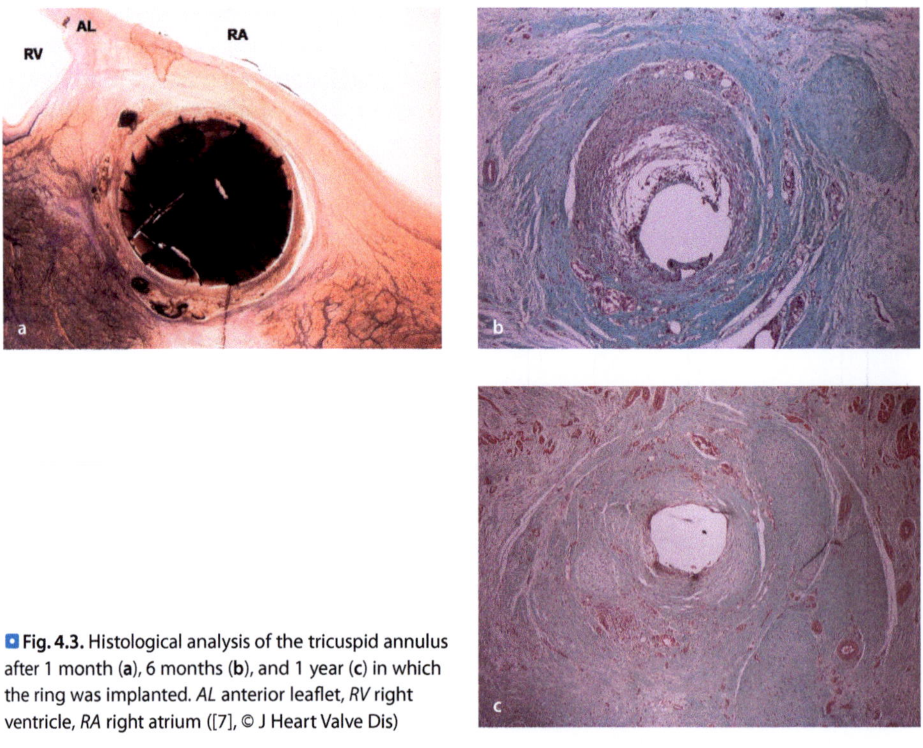

▣ **Fig. 4.3.** Histological analysis of the tricuspid annulus after 1 month (**a**), 6 months (**b**), and 1 year (**c**) in which the ring was implanted. *AL* anterior leaflet, *RV* right ventricle, *RA* right atrium ([7], © J Heart Valve Dis)

4.3 Surgical technique

The biodegradable ring, contrary to that of traditional rings implanted onto the native mitral or tricuspid annulus, is inserted into the native annulus to promote the inflammation process which will be converted into fibrous tissue, which incidentally prevents the release of degraded particles into the left atrial cavity. For mitral annuloplasty using the biodegradable ring, insertion starts at the level of the posterior commissure (2–3 mm from the insertion of the posterior leaflet on the annulus and 2–3 mm in depth) using the needle attached to one of the extremities of the prosthetic mitral ring. Insertion of the ring is begun by moving the inserted needle forward into the native annulus as far as possible and then pulling up the attached suture (*1* in ◘ Fig. 4.4a). The subsequent insertion of the needle is made through the first exit point of the first bite (*2* in ◘ Fig. 4.4a) allowing the ring to moving forward into the annulus up to the next exit point (*3* in ◘ Fig. 4.4a). By repeating the same steps of insertion and pulling up the suture material through the second exit point (*3* in ◘ Fig. 4.4a) up to the third one (close to the anterior commissure), the complete insertion of the ring within the native mitral annulus is achieved. The anterior suture material is then passed twice from the anterior trigone down to the anterior commissure, the first loop allowing for fixation of the anterior extremity of the ring to the anterior trigone and the second loop for tying the anterior suture material on itself. The posterior needle is then passed twice through the first entry point up to the posterior trigone twice, the first loop allowing for fixation of the posterior extremity of the ring to the posterior trigone and the second one for tying the posterior suture extension on itself (◘ Fig. 4.4a).

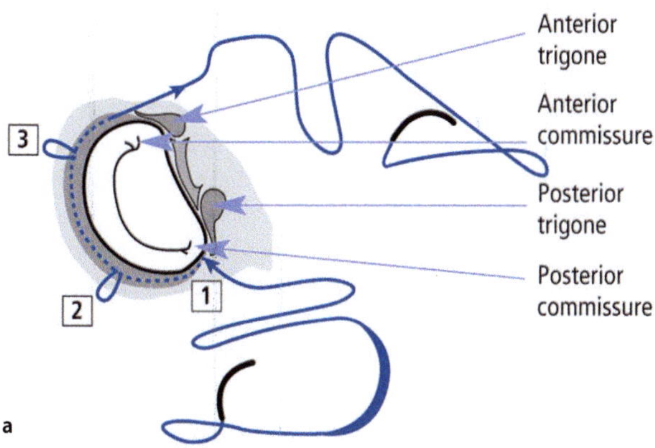

a

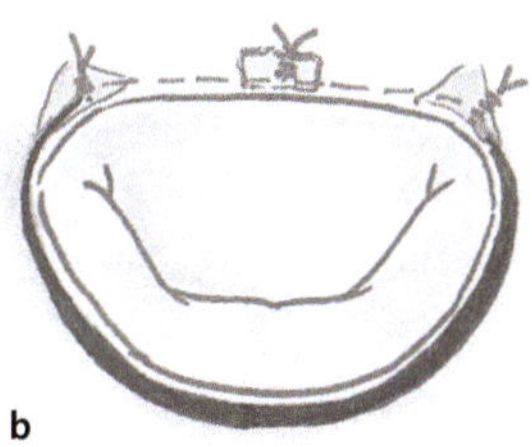

b

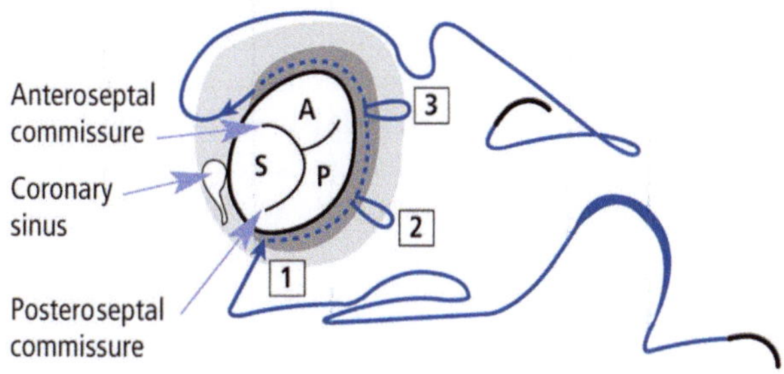

c

◘ **Fig. 4.4.** Implantation of the ring in the mitral position (**a**), complete ring position using the two extension sutures (**b**), and the tricuspid position (**c**). See text for details. *A* anterior leaflet, *P* posterior leaflet, *S* septal leaflet, *1* first entry point of the ring into the native annulus, *2* first exit and the second entry point of the ring, *3* second exit and third entry point of the ring. (**a** and **c** from [7], © J Heart Valve Dis)

The biodegradable ring–a partial ring in design–can also be converted into a complete ring by moving the suture material extensions to the midpoint of the anterior mitral annulus from both commissures and tying them together after fixing both extremities of the ring to the respective trigones with the first loop (◘ Fig. 4.4b). The complete insertion technique is especially recommended for the correction of ischemic mitral insufficiency and that associated with idiopathic dilated cardiomyopathy, as the resistance of the ring to tensile stretch is better distributed with the complete configuration, a factor crucial in preventing annular redilatation.

For tricuspid annuloplasty, ring implantation into the native annulus starts at the level of the posteroseptal commissure, advancing up to the anteroseptal commissure by respecting the same principles of insertion as for mitral annuloplasty: pulling up the suture material and progressively positioning the ring into the annulus, insertion is usually accomplished after only three bites (◘ Fig. 4.4c).

4.4 Midterm clinical results based on type of mitral valve disorder

4.4.1 Congenital malformations of the mitral valve

Preservation of growth potential of the native annulus is critical for long-term stability of valve repair procedures in a pediatric population. In an experimental study on a fast growing juvenile pig model, the growth potential of the tricuspid annulus was preserved with the biodegradable ring [7]. Based on this fact, we recently reviewed our pediatric cases with congenital mitral insufficiency which had undergone mitral valve repair using three different annuloplasty techniques over the past 15 years. These cases were divided into three groups: the first group included 18 cases (mean age: 25±12 months) which had undergone mitral repair with a posterior biodegradable suture annuloplasty using 5-0 or 4-0 PDS; the second group included 17 cases (mean age: 27±15 months) which had undergone mitral valve repair with a posterior pericardial annuloplasty band fixed onto the native annulus using interrupted 5-0 *U* polypropylene stitches; the third group included 22 cases (24±14 months) which had undergone mitral valve repair using the biodegradable ring.

During the follow-up period, echocardiographically obtained lateral and anteroposterior diameters of the mitral orifice were compared to those observed in healthy children, based on body surface areas according to King et al. [8]. In the first group, all cases developed recurrent mitral insufficiency of moderate or greater degrees over the follow-up period (60±22 months) because of subsequently dilated lateral and anteroposterior diameters of the mitral orifice. In the second group, 13 out of 17 cases developed recurrent mitral insufficiency of moderate or greater degrees (62±28 months) because of subsequent redilatation of the anteroposterior diameter and restriction of the lateral diameter of the mitral orifice, the latter probably due to the restrictive effect of the posterior pericardial band on the growth potential of lateral diameter. On repeat echocardiographic controls over the follow-up period, the lateral ellipsoidal shape of the mitral orifice in systole was transformed into a vertically ellipsoidal shape. Unlike the first two groups, the mitral valve repair group with the biodegradable ring showed homogeneous growing of the anteroposterior and lateral diameters of the mitral orifice, similar to that of physiological growth values, over the follow-up period of 57±12 months, with only two cases developing a moderate degree of recurrent mitral insufficiency (◘ Fig. 4.5). One case of ischemic mitral regurgitation due to an anomalous origin of the left coronary artery from the pulmonary trunk was also successfully managed using a biodegradable ring, with

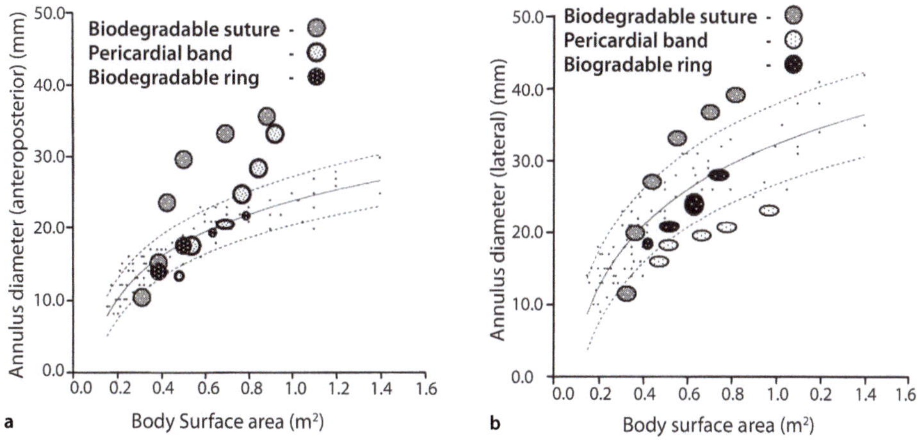

Fig. 4.5. Evolution of anteroposterior (**a**) and lateral diameters (**b**) of the mitral orifice over time compared to those obtained in healthy children based on the body surface area according to King et al. [8] in three different annuloplasty groups

no residual mitral insufficiency and a mean transmitral gradient estimated at 2 mmHg at the 2 year follow-up [9].

The biodegradable ring is also very useful in the correction of residual mitral and tricuspid insufficiency in atrioventricular canal defects which can persist after closure of the clefts [10]. In such cases, a ring, one size below that which corresponds to the surface of the anterior leaflet, is chosen and it is inserted into the native mitral annulus, taking particular care to avoid the area between the posterior trigone and the coronary sinus to prevent the risk of atrioventricular block. The posterior extremity of the ring is then attached to the premium interatrial septal defect closure patch, the »no patch technique« not being recommended in these cases with persistent mitral insufficiency after closure of the anterior mitral cleft. Contrary to the mitral position, the »no patch technique« does not preclude the conventional intraannular implantation of a biodegradable ring between the anteroseptal and posteroseptal commissures in the tricuspid position.

4.4.2 Rheumatic mitral valve disease in children

We have recently published our 13-year experience with mitral valve repair in rheumatic disease to determine the midterm results for the biodegradable annuloplasty ring as compared to that of the traditional rigid Carpentier–Edwards annuloplasty ring [11]. First, the biodegradable ring allowed us to successfully perform annuloplasty in 15% of these children with ring sizes under 26–sizes not available in traditional rings, hence, allowing for rheumatic valve repair in younger children. Transmitral gradients during the first postoperative year in both pure mitral insufficiency and mixed lesions (stenosis + insufficiency) groups were lower than those measured in the Carpentier–Edwards ring annuloplasty group. In addition, there was a smaller decrease in postoperative shortening fraction at 1 week compared to that of the Carpentier–Edwards annuloplasty group. We have speculated that the three-dimensional flexible nature of the biodegradable ring better preserves the three-dimensional dynamic geometry of the native mitral annulus. In fact, repeat echocardiographic controls over the follow-up period of 1 year showed no interference of the induced fibrous tissue with the dynamic behavior of the mitral annulus or with the mobility of posterior leaflet, contrary to traditional rings which hinder it. Another important aspect observed was the reduction in both aortic cross-clamping and cardiopulmonary bypass times of up to 10–12 min in the biodegradable ring group as compared to those of Carpentier–Edwards ring annuloplasty group.

4.4.3 Degenerative mitral insufficiency

From March 2005 to March 2007, we performed mitral valve repair in 102 consecutive cases of degenerative mitral insufficiency using the biodegradable ring. In a retrospective comparative study, these cases were matched with the preoperative characteristics of cases which had undergone mitral valve repair using a rigid Carpentier–Edwards ring during the same period. Three statistically important findings were observed over the first 3 postoperative years, the first one being the statistically significant lower transmitral gradients in the biodegradable ring group (3.0±1.2 mmHg versus 5.2±1.8 mmHg). These gradients remained stable in the Carpentier–Edwards group at 3 postoperative years (5.2±2.2 mmHg) and gradually decreased in the biodegradable ring group over the first 2 postoperative years, then remaining unchanged over the third postoperative year (2.3±0.4 mmHg). There was no significant difference between the two groups in terms of recurrent mitral insufficiency during this follow-up period. The second statistically significant finding was the smaller decrease in shortening fraction at 3 weeks after mitral valve repair in the biodegradable ring group as compared to that of the Carpentier–Edwards ring annuloplasty group. Incidentally, this same difference in decreased shortening fraction was also statistically significant in the rheumatic group. The third statistically significant finding was the variation of 15±3% of the anteroposterior diameter of the mitral orifice between diastole and systole at 1 year after mitral valve repair using biodegradable ring annuloplasty. These last two findings can be considered to be indirect signs of the preservation of the contractile geometry of the native annulus at 1 year in the biodegradable group (at 6 months the durable intraannular posterior fibrous tissue between the anterior and posterior trigones is present with complete degradation of the ring). There was no observed redilatation of the mitral orifice in adult cases, as the 2-0 polyvinyl nondegradable suture material in continuity over the entire portion of the biodegradable material is resistant to tensile stretches of up to 5 kg. Because of the resistant properties of this nondegradable component of the ring around which the fibrous reaction occurs, cardiac surgeons can be reassured about the long-term stability of mitral and tricuspid annuloplasty.

4.4.4 Mitral and tricuspid valve endocarditis

There is an obvious theoretical advantage of using the biodegradable ring in this infectious context, especially in acute cases of mitral or tricuspid involvement requiring urgent surgical intervention [12, 13]. As suggested by numerous surgeons, the use of synthetic material (including traditional rings implanted onto the native annulus) is not appropriate during the acute stage of active endocarditis, as there is a potential risk for recurrent infection by contamination of such synthetic material via circulating microorganisms. Moreover, the intraannular position of the biodegradable ring, inherently devoid of any synthetic material, allows it to remain isolated from any possibly circulating microorganisms. We did not observe any recurrent infection in the 17 cases of mitral and tricuspid valve repair for endocarditis between 2004 and 2009 [13].

4.5 Tricuspid annuloplasty

Early results for tricuspid annuloplasty using the biodegradable ring have already been published in a comparative study with the DeVega annuloplasty, in which functional tricuspid insufficiency was the predominant etiology of the tricuspid valve dysfunction [14]. In our experience in over 65 cases undergoing tricuspid annuloplasty with the biodegradable ring between 2005 and 2009, only 3 cases developed moderate to severe recurrent tricuspid insufficiency, all of whom had undergone annuloplasty for rheumatic involvement of the tricuspid valve in a context of multivalvular rheumatic lesions. The nondegradable component of the biodegradable ring–just as in mitral annuloplasty–prevents redilatation of the tricuspid annulus through permanent resistance against tensile stretch. Durable support of the tricuspid annulus in association with preservation of its growth potential has also been reported in a pediatric population over a follow-up period of 3 years [15]. The three-dimensional flexible structure of the ring also provides for simple and quick implantation in minimally invasive thoracoscopic and robotic surgery. Preliminary experience with these surgical approaches for tricuspid annuloplasty has confirmed the ease of implantation [16]. Moreover, it must be emphasized that contrary to traditional rings for which anticoagulation is recommended for the first 3 postoperative months, prophylactic anticoagulation following biodegradable ring annuloplasty is not necessary, provided that the patient has no other indications for it, as the intraannular position of the biodegradable ring protects against any »blood–biodegradable material« interaction.

Acknowledgment

I would like to sincerely thank Drs. Dominique Vala and Mustafa Cikirikcioglu for their invaluable editorial assistance.

References

1. Carpentier A (1983) Cardiac valve surgery–the »French correction« J Thorac Cardiovasc Surg 86:323–337
2. Duran CMG, Revuelta JM, Val Bernal F (1986) A new absorbable ring in the tricuspid position: An experimental study. Thorac Cardiovasc Surg 34:377–379
3. Chachques JC, Acar C, Latremouille C, Fontaliran F, Mihaileanu S, Chauvaud S, Tibi PR, Bilweis J, Carpentier A (1990) Absorbable rings for pediatric valvuloplasty. Circulation 82 (Suppl 5):IV82–IV88
4. Duran CMG, Balasundaram SG, Bianchi S, Herdson P (1992) The vanishing tricuspid annuloplasty: a new concept. J Thorac Cardiovasc Surg 104:796–801
5. Duran CM, Kumar N, Prabhakar G, Ge Z, Bianchi S, Gometza B (1991) Vanishing De Vega annuloplasty for functional tricuspid regurgitation. J Thorac Cardiovasc Surg 106:609–613
6. Miyamura H, Eguchi S, Watanabe H, Kanazawa H, Sugawara M, Tatebe S, Shinonaga M, Hayashi J (1994) Total circular annuloplasty with absorbable suture for the repair of left atrioventricular valve regurgitation in atrioventricular septal defect. J Thorac Cardiovasc Surg 107:1428–1431
7. Kalangos A, Sierra J, Vala D, Cikirikcioglu M, Walpoth B, Orrit X, Pomar J, Mestres C, Albanese S, Jhurry D (2006) Annuloplasty for valve repair with a new biodegradable ring: an experimental study. J Heart Valve Dis 15: 783–790

8. King DH, Smith EO, Huhta JC, Gutgesell HP (1985) Mitral and tricuspid valve anular diameter in normal children determined by two-dimensional echocardiography. Am J Cardiol 55:787–789
9. Myers P, Beghetti M, Kalangos A (2009) Biodegradable mitral annuloplasty for congenital ischemic mitral regurgitation. Thorac Cardiov Surg 57:363–371
10. Myers P, Cikirikcioglu M, Aggoun Y, Murith N, Kalangos A (2010) No-patch technique for complete atrioventricular canal repair. Ann Thorac Surg 90:317–319
11. Kalangos A, Christenson JT, Beghetti M, Cikirikcioglu M, Kamentsidis D, Aggoun Y (2008) Mitral valve repair for rheumatic valve disease in children: midterm results and impact of the use of a biodegradable mitral ring. Ann Thorac Surg 86:161–169
12. Kazaz H, Celkan MA, Ustunsoy H, Baspinar O (2005) Mitral annuloplasty with biodegradable ring for infective endocarditis: a new tool for the surgeon for valve repair in childhood. Interact Cardiovasc Thorac Surg 44:378–380
13. Pektok E, Sierra J, Cikirikcioglu M, Muller H, Myers P, Kalangos A (2010) Midterm results of valve repair with a biodegradable annuloplasty ring for acute endocarditis. Ann Thorac Surg 89:1180–1185
14. Burma O, Ustunsoy H, Davutoglu V, Celkan MA, Kazaz H, Pektok E (2007) Initial clinical experience with a novel biodegradable ring in patients with functional tricuspid insufficiency: Kalangos biodegradable tricuspid ring. Thorac Cardiovasc Surg 55:284–287
15. Mrowczynski W, Mrozinski B, Kalangos A, Walpoth BH, Pawelec-Wojtalik M, Wojtalik M (2011) A Biodegradable ring enables growht of the native tricuspid annulus. J Heart Valve Dis 20; in press
16. Panos A, Myers P, Kalangos A (2010) Thoracoscopic and robotic tricuspid valve annuloplasty with a biodegradable ring; initial experience. J Heart Valve Dis 19:201– 205

Hypertrophic obstructive cardiomyopathy and the mitral valve

B. Nasseri, C. Stamm, E.M. Delmo Walter, R. Hetzer

5.1 Introduction

Hypertrophic cardiomyopathy (HCM) is a complex congenital cardiac disease and belongs to the group of cardiomyopathies. The estimated prevalence is 1:500 [1]. Although it has unique pathophysiological characteristics, there is a great diversity of functional, clinical, morphological, and molecular findings. Therefore and because of the relatively low prevalence in general practice, therapy management decisions have been derived from nonrandomized and retrospective investigations [2].

HCM occurs in all races and equally effects men and women. It is the most common cause of sudden cardiac death in otherwise healthy young adults, including trained athletes [3–5], but it may cause death in all age groups.

Although HCM is usually asymmetric hypertrophy of the left ventricular wall >15 mm, any wall thickness, even those within the normal range, may be compatible with the presence of a HCM mutant gene [6, 7]. Over 200 gene defects of 10 genes that encode proteins of the cardiac sarcomere have been identified. Over 50% of these are structural defects of the ß-myosin heavy chain, cardiac troponin T, α-tropomyosin, and myosin-binding protein C [2, 8].

Despite normal left ventricular systolic function, symptomatic patients often complain of dyspnea, chest pain, syncope or presyncope, and dizziness. These are explained by a diastolic dysfunction with increased chamber stiffness and impaired left ventricular filling, especially in the presence of atrial fibrillation, but mainly due to abnormal relaxation, leading to an increased left ventricular end-diastolic pressure (LVEDP) and consequently to pulmonary congestion, also caused by mitral regurgitation and myocardial ischemia.

5.2 Obstructive form of hypertrophic cardiomyopathy

It is important to distinguish between the obstructive and the nonobstructive form of HCM. Obstruction may be present in midcavity or subaortic position and is the cause of left ventricular outflow tract (LVOT) gradients [8–10]. Although midcavity obstruction is rare, common findings are direct insertion of the anterolateral papillary muscle into the anterior mitral leaflet, or midventricular or papillary muscle hypertrophy and malalignment, causing muscular apposition [10, 11]. However, more common in symptomatic patients is subaortic septal hypertrophy with obstruction caused by systolic anterior motion (SAM) of the anterior mitral leaflet, causing it to come into contact with the hypertrophic septum [10, 12, 13].

LVOT obstruction in HCM and therewith outflow gradients are typically dynamic. While during early systole blood is ejected from the left ventricle, LVOT obstruction and gradient reach their peak during mid- and end-systole. This peak gradient varies considerably with physiological alterations and is inducible with various maneuvers, such as the Valsalva maneuver. The dynamic characteristics of the LVOT obstruction and gradient make categorization into hemodynamic subgroups difficult. Nevertheless, three subgroups based on continuous wave Doppler echocardiography (current clinical convention) were characterized by the ACC/ESC Expert Consensus Document on Hypertrophic Cardiomyopathy [2]:

- Obstructive gradient under basal (resting) conditions >30 mmHg (2.7 m/s by Doppler)
- Latent (provocable) obstructive gradient <30 mmHg under basal conditions and >30 mmHg with provocation
- Nonobstructive gradient <30 mmHg under both basal and provocable conditions.

5.3 Mechanism of LVOT obstruction

As mentioned above, SAM is the major cause of LVOT obstruction [14] but also of the mitral valve regurgitation [15] regularly seen in hypertrophic obstructive cardiomyopathy (HOCM) patients. Mitral regurgitation caused by SAM is usually mild to moderate in degree and the regurgitation jet is directed posteriorly into the left atrium [16]. Mechanisms of SAM and, therefore, of LVOT obstruction and mitral regurgitation in subaortic septal hypertrophy patients are due to an early systolic high velocity blood flow forced by a hyperkinetic LV and the Venturi phenomenon [17]. Subaortic septal hypertrophy directs blood flow toward the mitral valve and drags the anterior mitral leaflet [18] into the LVOT, producing SAM. Furthermore, SAM and, therefore, mitral regurgitation may be amplified by an abnormal mitral valve apparatus including an abnormal leaflet–especially the A2 portion of the anterior mitral leaflet (AML)–and/or chordal length and laxity, as well as malinsertion and/or malalignment of the papillary muscles [19].

5.4 Sudden cardiac death in HCM

Unexpected sudden cardiac death is a fatal complication in HCM patients and can be the initial manifestation of HCM [5, 20]. Although different symptoms of HCM have been studied for risk stratification of sudden cardiac death, the question of precise identification of all high-risk patients is not resolved. Nevertheless, the highest risks for sudden cardiac death summarized by the ACC/ESC Expert Consensus Document on Hypertrophic Cardiomyopathy are shown in ◘ Table 5.1.

Nowadays, most clinicians would recommend an implantable cardioverter/defibrillator in the absence of an LVOT gradient >30 mmHg and the avoidance of competitive sports to prevent sudden cardiac death in these patients. Historically, drug therapy with β-adrenergic blockers, verapamil, and type I-A antiarrhythmic agents were prophylactically recommended. Nevertheless, most clinical markers of sudden cardiac death have a low positive but a high negative predictive value (90%). For this reason the ACC/ESC Expert Consensus Document

◘ **Table 5.1.** Patients at high-risk of sudden cardiac death [2]

1	Prior cardiac arrest or spontaneously occurring and sustained ventricular tachycardia
2	Family history of a premature hypertrophic cardiomyopathy-related sudden cardiac death particular if sudden death, in a close relative, or if multiple in occurrence
3	Identification of high-risk mutant gene
4	Unexplained syncope, particularly in young patients or when exertional or recurrent
5	Nonsustained ventricular tachycardia (of 3 beats or more and at least 120 beats/min) evident on ambulatory (Holter) electrocardiogram recording
6	Abnormal blood pressure response during upright exercise which is attenuated or hypotensive
7	Extreme left ventricular hypertrophy with maximum wall thickness of 30 mm or more, particularly in adolescents and young adults

Table 5.2. Patients at low-risk of sudden cardiac death [2]

1	No or only mild symptoms of chest pain or exertional dyspnea (NYHA functional classes I and II)
2	Absence of family history of premature death from hypertrophic cardiomyopathy
3	Absence of syncope judged to be hypertrophic cardiomyopathy related
4	Absence of nonsustained ventricular tachycardia during ambulatory (Holter) electrocardiogram
5	Left ventricular outflow gradient at rest of <30 mmHg
6	Normal or relatively mild increase in atrial size (<45 mm)
7	Normal blood pressure response to upright exercise
8	Mild left ventricular hypertrophy (wall thickness <20 mm)

on Hypertrophic Cardiomyopathy states adult patients to be at low risk for sudden cardiac death or other adverse events if they demonstrate the criteria given in Table 5.2.

Although ventricular tachycardia is the arrhythmia leading to sudden cardiac death, atrial fibrillation is the most common sustained arrhythmia in HCM and justifies aggressive therapeutic strategies [21, 22], due to reduced left ventricular diastolic filling in the absence of sinus rhythm and its major complications, such as thromboembolism. Atrial fibrillation in HCM should be managed in accordance with the ACC/AHA guidelines [23].

While the clinical course of HCM patients is variable with many having a normal life expectancy, symptomatic patients in general experience, according to the ACC/ESC Expert Consensus Document on Hypertrophic Cardiomyopathy, one or more of the following adverse clinical courses [2]:

- High risk for premature sudden and unexpected death
- Progressive symptoms largely of exertional dyspnea, chest pain (either typical of angina or atypical in nature), and impaired consciousness, including syncope, near-syncope or presyncope (i.e., dizziness/lightheadedness), in the presence of preserved left ventricular systolic function
- Progression to advanced congestive heart failure (the »end-stage« phase) with left ventricular remodeling and systolic dysfunction
- Complications attributable to atrial fibrillation, including embolic stroke

These clinical courses may be influenced by other cardiac diseases, such as coronary artery disease and/or systemic hypertension.

5.5 Pharmacological therapy

Pharmacological therapy is traditionally initiated when symptoms occur. However, so far there have been no randomized clinical trials comparing the effect of different drugs in these patients. β-Adrenergic blocking agents were the first drugs introduced for symptomatic HCM patients in the mid-1960s. Another negative inotropic agent often used in the treatment of HCM is the calcium antagonist verapamil, as well as disopyramide, which has an additional antiarrhythmic effect. Due to the lack of data, the value of prophylactic therapy for asymptomatic patients is arguable.

5.6 Surgical treatment

Different treatment options for drug-refractory, symptomatic HOCM patients, e.g., dual-chamber pacing and percutaneous alcohol septal ablation, have been introduced and are performed by cardiologists, but surgery is still the treatment of choice. These patients often have LVOT gradients of 50 mmHg or above under resting conditions and/or with provocation and are in NYHA class III or IV with severe chest pain and dyspnea despite maximal drug therapy. After Morrow pioneered and introduced the ventricular septal myectomy operation (known as the Morrow procedure) in 1964 [24] and it was successfully carried out in many centers throughout the world, it became the gold standard for HOCM patients with failed drug therapy. The surgical approach for the Morrow procedure is through an aortotomy and involves the resection of the hypertrophic subaortic septum through the aortic valve as described by Morrow [25]. Briefly, two vertical incisions are made (one 2–3 mm to the right of the center of the right coronary leaflet and one 10–12 mm left of and parallel to the first incision) directly opposite the anterior mitral leaflet. These vertical incisions are connected with transverse incisions directly below the aortic annulus and in the apical direction beyond the point of anterior mitral leaflet–septal contact. After resection of this muscular block, a rectangular channel has been created (Fig. 5.1). In about 90% of cases, this procedure abolishes LVOT gradients [25–35], while in about 70% of the patients, it achieves substantial and persistent mid- and long-term symptomatic improvement [27–35]. Simultaneously operative mortality is less than 2% at highly experienced centers [17, 28, 30, 32, 34, 35]. The 5-year actuarial survival rate has been as good as 84±4% and decreases in elderly patients and patients undergoing concomitant procedures [35–38]. Other surgical approaches to relieve LVOT obstruction, e.g., the left ventricular apical approach [39, 40] or right-sided septal resection [41, 42], have been introduced.

Even though the amount of SAM and mitral regurgitation improves in most patients once the hypertrophic septum has been resected, the abnormal mitral valve apparatus still exists and, therefore, SAM and mitral regurgitation may still be present and may lead to unresolved symptoms.

5.7 Mitral valve replacement

To solve these problems, mitral valve replacement without additional subaortic septal myectomy was introduced by Cooley [25, 43, 44]. Surgeons at the National Institute of Health reported in 53 patients a 30-day and mid-term (average 22.3 months) mortality of 8.6% and 11.3% after mitral valve replacement, respectively, with an actuarial survival of about 65% at 4.8 years [45]. In 1984, Fighali et al. [46] published their results in 36 patients comparing three groups: mitral valve replacement without myectomy, myectomy without mitral valve replacement, and a combination of both. The reduction of LVOT gradients was more impressive after mitral valve replacement with or without septal myectomy than after septal myectomy alone. Nevertheless, mitral valve replacement has been abandoned by most surgeons due to the high risk of thromboembolism, bleeding, endocarditis, and prosthesis destruction, and it is reserved for patients in whom mitral valve repair fails.

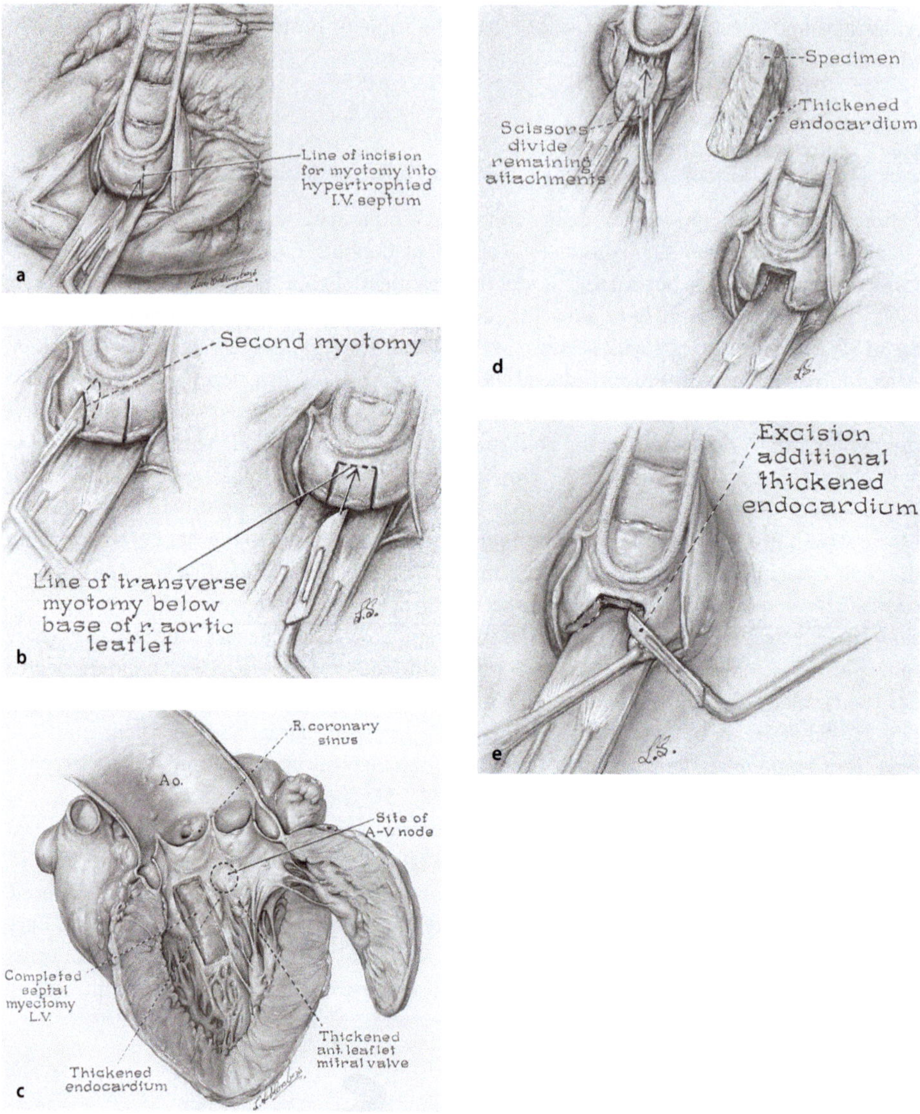

◘ Fig. 5.1. Morrow procedure: **a** Site of 1st myotomy incision: 2–3 mm to the right (clockwise) of the center of the right coronary leaflet. **b** A 2nd vertical myotomy is made 10–12 mm to the left of and parallel to the 1st one. A transverse incision is then made, connecting the vertical ones at the base of the right coronary leaflet. With this knife, angled on the flat, the bar of muscle between the vertical myotomies is largely detached from the septum. **c** The tip of the cloth-covered retractor is passed into the left vertical, and any remaining attachments of the muscle bar to the septum are divided under direct vision with straight Potts scissors. After completion of the resection, a rectangular channel 1 cm x 1.5 cm extends from the valve ring toward the apex for about 4.5 cm. **d** Additional thickened and scarred endocardium is trimmed from the edge of the channel created. Before the aorta is closed, the left ventricle is lavaged with saline solution to remove any particulate matter. **e** Semidiagrammatic representation of the left ventricle after completion of the septal resection. The relations of the channel to the valve leaflet and to the adjacent membranous septum (and conduction tissue) are shown. The apical end of the floor of the channel blends smoothly onto the wall of the distal left ventricle ([53]; © Elsevier)

5.8 Combined mitral valve repair and myectomy

Different methods to repair the mitral valve combined with the Morrow procedure in HOCM patients have been introduced to the surgical community [47–51].

5.8.1 Mitral leaflet plication plasty

In 1992, combined myectomy and plication of the anterior mitral leaflet were proposed as an alternative to mitral valve replacement [48]. Plication of the anterior mitral leaflet was performed through the aortic valve (◻ Fig. 5.2). After identification of the contact point of

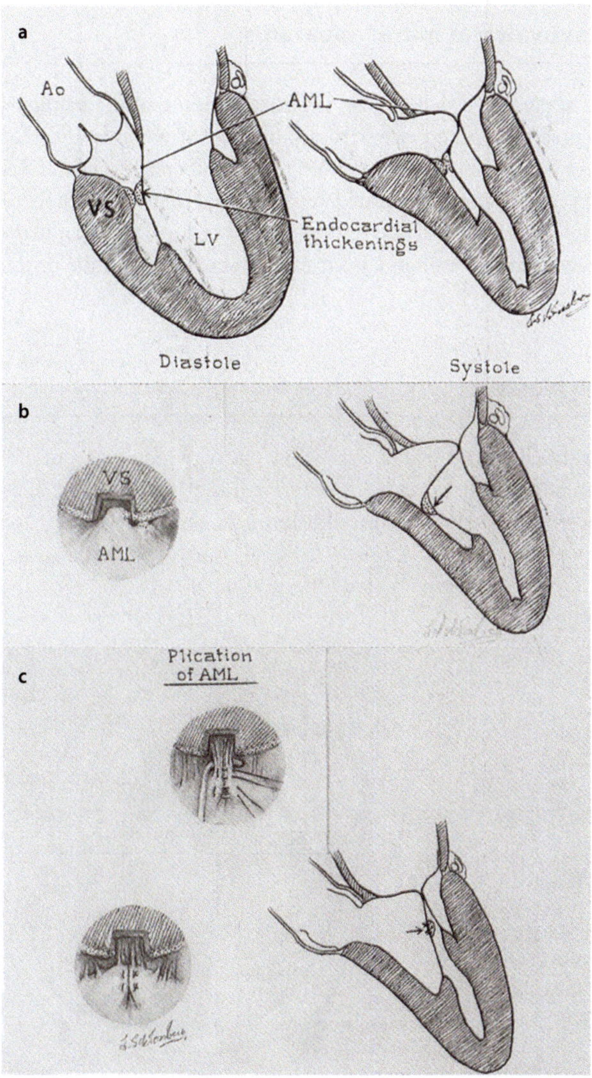

◻ **Fig. 5.2.** Illustration of surgical technique used in suture plication of the anterior mitral leaflet. **a** Before surgery: Systolic anterior mitral valve motion with the typical acute-angeled bend (drawing on right); endocardial thickening of anterior mitral leaflet (*AML*) and ventricular septum (*VS*) shown by stippling. **b** After ventricular septal myotomy–myectomy (but without mitral valve plication) showing the circumstance in which an enlarged and elongated anterior leaflet prolapses into the myectomy trough (*arrow*) and produces systolic anterior motion (SAM) and septal contact. Drawing on left shows myectomy trough as viewed through aortotomy with persistent SAM and mitral–septal contact; drawing on right shows long-axis plane. **c** After plication: Anterior mitral leaflet shows limited systolic anterior motion (and no longer approaches the septum). Upper left drawing shows plication procedure in which dull nerve hook retracts the chordae tendineae of the anterior leaflet; plication with two sutures starts at the insertion of chordae into the leaflet near endocardial contact lesion; drawings at bottom left and right show the completed plication (*arrow*). *Ao* aorta, *LV* left ventricle ([48]; © American Heart Association)

the anterior mitral leaflet with the ventricular septum, this fibrous region was plicated with single or multiple 4-0 Prolene sutures. The sutures were placed perpendicular to the long axis of the leaflet in a mattress fashion, involving an area of about 1 cm x 2 cm. Leaflet tissue was not resected. In a study of 36 patients, resting and provocative LVOT gradients decreased significantly and SAM could be limited without creating mitral valve stenosis or regurgitation. In addition, the authors compared the group with combined myectomy and plication with a group of patients receiving myectomy or mitral valve replacement alone. No differences regarding LVOT gradient or left ventricular end-diastolic pressure reduction were seen compared with myectomy alone. However, patients with mitral valve replacement alone showed the most substantial improvement of gradient and end-diastolic reduction. Nevertheless, the authors concluded that mitral valve replacement and its potential complications make the plication technique a good alternative to mitral valve replacement.

5.8.2 Reconstruction of the subvalvular mitral apparatus

Reconstruction of the subvalvular apparatus was based on the observation that the papillary muscles may be displaced by malpositioning and hypertrophy in HOCM patients and that these anomalies produce SAM. For reconstruction after myectomy, both papillary muscles were mobilized down to the apex, and all hypertrophied portions and muscular trabeculae were resected [49]. The authors stated that »at the end of the procedure, both papillary muscles should be clearly separated from the wall and from each other in the middle of the ventricle« [52].

5.8.3 Mitral leaflet extension plasty

Kofflard et al. [50] adapted a modified mitral leaflet extension plasty, which was initially described by Carpentier for rheumatic mitral valves with anterior leaflet shrinkage or leaflet perforation resulting from bacterial endocarditis, in addition to a septal myectomy for

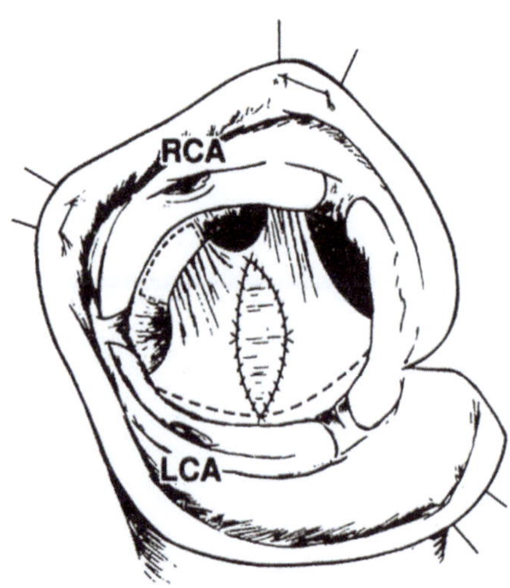

Fig. 5.3. Schematic presentation of mitral leaflet extension. The pericardial patch is clearly seen in the middle of the drawing, within the anterior mitral leaflet. The area of the myectomy is seen in the interventricular septum, demarcated by dots. The ostia of both the left (*LCA*) and right (*RCA*) coronary arteries are indicated for orientation purposes ([51]; © American College of Cardiology Foundation)

HOCM patients. They used a 3 cm x 2.5 cm oval-shaped glutaraldehyde-treated autologous pericardial patch. The anterior mitral leaflet was exposed through the aortic valve and, after the Morrow procedure, a longitudinal incision from its subaortic hinge point to the rough zone was performed. The patch was sewn onto the ventricular surface of the leaflet at the site of the incision using three running polypropylene monofilament sutures (◘ Fig. 5.3). In a series of 20 patients (8 with combined myectomy and leaflet extension plasty and 12 with myectomy alone), there was no perioperative mortality. However, 2 patients from the group with myectomy alone died after 2 and 6 years, respectively. Although preoperative SAM and mitral regurgitation were significantly worse in the combined group, during follow-up SAM and mitral regurgitation were significantly better. Furthermore, patients with the combined surgical treatment had more improvement in functional NYHA class and greater reduction of drugs prescribed than patients with myectomy alone. The authors claim that these positive effects of the technique are due to the increased width (horizontal dimension) of the anterior mitral leaflet erecting lax chordae of the central portion (A2) and, thus, preventing buckling into the LVOT.

5.8.4 Anterior mitral valve leaflet retention plasty

At our institute, we prefer to reconstruct the mitral valve in HOCM patients via a left atriotomy and an anterior mitral leaflet retention plasty (ALRP), developed by Roland Hetzer. This procedure was first described by Delmo Walter in 2009 in 12 pediatric patients [51]. Briefly, after performing a Morrow procedure through the aortic valve to avoid iatrogenic ventricular septal defect or atrial ventricular blockage, especially in small children, the left atrium is entered below the interatrial groove. Mitral valve apparatus mobility and morphology are inspected. With pledgeted polypropylene mattress sutures, the anterior mitral leaflet closest to the trigones is sutured to the corresponding posterior annulus (◘ Fig. 5.4). For the pledgets, autologous untreated pericardium is used. Following the concept that the anterior mitral leaflet is abnormal in the sense that the leaflet is lengthened and lax, and protrudes into the left ventricular outflow tract, the anterior mitral leaflet becomes stretched by the ALRP, especially in its central part (A2) and the mobility of the anterior mitral leaflet becomes limited. The retained anterior mitral leaflet appears tightened in systole and is pushed toward the left atrium, anticipating SAM and mitral regurgitation. If other mitral valve anomalies are present, different mitral valve reconstruction techniques, e.g., Gerbode plasty or anuloplasty, may be easily performed via this mitral valve approach.

So far, we have used combined ALRP and myectomy in 37 patients, 12 children, and 25 adults. During a mean follow-up of 11.85±1.22 years, there was no early or late mortality or reoperation for repeat myecotomy or mitral valve operation in the pediatric group. SAM disappeared completely after the operation, and the left ventricular outflow tract gradient and mitral regurgitation were significantly reduced. Over time, the NYHA class improved. No iatrogenic ventricular septal defect or atrial ventricular blockage was observed [51].

In the adult group, all patients survived the operation and only 10% showed mild SAM at follow-up. Survival after 1, 5, and 10 years was 100%, 82.2±6.6%, and 60.9±7.7%, and freedom from reoperation after 30 days, 1 and 5 years was 92±5.4%, 87.8±6.6%, and 83.2±7.7%, respectively. Mean LVOT pressure gradient decreased from 84±32 mmHg to 19±11 mmHg postoperatively ($p<0.001$). Mitral regurgitation and NYHA classification improved signifi-

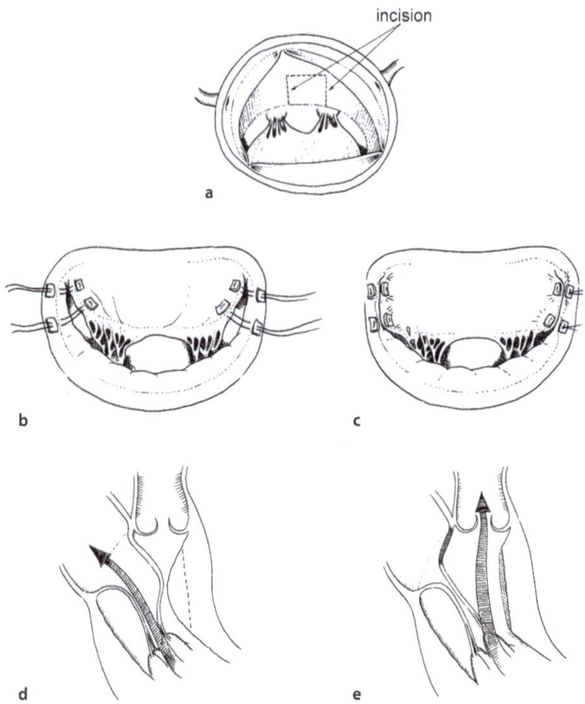

Fig. 5.4. Hetzer's septal myectomy (aortic view, **a**) opposite anterior mitral valve leaflet (dashed lines indicate myocardial septal incisions), **b** Hetzer's ALRP for hypertrophic obstructive cardiomyopathy (HOCM) and systolic anterior motion (SAM), **c** completed repair (atrial view), **d** mitral insufficiency in HOCM and SAM before repair, and **e** redirection of mitral insufficiency following septal myectomy and ALRP ([51]; © Elsevier)

cantly at follow-up. Iatrogenic mitral stenosis from ALRP, ventricular septal defect, or atrial ventricular blockage was not observed.

We believe that ALRP is an easy technique to abolish SAM and mitral regurgitation in HOCM patients, especially in small children, in whom it may be difficult and dangerous to perform sufficient myectomy or one of the other techniques of mitral valve reconstruction to adequately decrease LVOT gradients and SAM.

5.9 Conclusion

Although HCM in most people is asymptomatic or may be adequately treated by drug therapy or prophylactic implantation of a defibrillator to prevent sudden cardiac death, in a small number of patients hypertrophic obstruction occurs and they become symptomatic. If the LVOT gradient reaches 50 mmHg under resting conditions and/or with provocation and/or patients are in NYHA class III or IV with severe chest pain and dyspnea despite maximal drug therapy, surgery is the treatment of choice.

Subaortic septal myectomy–the Morrow procedure–has become the gold standard in these patients. Because mitral apparatus abnormalities are not addressed by myectomy, and SAM as well as mitral regurgitation may still be present and LVOT gradients and heart failure remain, mitral valve surgery abolishes these circumstances. After an initial era of mitral valve replacement, this has been abandoned by most surgeons due to the high risk of thromboembolism, bleeding, endocarditis, and prosthesis destruction, and it is now reserved for patients in whom mitral valve repair fails. Mitral valve reconstruction techniques have been introduced and seem to produce good results. However, reports of the individual reconstruction techniques are based on limited experience with small patient numbers; they also seem to be time consuming and not applicable for children.

The technique of combined myectomy and anterior leaflet retention plasty (ALRP) is an easy, time-saving approach. It allows the performance of other reconstruction procedures on the mitral valve, which may be necessary, especially when the mitral annulus is dilated due to heart failure. It can be performed with good mid- and long-term results in children and adults.

Acknowledgment

We thank Anne Gale, Editor in the Life Sciences, for editorial assistance.

References

1. Maron BJ, Gardin JM, Flack JM, Gidding SS, Kurosaki TT, Bild DE (1995) Prevalence of hypertrophic cardiomyopathy in a general population of young adults. Echocardiographic analysis of 4111 subjects in the CARDIA Study. Coronary Artery Risk Development in (Young) Adults. Circulation 92(4):785–789
2. Maron BJ, McKenna WJ, Danielson GK, Kappenberger LJ, Kuhn HJ, Seidman CE, Shah PM, Spencer WH 3rd, Spirito P, Ten Cate FJ, Wigle ED; Task Force on Clinical Expert Consensus Documents. American College of Cardiology; Committee for Practice Guidelines. European Society of Cardiology (2003) American College of Cardiology/European Society of Cardiology clinical expert consensus document on hypertrophic cardiomyopathy: a report of the American College of Cardiology Foundation Task Force on Clinical Expert Consensus Documents and the European Society of Cardiology Committee for Practice Guidelines. J Am Coll Cardiol 42(9):1687–1713
3. Elliott PM, Poloniecki J, Dickie S, Sharma S, Monserrat L, Varnava A, Mahon NG, McKenna WJ (2000) Sudden death in hypertrophic cardiomyopathy: identification of high risk patients. J Am Coll Cardiol 36(7):2212–2218
4. Maron BJ, Shirani J, Poliac LC, Mathenge R, Roberts WC, Mueller FO (1996) Sudden death in young competitive athletes. Clinical, demographic, and pathological profiles. JAMA 276(3):199–204
5. Spirito P, Bellone P, Harris KM, Bernabo P, Bruzzi P, Maron BJ (2000) Magnitude of left ventricular hypertrophy and risk of sudden death in hypertrophic cardiomyopathy. N Engl J Med 342(24):1778–1785
6. Seidman JG, Seidman C (2001) The genetic basis for cardiomyopathy: from mutation identification to mechanistic paradigms. Cell 104(4):557–567
7. Maron BJ, Niimura H, Casey SA, Soper MK, Wright GB, Seidman JG, Seidman CE (2001) Development of left ventricular hypertrophy in adults in hypertrophic cardiomyopathy caused by cardiac myosin-binding protein C gene mutations. J Am Coll Cardiol 38(2):315–321
8. Spirito P, Seidman CE, McKenna WJ, Maron BJ (1997) The management of hypertrophic cardiomyopathy. N Engl J Med 336(11):775–785
9. Maron BJ (2002) Hypertrophic cardiomyopathy: a systematic review. JAMA 287(10):1308–1320
10. Wigle ED, Sasson Z, Henderson MA, Ruddy TD, Fulop J, Rakowski H, Williams WG (1985) Hypertrophic cardiomyopathy. The importance of the site and the extent of hypertrophy. A review. Prog Cardiovasc Dis 28(1):1–83
11. Klues HG, Roberts WC, Maron BJ (1991) Anomalous insertion of papillary muscle directly into anterior mitral leaflet in hypertrophic cardiomyopathy. Significance in producing left ventricular outflow obstruction. Circulation 84(3):1188–1197
12. Pollick C, Rakowski H, Wigle ED (1984) Muscular subaortic stenosis: the quantitative relationship between systolic anterior motion and the pressure gradient. Circulation 69(1):43–49
13. Shah PM, Taylor RD, Wong M (1981) Abnormal mitral valve coaptation in hypertrophic obstructive cardiomyopathy: proposed role in systolic anterior motion of mitral valve. Am J Cardiol 48(2):258–262

14. Henry WL, Clark CE, Glancy DL, Epstein SE (1973) Echocardiographic measurement of the left ventricular outflow gradient in idiopathic hypertrophic subaortic stenosis. N Engl J Med 288(19):989–993
15. Spirito P, Maron BJ, Rosing DR (1984) Morphologic determinants of hemodynamic state after ventricular septal myotomy-myectomy in patients with obstructive hypertrophic cardiomyopathy: M mode and two-dimensional echocardiographic assessment. Circulation 70(6):984–995
16. Grigg LE, Wigle ED, Williams WG, Daniel LB, Rakowski H (1992) Transesophageal Doppler echocardiography in obstructive hypertrophic cardiomyopathy: clarification of pathophysiology and importance in intraoperative decision making. J Am Coll Cardiol 20(1):42–52
17. Wigle ED, Rakowski H, Kimball BP, Williams WG (1995) Hypertrophic cardiomyopathy. Clinical spectrum and treatment. Circulation 92(7):1680–1692
18. Sherrid MV, Chu CK, Delia E, Mogtader A, Dwyer EM Jr (1993) An echocardiographic study of the fluid mechanics of obstruction in hypertrophic cardiomyopathy. J Am Coll Cardiol 22(3):816–825
19. Klues HG, Maron BJ, Dollar AL, Roberts WC (1992) Diversity of structural mitral valve alterations in hypertrophic cardiomyopathy. Circulation 85:1651–1660
20. Cecchi F, Maron BJ, Epstein SE (1989) Long-term outcome of patients with hypertrophic cardiomyopathy successfully resuscitated after cardiac arrest. J Am Coll Cardiol 13(6):1283–1288
21. Robinson K, Frenneaux MP, Stockins B, Karatasakis G, Poloniecki JD, McKenna WJ (1990) Atrial fibrillation in hypertrophic cardiomyopathy: a longitudinal study. J Am Coll Cardiol 15(6):1279–1285
22. Olivotto I, Cecchi F, Casey SA, Dolara A, Traverse JH, Maron BJ (2001) Impact of atrial fibrillation on the clinical course of hypertrophic cardiomyopathy. Circulation 104(21):2517–2524
23. Fuster V, Rydén LE, Cannom DS, Crijns HJ, Curtis AB, Ellenbogen KA, Halperin JL, Le Heuzey JY, Kay GN, Lowe JE, Olsson SB, Prystowsky EN, Tamargo JL, Wann S; Task Force on Practice Guidelines, American College of Cardiology/American Heart Association; Committee for Practice Guidelines, European Society of Cardiology; European Heart Rhythm Association; Heart Rhythm Society (2006) ACC/AHA/ESC 2006 guidelines for the management of patients with atrial fibrillation-executive summary: a report of the American College of Cardiology/American Heart Association Task Force on Practice Guidelines and the European Society of Cardiology Committee for Practice Guidelines (Writing Committee to Revise the 2001 Guidelines for the Management of Patients with Atrial Fibrillation). Eur Heart J 27(16):1979–2030
24. Morrow AG, Lambrew CT, Braunwald E (1964) Idiopathic hypertrophic subaortic stenosis. II. Operative treatment and the results of pre- and postoperative hemodynamic evaluations. Circulation 30(Suppl 4):120–151
25. Cooley DA, Leachman RD, Hallman GL, Gerami S, Hall RJ (1971) Idiopathic hypertrophic subaortic stenosis. Surgical treatment including mitral valve replacement. Arch Surg 103(5):606–609
26. Morrow AG, Reitz BA, Epstein SE, Henry WL, Conkle DM, Itscoitz SB, Redwood DR (1975) Operative treatment in hypertrophic subaortic stenosis. Techniques, and the results of pre and postoperative assessments in 83 patients. Circulation 52(1):88–102
27. Maron BJ, Merrill WH, Freier PA, Kent KM, Epstein SE, Morrow AG (1978) Long-term clinical course and symptomatic status of patients after operation for hypertrophic subaortic stenosis. Circulation 57(6):1205–1213
28. Williams WG, Wigle ED, Rakowski H, Smallhorn J, LeBlanc J, Trusler GA(1987) Results of surgery for hypertrophic obstructive cardiomyopathy. Circulation 76(5 Pt 2):V104–108
29. McIntosh CL, Maron BJ (1988) Current operative treatment of obstructive hypertrophic cardiomyopathy. Circulation 78(3):487–495
30. Cohn LH, Trehan H, Collins JJ Jr (1992) Long-term follow-up of patients undergoing myotomy/myectomy for obstructive hypertrophic cardiomyopathy. Am J Cardiol 70(6):657–660
31. Schulte HD, Bircks WH, Loesse B, Godehardt EA, Schwartzkopff B (1993) Prognosis of patients with hypertrophic obstructive cardiomyopathy after transaortic myectomy. Late results up to twenty-five years. J Thorac Cardiovasc Surg 106(4):709–717
32. ten Berg JM, Suttorp MJ, Knaepen PJ, Ernst SM, Vermeulen FE, Jaarsma W (1994) Hypertrophic obstructive cardiomyopathy. Initial results and long-term follow-up after Morrow septal myectomy. Circulation 90(4):1781–1785
33. Heric B, Lytle BW, Miller DP, Rosenkranz ER, Lever HM, Cosgrove DM (1995) Surgical management of hypertrophic obstructive cardiomyopathy. Early and late results. J Thorac Cardiovasc Surg 110(1):195–206; discussion 206–208
34. Robbins RC, Stinson EB (1996) Long-term results of left ventricular myotomy and myectomy for obstructive hypertrophic cardiomyopathy. J Thorac Cardiovasc Surg 111(3):586–594
35. McCully RB, Nishimura RA, Tajik AJ, Schaff HV, Danielson GK (1996) Extent of clinical improvement after surgical treatment of hypertrophic obstructive cardiomyopathy. Circulation 94(3):467–471

36. Mohr R, Schaff HV, Danielson GK, Puga FJ, Pluth JR, Tajik AJ (1989) The outcome of surgical treatment of hypertrophic obstructive cardiomyopathy. Experience over 15 years. J Thorac Cardiovasc Surg 97(5):666–674
37. Cooper MM, McIntosh CL, Tucker E, Clark RE (1987) Operation for hypertrophic subaortic stenosis in the aged. Ann Thorac Surg 44(4):370–378
38. Siegman IL, Maron BJ, Permut LC, McIntosh CL, Clark RE (1989) Results of operation for coexistent obstructive hypertrophic cardiomyopathy and coronary artery disease. J Am Coll Cardiol 13(7):1527–1533
39. Agnew TM, Barratt-Boyes BG, Brandt RWT, Roche AHG, Lowe JB, O'Brien KP (1977) Surgical resection in idiopathic hypertrophic subaortic stenosis with a combined approach through aorta and left ventricle. J Thorac Cardiovasc Surg 74:307–316
40. Senning A (1976) Transventricular relief of idiopathic hypertrophic subaortic stenosis. J Cardiovasc Surg (Torino) 17:371–375
41. Cooley DA, Beall AC Jr, Hallman GL (1965) Obstructive lesions of the left ventricular outflow tract: surgical treatment. Circulation 31:612–621
42. Colley DA, Bloodwell RD, Hallman GL, LaSorte A, Leachman RD, Chapman DW (1967) Surgical treatment of muscular subaortic stenosis: results from septectomy in 26 patients. Circulation 35(Suppl 1):124–132
43. Cooley DA, Leachman RD, Wukasch DC (1973) Diffuse muscular subaortic stenosis: surgical management. Am J Cardiol 31:1–6
44. Colley DA, Wukasch DC, Leachman RD (1976) Mitral valve replacement for idiopathic hypertrophic subaortic stenosis: results in 27 patients. J Cardiovasc Surg (Torino) 17:380–387
45. McIntosh CL, Greenberg GJ, Maron BJ, Leon MB, Cannon III RO, Clark RE (1989) Clinical and hemodynamic results after mitral valve replacement in patients with obstructive hypertrophic cardiomyopathy. Ann Thorac Surg 47:236–246
46. Fighali S, Krajcer Z, Leachman RD (1984) Septal myomectomy and mitral valve replacement for idiopathic hypertrophic subaortic stenosis: short- and long-term follow-up. J Am Coll Cardiol 3(5):1127–1134
47. Roberts WC (1973) Operative treatment of hypertrophic obstructive cardiomyopathy: the case against mitral valve replacement. Am J Cardiol 32.377–381
48. McIntosh CL, Maron BJ, Cannon RO 3rd, Klues HG (1992) Initial results of combined anterior mitral leaflet plication and ventricular septal myotomy-myectomy for relief of left ventricular outflow tract obstruction in patients with hypertrophic cardiomyopathy. Circulation 86(5 Suppl):II60–67
49. Messmer BJ (1994) Extended myectomy for hypertrophic obstructed cardiomyopathy. Ann Thorac Surg 58:575–577
50. Kofflard MJ, van Herwerden LA, Waldstein DJ, et al. (1996) Initial results of combined anterior mitral leaflet extension and myectomy in patients with obstructive hypertrophic cardiomyopathy. J Am Coll Cardiol 28(1):197–202
51. Delmo Walter EM, Siniawski H, Hetzer R (2009) Sustained improvement after combined anterior mitral valve leaflet retention plasty and septal myectomy in preventing systolic anterior motion in hypertrophic obstructive cardiomyopathy in children. Eur J Cardiothorac Surg 36(3):546–552
52. Schoendube FA, Klues HG, Reith S, Flachskampf FA, Hanrath P, Messmer BJ (1995) Long-term clinical and echocardiographic follow-up after surgical correction of hypertrophic obstructive cardiomyopathy with extended myectomy and reconstruction of the subvalvular mitral apparatus. Circulation 92(9 Suppl):II122–127
53. Morrow AG (1978) Hypertrophic subaortic stenosis. Operative methods utilized to relieve left ventricular outflow obstruction. J Thorac Cardiovasc Surg 76(4):423–430

Modified tricuspid repair in patients with Ebstein's anomaly

N. Nagdyman

6.1 Background

Ebstein's anomaly is an unusual congenital heart lesion notable for its extremely variable anatomy [3]. One characteristic is the differing degree of dysplasia and displacement of the proximal attachments of the septal and posterior leaflets from the true atrioventricular junction. The anterior leaflet is normally attached to the tricuspid annulus but is usually larger than normal, with a sail-like aspect and various degrees of interchordal space obliteration and adherence to the ventricular wall. In Ebstein's anomaly, the valve divides the right ventricle into a proximal part between the atrioventricular junction and the displaced valve, called the atrialized portion of the right ventricle, and a distal part, called the functional right ventricle. Between 10% and 15% of these patients have accessory conduction pathways, while Wolff–Parkinson–White syndrome is the most frequent [15]. An atrial septal defect is present in most of the patients [23] and may result in a right-to-left shunt with cyanosis.

Various surgical techniques have been developed for the repair of Ebstein's anomaly and standard valvuloplastic repair usually included annuloplasty with the exclusion of the atrialized portion of the right ventricular chamber. Danielson et al. [9] introduced a modification of the Hardy technique [13] with transversal plication of the atrialized chamber, which was reproducibly effective and became a standard repair technique. Carpentier [4] and Chauvaud [6] favored a different form of repair, involving temporary detachment of the anterior tricuspid valve leaflet to achieve its complete mobilization, longitudinal plication of the atrialized right ventricle, and clockwise advancement of the anterior leaflet and posterior tricuspid annuloplasty with a prosthetic ring which resulted in a monocusp valve. Another modification without a prosthetic ring was proposed by Quaegebeur [20] and Chen [8]. The concept of annuloplasty at the level of the displaced tricuspid leaflets with plication of the atrialized right ventricle above the level of the reconstructed valve was introduced by Vargas and coworkers [22]. The value of plication of the atrialized chamber is still under discussion.

At some institutions–including our own–a repair technique without ventricular placation is preferred [1, 12, 14]. However, when a severe form of Ebstein's anomaly is present and the mobility of the anterior leaflet is significantly restricted, the best way to achieve tricuspid valve competence and good performance of the right ventricle is still being debated. We would like to contribute to this discussion by presenting our mid- and long-term results of repair without plication and the modifications applied to increase valve competence even in severe cases of Ebstein's anomaly.

6.2 Patients and methods

Between 1988 and 2008, 50 patients (33 female, 27 male; age 0.6–60 years, median 22 years) with Ebstein's anomaly underwent surgical repair at our hospital by a single surgeon (Roland Hetzer). The so-called »conventional technique« was used for tricuspid valve reconstruction (◘ Fig. 6.1) according to the Hetzer method [14] in 31 patients and, since 2004, with some modifications of the method in 19 patients. Indications for surgery were increasing signs of cardiac failure, cyanosis, severe tricuspid regurgitation, cardiomegaly (cardiothoracic ratio >65%) and rhythm disturbances.

The »conventional technique« used so far restructures the valve mechanism at the level of the true tricuspid annulus by using the most mobile leaflet for valve closure without plication of the atrialized chamber (Fig. 6.1). This results in the reconstruction of a monocusp valve as demonstrated in Fig. 6.2.

Since 2004, additional attachment of the anterior right ventricle wall to the interventricular septum (using the so-called »Sebening stich«) [1] and reconstruction of a tricuspid valve as a double orifice valve were performed in 19 patients (Figs. 6.3 and 6.4). After approximation of the center of the natural tricuspid annulus to the opposite site with mattress sutures, two orifices are created. Then, by injecting saline solution into the cavity of the ventricle, the

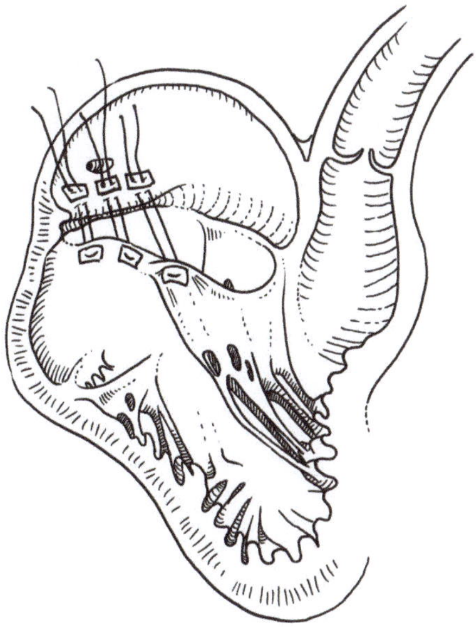

Fig. 6.1. »Conventional« technique of the reconstruction of the tricuspid valve in patients with Ebstein's anomaly. The principle is the use of the most mobile leaflet for valve closure, which results in a monocusp valve

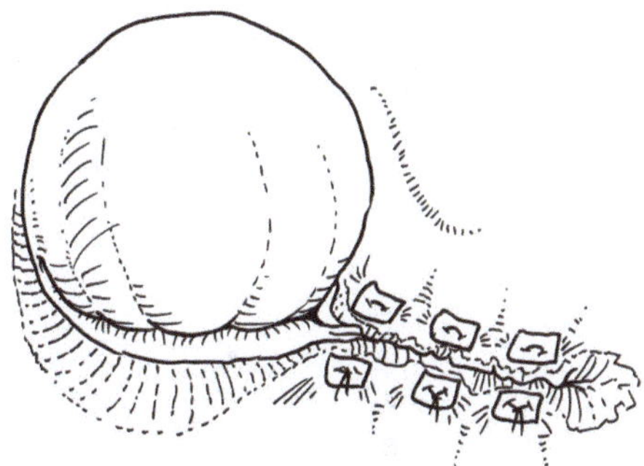

Fig. 6.2. Schematic view of the reconstructed monocusp valve after »conventional« reconstruction

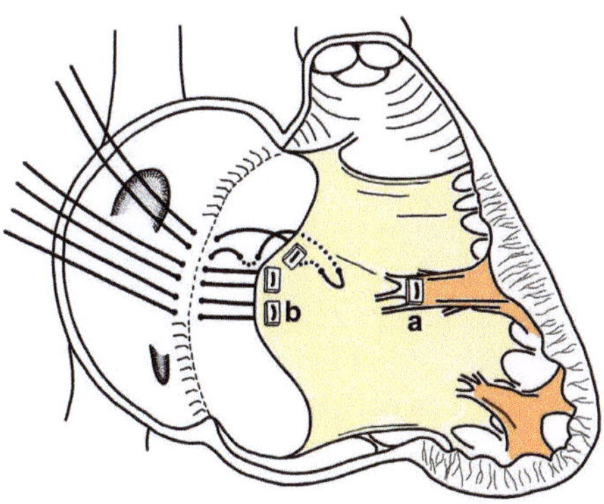

Fig. 6.3. Schematic view of the modified Hetzer surgical technique. Additional attachment of the anterior right ventricle wall to the interventricular septum by the Sebening stich (*a*) and reconstruction of the tricuspid valve as a double orifice valve (*b*) were performed as modifications

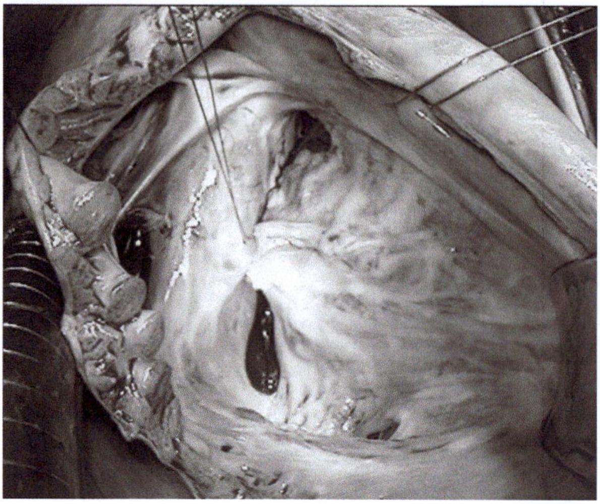

Fig. 6.4. Intraoperative view of the reconstructed tricuspid valve with two orifices after approximation of the center of the natural tricuspid annulus to the opposite side

6

Table 6.1. Operations performed in 50 patients with Ebstein's anomaly

Procedure	*n*
Posterior annulorhaphy	26
Anterior annulorhaphy	1
Bilateral annulorhaphy	4
Double orifice valve and Sebening stich	19
Additional Glenn anastomosis	3

competence of both »new« valves is tested. If the posterior orifice, which is usually smaller, still shows significant incompetence, the orifice is completely closed if the anterior orifice is large enough. If both orifices are competently closed by valve tissue, the reconstructed tricuspid valve functions as a so-called »double orifice« valve. The other modification introduced, the Sebening stich, helps to support the competence of the anterior leaflet. A mattress suture is placed between the papillary muscle tip and the fibrous remnants of the septal leaflet at the ventricular septum at the opposite site (Fig. 6.3).

Additional closure of atrial septal defect was necessary in 76% of the patients and associated congenital cardiac anomalies included the following: partial anomalous pulmonary venous return and ventricular septal defect (n=1), Chiari network malformation (n=1), pulmonary valve stenosis treated by balloon valvuloplasty several years before operation on the tricuspid valve (n=1), and mitral valve insufficiency (n=2). Table 6.1 gives an overview of the operations performed. According to the Carpentier classification system [4], 12 patients were graded as having type A, 19 patients type B, 12 patients type C, and 7 patients type D form of Ebstein's anomaly. Glenn anastomosis was additionally performed in 3 patients (2 patients with type C and 1 patient with type D). Survival rate, reoperations, NYHA classification, maximal oxygen uptake (VO_{2max}), right ventricular function measured by the pulmonary flow velocity integral, and tricuspid valve incompetence were evaluated. The median follow-up time was 68 (5–238) months.

6.3 Results

There were no intraoperative deaths. The early (30 day) mortality rate was 7.1% and late mortality rate 2.4%; since 2004 no further patients have died. Univariate analysis for death revealed that patients older than 50 years and in NYHA functional class III or IV were at risk. In our series, 2 patients with type C, 1 patient with type D, and 1 patient with type B died. Four reoperations in 3 patients were necessary: 1 patient had a re-do procedure 6 years after the first operation, 1 patient after 12 years, and 1 patient 7 and 12 months after the primary operation.

We observed an improvement in functional NYHA class from mean 3.1 preoperatively to mean 1.8 postoperatively ($p<0.001$), and these results were constant during the whole follow-up period. Exercise testing ($n=39$ patients) demonstrated an improvement in VO_{2max} ($p<0.02$).

The echocardiographic examinations revealed an improvement in the degree of tricuspid valve regurgitation directly after the operation from a mean 3.2 to a mean 1.9 ($p<0.001$) which remained stable in the following check-up examinations. We did not observe any tricuspid valve stenosis by Doppler echocardiography.

Type C and D patients demonstrated encouraging results 1 year postoperatively: at least 83% of patients with type C had the same grade of tricuspid valve incompetence as in the early postoperative period, and only 8.3% demonstrated a further decrease in their valve competence. In the group of type D patients, 71% demonstrated stable tricuspid valve function in echocardiography, while at least 28% had a progressive decrease in their competence.

Long-term analysis of the patients with »conventional« reconstruction demonstrated constant echocardiographic results in 72% of all patients; 16% had an improvement of their valve competence and 16% had a decrease in the degree of competence. After operations with modifications of this conventional technique, 88% of all patients had stable echocardiographic findings and only 12% had an increase of their tricuspid valve regurgitation.

Right ventricular function measured indirectly by pulmonary flow velocity integral improved significantly ($p<0.001$). Neither aneurysmal nor thrombotic formation of the former atrialized right ventricle was observed.

6.4 Discussion

Surgeons who operate on patients with Ebstein's malformation are confronted with a rare congenital heart defect with a wide spectrum of anatomical variations [11]. Over the past 30 years, various surgical techniques have been developed. For example, there are differences in the various techniques including the management of the atrialized right chamber, such as no plication [1, 12, 14, 21], or plication in horizontal [9, 13] or longitudinal direction [4, 20] or even longitudinal resection [24]. Most techniques work on the same principle–to obtain valve competence, namely using the large anterior leaflet as a functional monocusp valve [1, 4, 9, 12–14, 20]. Recently, new variations of repair techniques have been reported. They involve, for example, the mobilization of all tricuspid leaflets and transposition of the septal and posterior leaflets to the true annulus, without plication [21]. Results obtained after repairing severe forms of Ebstein's anomaly can be considerably improved if the right ventricle is unloaded by a concomitant Glenn shunt, which represents »one and a half ventricle repair« [5, 19] and some hospitals even prefer Fontan palliation [16, 18]. Therefore, there is currently still no *single* or *best* operation technique that offers optimal results.

Our reconstructive technique without plication of the atrialized right chamber and its modifications seem to provide encouraging results. The main characteristic of this technique is the incorporation of the atrialized chamber into the functional right ventricle while using the most mobile tricuspid leaflet for valve competence. This results in either a single orifice valve, where mostly the posterior part is closed, or in a »double orifice« valve. As a rule we have, since 2004, performed the Sebening stich as a supportive measure to alleviate tension on the sutures which approximate the anterior and septal annulus.

6

Table 6.2 gives an overview of the results of reconstructive techniques and shows that our results are comparable to those of other institutions. It is noteworthy that, since 2004, inhospital mortality has decreased to zero at our hospital. It remains open whether this is a direct result of the modifications of our operation technique or of better patient selection or both. The late mortality is very low and the analysis of the deceased patients showed that they were all operated on at ages above 50 years and were in at least functional NYHA class III or IV. They suffered from moderate to severe forms of Ebstein's anomaly with progressive heart failure, which leads to the question of whether they were operated upon too late. In these cases, several authors discuss the view that the indication for the operation should be prior to a patient reaching functional NYHA class III [1, 17]. We share this opinion and for this reason we perform annual exercise testing to detect any deterioration in exercise tolerance.

Two patients needed reoperation 6 and 12 years, respectively, after the initial procedure. Another patient received his first reoperation already 7 months after the primary repair, but in this re-do operation no valve reconstruction was possible. This patient received a biological valve, which became severely incompetent 5 months later without any obvious reasons. Thus, in a second reoperation, this patient received a mechanical tricuspid valve.

The postoperative improvement in NHYA class is associated with an increase in VO_{2max}. We did not detect any aneurysm formation or any thrombosis in the formerly atrialized right chamber. We believe that the formerly atrialized right ventricle assumes a part of the right ventricular contraction. The documented increase in the pulmonary flow velocity integral after the operation supports this suggestion of improved right ventricular function.

Table 6.2. Results of surgical techniques for Ebstein's anomaly

Operation	Follow-up (mean, years)	Number of patients	Early mortality (%)	Late mortality (%)	Re-operation (%)
Mayo Clinic [10] (1972–2005)	25	540	5.4	7.6	16
Carpentier technique [7] (1980–2002)	4.8	191	9	5.2	4.7
Sebening [2] technique	7.6	65	2.9	8.7	14.5
Hetzer technique (1988–2008)	5.6	50	6	2	8

6.5 Conclusion

Our mid-term and long-term results of surgical repair of Ebstein's anomaly by our operative technique are encouraging. A longer observation period is necessary to reveal the advantages of the modifications over the »conventional« Hetzer technique.

Acknowledgment

The author thanks Anne M. Gale for editorial assistance.

References

1. Augustin N, Schmidt-Habelmann P, Wottke M, Meisner H, Sebening F (1997) Results after surgical repair of Ebstein's anomaly. Ann Thorac Surg 63:1650–1656
2. Augustin N, Schreiber C, Wottke M, Meisner H (1998) [Ebstein's anomaly: when should a patient have operative treatment?] Herz 23:287–292
3. Becker AE, Becker MJ, Edwards JE (1971) Pathological spectrum of dysplasia of the tricuspid valve: features in common with Ebstein's malformation. J Pathol 103:Pxix–xx
4. Carpentier A, Chauvaud S, Mace L, et al. (1988) A new reconstructive operation for Ebstein's anomaly of the tricuspid valve. J Thorac Cardiovasc Surg 96:92–101
5. Chauvaud S, Fuzellier JF, Berrebi A, et al. (1998) Bi-directional cavopulmonary shunt associated with ventriculo and valvuloplasty in Ebstein's anomaly: benefits in high risk patients. Eur J Cardiothorac Surg 13:514–519
6. Chauvaud S (2000) Ebstein's malformation. Surgical treatment and results. Thorac Cardiovasc Surg 48:220–223
7. Chauvaud S, Berrebi A, d'Attellis N, Mousseaux E, Hernigou A, Carpentier A (2003) Ebstein's anomaly: repair based on functional analysis. Eur J Cardiothorac Surg 23:525–531
8. Chen JM, Mosca RS, Altmann K, et al. (2004) Early and medium-term results for repair of Ebstein anomaly. J Thorac Cardiovasc Surg 127:990–998; discussion 998–999
9. Danielson GK, Maloney JD, Devloo RA (1979) Surgical repair of Ebstein's anomaly. Mayo Clin Proc 54:185–192
10. Dearani JA, Danielson GK (2005) Surgical management of Ebstein's anomaly in the adult. Semin Thorac Cardiovasc Surg 17:148–154
11. Frescura C, Angelini A, Daliento L, Thiene G (2000) Morphological aspects of Ebstein's anomaly in adults. Thorac Cardiovasc Surg 48:203–208
12. Hancock Friesen CL, Chen R, Howlett JG, Ross DB (2004) Posterior annular plication: tricuspid valve repair in Ebstein's anomaly. Ann Thorac Surg 77:2167–2171
13. Hardy KL, May IA, Webster CA, Kimball KG (1964) Ebstein's anomaly: a functional concept and successful definitive repair. J Thorac Cardiovasc Surg 48:927–940
14. Hetzer R, Nagdyman N, Ewert P, et al. (1998) A modified repair technique for tricuspid incompetence in Ebstein's anomaly. J Thorac Cardiovasc Surg 115:857–868
15. Kastor JA, Goldreyer BN, Josephson ME, et al. (1975) Electrophysiologic characteristics of Ebstein's anomaly of the tricuspid valve. Circulation 52:987–995
16. Kaulitz R, Ziemer G (1995) Modified Fontan procedure for Ebstein's anomaly of the tricuspid valve–an alternative surgical approach preserving Ebstein's anatomy. Thorac Cardiovasc Surg 43:275–279
17. Kupilik N, Simon P, Moidl R, et al. (1999) Valve-preserving treatment of Ebstein's anomaly: perioperative and follow-up results. Thorac Cardiovasc Surg 47:229–234
18. Marcelletti C, Duren DR, Schuilenburg RM, Becker AE (1980) Fontan's operation for Ebstein's anomaly. J Thorac Cardiovasc Surg 79:63–66
19. Marianeschi SM, McElhinney DB, Reddy VM, Silverman NH, Hanley FL (1998) Alternative approach to the repair of Ebstein's malformation: intracardiac repair with ventricular unloading. Ann Thorac Surg 66:1546–1550
20. Quaegebeur JM, Sreeram N, Fraser AG, et al. (1991) Surgery for Ebstein's anomaly: the clinical and echocardiographic evaluation of a new technique. J Am Coll Cardiol 17:722–728
21. Ullmann MV, Born S, Sebening C, Gorenflo M, Ulmer HE, Hagl S (2004) Ventricularization of the atrialized chamber: a concept of Ebstein's anomaly repair. Ann Thorac Surg 78:918–924; discussion 924–915

22. Vargas FJ, Mengo G, Granja MA, Gentile JA, Rannzini ME, Vazquez JC (1998) Tricuspid annuloplasty and ventricular plication for Ebstein's malformation. Ann Thorac Surg 65:1755–1757
23. Watson H (1974) Natural history of Ebstein's anomaly of tricuspid valve in childhood and adolescence. An international co-operative study of 505 cases. Br Heart J 36:417–427
24. Wu Q, Huang Z (2004) A new procedure for Ebstein's anomaly. Ann Thorac Surg 77:470–476; discussion 476

III Degenerative mitral valve disease

Introduction to the keynote lecture by Robert W.M. Frater, M.B., CH.B.*

J.S. Rankin

* The video presentation associated with this paper is available for download from: http://www.jsrmd.com/ftp/25_Frater_Intro.m4v

Dr. Robert William Mayo Frater was born in Cape Town, South Africa, and obtained his medical degree from the University of Cape Town. You might wonder how Dr. Frater came to be named after Will Mayo: his father was the first South African to train in surgery at the Mayo Clinic, while his mother was the first Englishwoman to train there. They met in Rochester, MN, married in St. Paul, and then moved back to South Africa to practice surgery. Thus, it was natural that when Bob finished basic surgery training in England, he would go to the Mayo Clinic from 1955–1962 to train in the new specialty of cardiothoracic surgery.

The Mayo Clinic Department of Surgery had numerous well-known and excellent mentors for Dr. Frater, including Dr. Jim Clagett and Dr. John Kirklin, who at the time was doing the first series of intracardiac operations using the pump oxygenator–it was quite an era to be there. Photos of Dr. Frater taken during those years shows a young man with a look of determination (Fig. 7.1).

Dr. Clagett's assessment of Bob's performance was as follows: »A very outstanding man. Wonderful basic knowledge. Inspires confidence in patients. Excellent judgment and unusually good technical skills. This man is really very superior in every respect. Grade: A^{+}«. Later, Dr. F. Henry Ellis, who became a mentor to Bob, said: »Best first assistant I have had. Good staff material. Outstanding in every way. Grade: A^{+}«. When Bob began working with Dr. Ellis in the laboratory, they published a seminal paper in 1961 on problems with mitral valve replacement in Dr. Merendino's book [1]. Note the flexible monocusp valve, and the tricuspid annuloplasty ring (Fig. 7.2).

The following year [2], Bob proposed repairing mitral valves with autologous pericardial patches and pericardial chordal replacement (Fig. 7.3), which was revolutionary for the time! Bob then put a letter in *The Lancet* in 1962 [3]: »...these comments are made to emphasize that the patient with a mitral prosthesis is a patient for life. There is a need for satisfactory

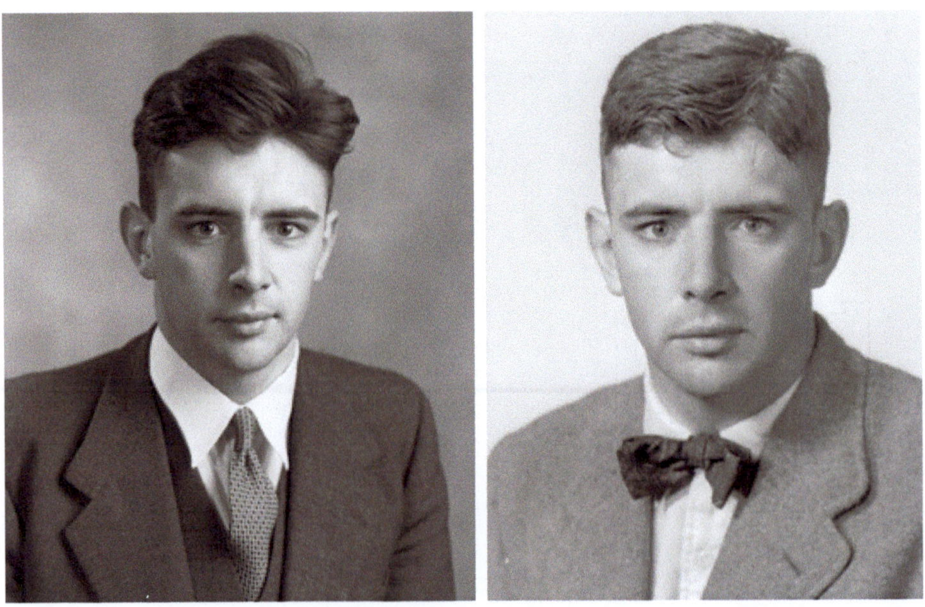

Fig. 7.1. Photos of Dr. Robert W.M. Frater, taken while he was at the Mayo Clinic (1955–1962)

techniques of repair of the valves that fall between those suitable for annuloplasty procedures and those for which replacement is mandatory. Procedures using pericardial autografts are promising in this regard«. He then went on to describe pericardial augmentation of the posterior leaflet [4]. In a 1964 *Thorax* paper [5], he reported performing these types of reparative procedures in patients in South Africa, using autologous pericardial patches and pericardial chordal replacement. That work ultimately led to the development of ePTFE artificial chordal replacement with Herb Vetter in 1986 [6]. Bob's initial clinical series of ePTFE chordal replacements were published in 1989 and 1990 [7, 8] and, as is said, »the rest is history«.

Bob spent most of his career at Albert Einstein Medical School, Montefiore Hospital, where he served both as Division Chief of Cardiothoracic Surgery and Chairman of the

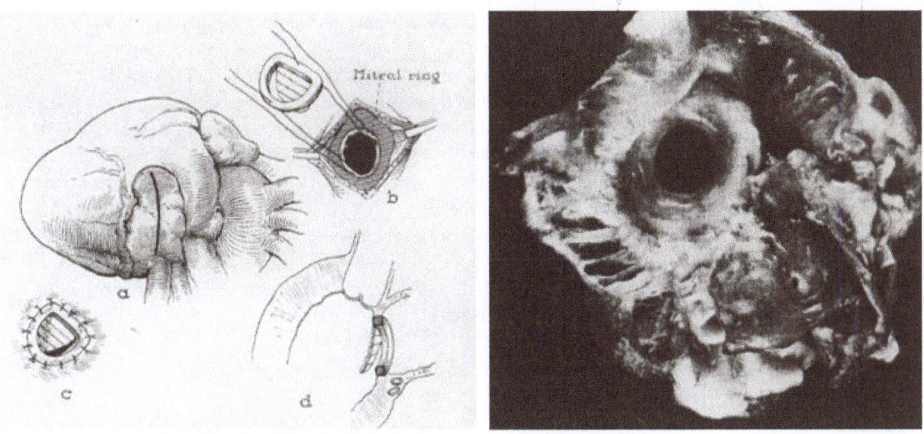

Fig. 7.2. Illustrations of experimental mitral valve replacement and tricuspid annuloplasty taken from a seminal paper published in 1961 ([1]; © Charles C. Thomas Publisher)

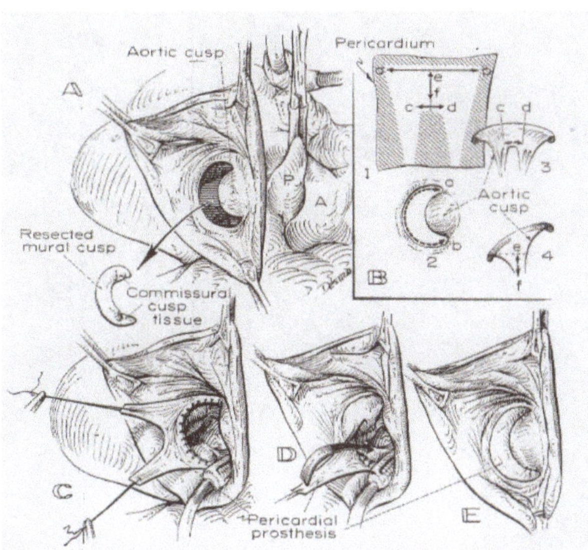

Fig. 7.3. Repair of mitral valves using autologous pericardial patches and pericardial chordal replacement in 1962 ([2]; © Surgery)

Department of Surgery. He ran a world-class cardiac physiology lab with Dr. Ed Yellin, Herb Vetter, and Octavio Pajaro. Very few individuals have made as many basic and clinical contributions as Dr. Robert Frater, and certainly, his concepts about mitral valve surgery have now become mainstream.

References

1. Frater RWM, Ellis FH Jr (1961) Problems in the development of a mitral-valve prosthesis. In: Merendino KA (ed) Prosthetic valves for cardiac surgery. Charles C Thomas Publisher, Springfield, IL, pp 244–265
2. Frater RWM, Berghuis J, Brown AL, Ellis FH Jr (1962) Autogenous pericardium for posterior mitral leaflet replacement. Surgery 84:260–268
3. Frater RWM(1962) Artificial heart valves. Lancet 2:1171
4. Frater RWM, Berghuis J, Brown AL, Ellis FH Jr (1963) Autogenous pericardium for posterior mitral leaflet replacement. Surgery 84:260–268
5. Frater RWM (1964) Anatomical rules for plastic repair of the diseased mitral valve. Thorax 19: 458
6. Vetter H, Burack J, Factor S, Macaluso F, Frater RWM (1986) Replacement of chordae tendineae of the mitral valve using the new expanded PTFE suture in sheep. In: Bodnar E, Yacoub M (eds) Biologic bioprosthetic valves. Yorke Medical Books, New York, pp 772–784
7. Zussa C, Frater RWM, Polesel E, Galloni M, Valfre C (1990) Artificial mitral valve chordae: experimental and clinical experience. Ann Thor Surg 50:367–373
8. Frater RWM, Vetter HO, Zussa C, Dahm M (1990) Chordal replacement in mitral valve repair. Circulation 82 (Suppl IV):125–130
9. Nikolic SD, Feneley MP, Pajaro OE, Rankin JS, Yellin EL (1995) Origin of regional pressure gradients in the left ventricle during early diastole. Am J Physiol 268:H550–557

Chordae: 1959–2009

R.W.M. Frater

8.1 Introduction

In October 1955, I started training in General Surgery at the Mayo Clinic (Rochester, MN). On the third Saturday afternoon in October, I observed John Kirklin performing an open heart operation using extracorporeal circulation. On Monday, I visited the Fellowship Office and requested the addition of Thoracic Training to my studies. This was added and carried with it the requirement of writing a thesis. For this task, my advisor Dr. Bunky Ellis gave me a project: development of a mitral valve prosthesis. This was a virgin field at the time and I first asked myself the question: how does the mitral valve work? In 1959, I started my thesis in the classical manner by studying the anatomy of any mitral valve I could get my hands on. I dissected the hearts of humans, dogs, deer, guinea pigs, beaver, etc. My major conclusion from this effort was that mitral valve anatomy was dominated by irregularity.

8.2 Anatomy and function of chordae

There was always a large anterior leaflet with a straight fibrous base from trigone to trigone and opposite it was the posterior leaflet. The deepest part of the posterior leaflet was opposite the middle of the anterior leaflet and frequently in the form of a distinct scallop. Both the anterior leaflet and this central scallop were supported on each side by chordae from the left and right papillary muscles. Between the anterior leaflet and the central scallop on both sides, there were sometimes smooth slopes but most often 1–3 scallops of protruding tissue. ▪ Fig. 8.1 shows a canine mitral valve from 1959; there is a straight-sided anterior leaflet and a similar posterior central scallop, three right-sided posterior scallops, and one left-sided scallop. Chordae are of many different lengths and arise from the top and sides of the papillary muscles. ▪ Fig. 8.2 shows a human valve from 1959; the rounded anterior leaflet and central scallop have wide bases occupying the greater part of the annular length. There is no scallop between the anterior leaflet and the posterior central scallop on the left side and one small right-sided scallop. The chordae are of many different lengths and arise from high and low on the multiheaded papillary muscles.

The chordae of the anterior leaflet from a dog and a human are shown in ▪ Fig. 8.3. Tandler [1] had made sense of the insertion of the cords: 1st order into the free edge and 2nd order into the body of the leaflet. In the dog's valve, the chordae are numbered I and II and, in the human valve, a silk suture has been passed between the leaflet and the 2nd order chordae. Especially in the case of the anterior leaflet, there is an area between the last of the 2nd order chordae and the annulus that is bare of chordal insertions. In the middle of the anterior leaflet and the middle of the central scallop, there is a division between the left and right sides of the leaflet tissue. To the left, all the inserted chordae have arisen from the left papillary muscle and, to the right, all the chordae have arisen from the right papillary muscle. The 2nd order chordae arise either from a papillary muscle or from another 2nd order chorda. They are thicker than 1st order cords. The 1st order cords may arise directly from a papillary muscle, from a 2nd order cord, or from a 1st order cord. The sites of papillary origins were also irregular so that the distance from the origin to insertion could be grossly different for cords inserted close to each other at the leaflet level. Papillary muscles were also irregular with conical, multiheaded, sessile and wedge shapes. Despite these variations, there was a very distinct pattern with the anterior leaflet being supported from the anterior half of a papillary muscle and the posterior leaflet from the posterior half.

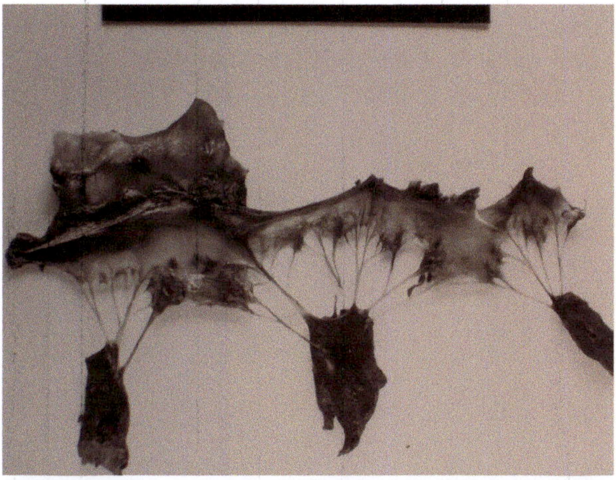

Fig. 8.1. Canine mitral valve dissected in 1959. Viewed from the ventricular side. Right papillary muscle divided. Square-shaped anterior leaflet and posterior central scallop

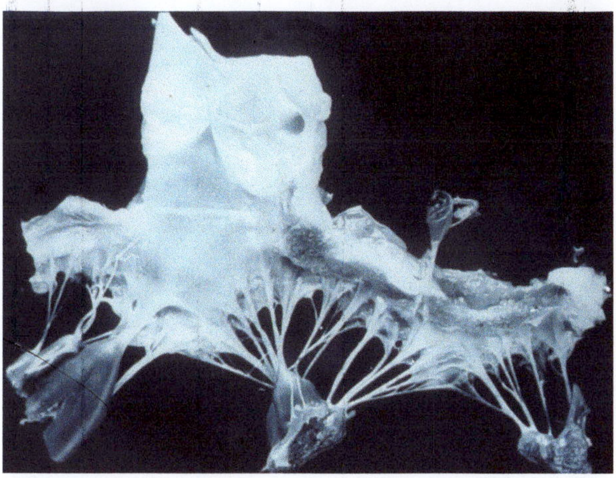

Fig. 8.2. Human mitral valve dissected in 1959. Right papillary muscle divided. Wide based anterior leaflet and central scallop. Only one small right sided scallop. Chordae of many different lengths arising from high and low on the multiheaded papillary muscles

8.3 Studying the valve in action

Without feeling and seeing the mitral valve in action, it was difficult to understand why it is normally competent. The first critical experience was to have my finger in the valve of a living dog. I could feel the squeeze of the mural annulus and the considerable area of leaflet that closed around my finger. It was very clear that the annulus was dynamic, opening for flow and narrowing for closure. I also had the enormous benefit of observing the valve working in a live beating heart. Essex, Smith, and Baldes, two physiologists and a cardiologist, were trying to prove the origin of the first heart sound (there were two theories at the time: one that the noise came from contracting muscle and another that it was from the smacking together of the leaflets). The atrium was secured to a flat circular Plexiglas® box through which the valve could be filmed and observed. The ascending aorta opened into a tube that returned the clear oxygenated Ringer–Locke solution, which kept the heart beating, back into the side of the atrial chamber. There was a resistance in the tube that allowed physiologic pressures to be maintained, while the valves were observed and the heart sounds recorded. I saw the experiments live and watched the films that were taken. After visiting the Mayo Clinic's archives a few years ago, it was found that the films had unfortunately deteriorated to a point that they could not be reproduced.

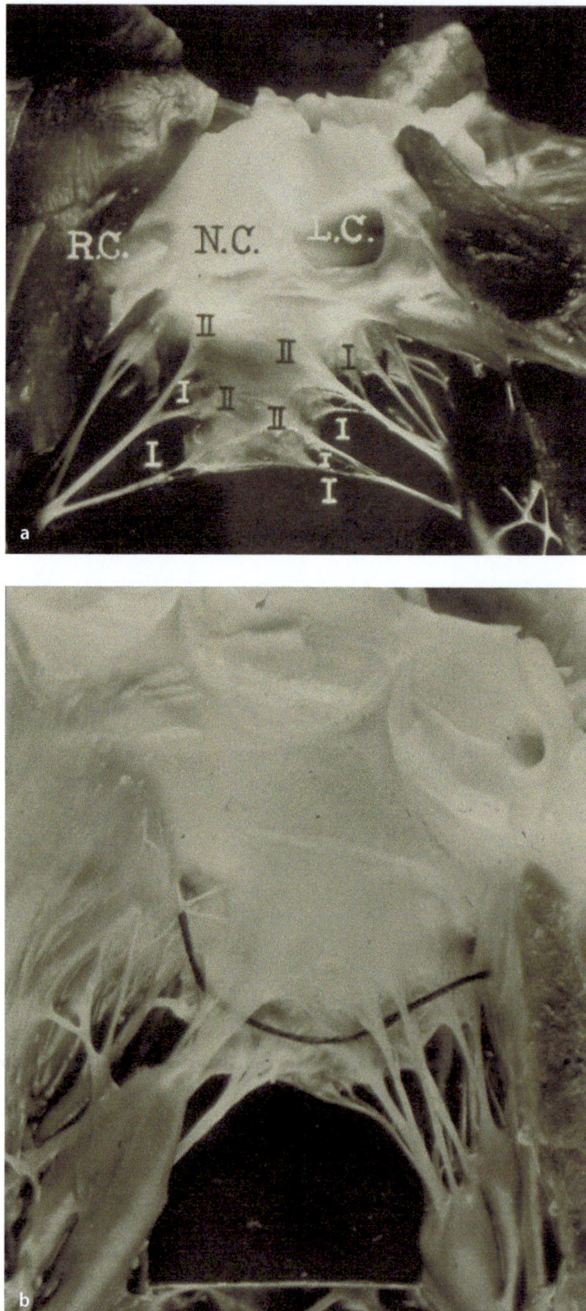

Fig. 8.3. a Canine anterior leaflet with 1st and 2nd order chordae numbered. **b** Human anterior leaflet with a silk suture between the leaflet and the 2nd order insertions. See text for an analysis of chordal origins and insertions

Further studies included hanging dead hearts by the atrium and aorta and enclosing them in a watertight fluid-filled box. The ventricle was subjected to phasic pressure from outside that produced a passable imitation of systole and diastole. The clear fluid inside the heart was pumped past a resistance back into the atrial chamber. The pressures imitated nature.

In studies on the live heart, the main chordae were seen to remain straight throughout diastole with the clear implication that they must be under some tension even during diastole. This observation was confirmed in the suspended dead heart model. During systole, the shortening of the mural annulus closed the spaces between the »cusps« or scallops, as we now call them, compressing them into a shelf. The more mobile anterior leaflet met this shelf over a depth of coaptation (◘ Fig. 8.4).

All the way along the semicircular line of contact between the anterior and posteior leaflets, the free edges, wherever they meet, when gently pulled with hooks, would be found to be parallel. Wherever the free edges of anterior and posterior leaflets are in contact, they are parallel. Despite the irregularity of chordal origins, wherever the anterior and posterior leaflets make contact, those 1st order chordae supporting them *at that point* are exactly the right length to keep the free edges parallel. ◘ Fig. 8.5 is an illustration from an article with a bold title that was published in *Thorax* in 1964 [2]. In the two drawings on the left, the parallel relationship of the anterior and posterior leaflet edges in diastole and systole, the coaptation over a depth of leaflets, and the atrial limit of the coaptation below the atrioventricular plane are shown [2].

We used the external pulse duplicator to try to differentiate between the function of the 1st and 2nd order chordae by cutting them selectively and observing the behavior of the leaflets under cyclic pressure. »When the second order chordae are cut, the line of closure is maintained, although the aortic cusp bulges more than usual into the atrium and probably more of the tissue comes into view than usual« [3]. When only one of the 1st order chordae was cut, our observation was: »the leading edge of the cusp inverts during systole« and »there is immediate insufficiency« in the region of the cut chorda.

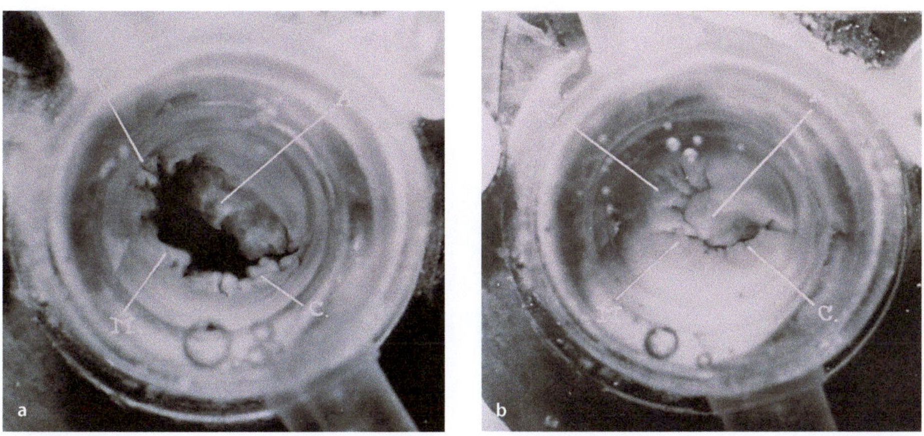

◘ **Fig. 8.4.** Canine mitral valve viewed through the atrial window of the external pulse duplicator. **a** During diastole, the anterior leaflet (*A*) , the posterior leaflet central scallop (*M*), and multiple scallops (*C*) are visible. **b** During systole, all the scallops of the posterior leaflet have been compressed together into a shelf by shortening of the posterior annulus. The anterior leaflet has met the shelf. The coapted areas which are not visible are about half of the posterior leaflet and a third of the anterior leaflet

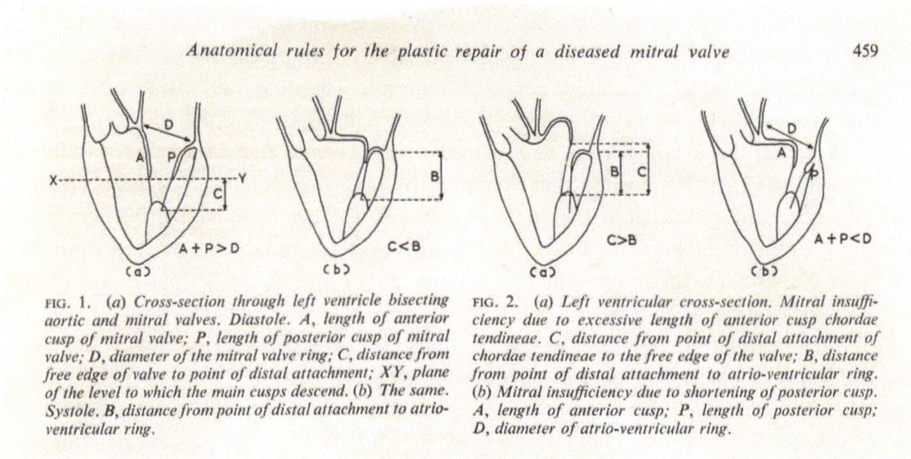
Anatomical rules for the plastic repair of a diseased mitral valve 459

FIG. 1. (*a*) *Cross-section through left ventricle bisecting aortic and mitral valves. Diastole. A, length of anterior cusp of mitral valve; P, length of posterior cusp of mitral valve; D, diameter of the mitral valve ring; C, distance from free edge of valve to point of distal attachment; XY, plane of the level to which the main cusps descend.* (*b*) *The same. Systole. B, distance from point of distal attachment to atrio-ventricular ring.*

FIG. 2. (*a*) *Left ventricular cross-section. Mitral insufficiency due to excessive length of anterior cusp chordae tendineae. C, distance from point of distal attachment of chordae tendineae to the free edge of the valve; B, distance from point of distal attachment to atrio-ventricular ring.* (*b*) *Mitral insufficiency due to shortening of posterior cusp. A, length of anterior cusp; P, length of posterior cusp; D, diameter of atrio-ventricular ring.*

Fig. 8.5. Illustration from *Thorax* article published in 1964. See text for details ([2]; © Thorax)

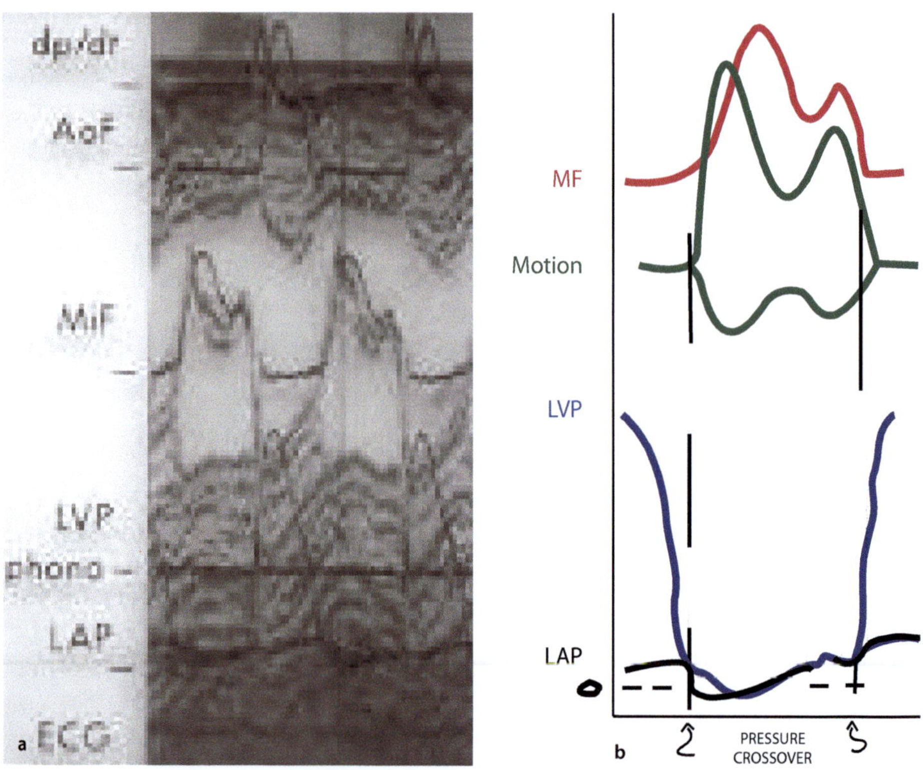

Fig. 8.6. a Simultaneous recording of M-mode echocardiography, mitral and aortic flow, mitral leaflet and ventricular motion, ventricular and aortic pressure. **b** Explanation of images in **a**. Mitral flow is shown by the *red* line, the motion of the anterior and posterior leaflets are indicated by the *green* lines which separate during diastole, and the left ventricular and left atrial pressures are indicated by the *black* and *blue* lines, respectively, which cross each other at the beginning and end of diastole

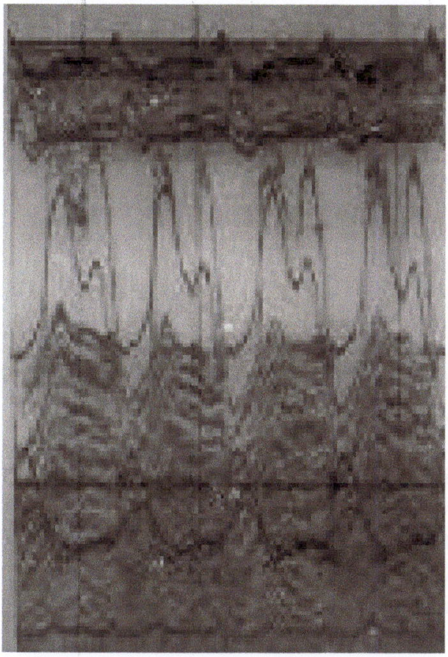

Fig. 8.7. Demonstration of important restraining function of the chordae which induces the leaflets to respond to the forces produced by the fluid flowing past them. Papillary muscle support of the anterior leaflet had been separated from the ventricular wall and then sewn back. The sutures tore loose and without support the anterior leaflet hit the septum in early diastole and then again with atrial contraction. The upper part of the M-mode echocardiograph shows the leaflet making contact with the septum during diastole

Without modern imaging, our observations of living beating hearts led us to conclusions in 1959 which proved to be valid [2–4]. We could see that the ventricle lengthened in diastole and shortened in systole. The papillary muscles, which are shorter than the posterior ventricular wall, must also lengthen in diastole and shorten in systole. The net effect must be to move the chordal origins away from the annulus in diastole and towards it in systole. Since the anterior and posterior chordae arose separately from the anterior and posterior halves of each papillary muscle, this movement, contrary to the beliefs at the time, had to pull the valve open in diastole and allow it to close in systole.

In the 1960s, we became more sophisticated and simultaneously recorded mitral flow (using an electromagnetic flow probe in the atrium that did not interfere with annular motion), atrial, ventricular and aortic pressures (catheter tip pressure transducers), and M-mode echocardiography of ventricular and leaflet motion (Fig. 8.6). Flow started just before the pressure crossover and accelerated very rapidly as a result of the sucking action of the ventricle. The leaflet opening was also rapid but, remarkably, while flow was still accelerating, the leaflets began to move together again. With atrial contraction, they separated and the forward flow once more accelerated and decelerated. The leaflets moved rapidly together as the »atrial kick« subsided and by the end of diastole they were almost touching, ready to snap shut as the ventricular–atrial pressure crossover occurred.

We recognized that fluid dynamic forces exerted on the leaflets in diastole had something to do with this leaflet behavior. Bellhouse [5] had described a vortex behind the anterior leaflet in a model with a transparent ventricle. Serendipity showed us the importance of chordal restraint in these movements. In an experiment in which, after the anterior part of a papillary muscle was detached and then resutured back in place, the sutures tore through. In diastole, the flail anterior leaflet moved across to hit the septum and hit it again with atrial contraction (Fig. 8.7). For normal leaflet movement, the restraint provided by the chordal insertions was essential. Ed Yellin, who ran our laboratory, explained this behavior using fluid dynamic theory and Charles Peskin, a MD/PhD student, used the Cray super computer to produce dynamic moving pictures of leaflet and blood interactions [6]. It was clear that the leaflets, like the sails of a yacht in wind, needed to be restrained for these interactions to take place. Peskin was subsequently awarded a Macarthur Prize and is the professor of Biomathematics at the Courant Institute of Mathematics in New York City.

8.4 Clinical applications

8 At the same time as we were trying to understand the function of normal chordae, we were operating on patients with valvular heart disease. Rheumatic fever was the dominant etiology. There was a vast reservoir of these patients, many with insufficiency. These cases invariably had fusion of the posterior scallops producing a fixed shelf. It seemed that the annulus was dilated as a consequence of rheumatic carditis. The anterior leaflet commonly remained pliable but its chordae were quite often elongated, again probably as a result of a change in chordal integrity produced by rheumatic inflammation. On the right in Fig. 8.5, elongated anterior chordae are illustrated and a shrunken posterior leaflet in the other. Fig. 8.8 shows a repair used for a case of rheumatic mitral insufficiency, in which annular dilatation, elongated anterior chordae on the right side, and a shrunken, fused posterior leaflet caused the insufficiency. Note the restoration of competence by separating the shrunken posterior leaflet from the annulus, bringing the prolapsing right anterior leaflet to a proper depth by attaching to it the posterior leaflet with its normal length chordae, and then inserting a gusset of pericardium in the posterior leaflet to reestablish a proper degree of anterior–posterior leaflet coaptation.

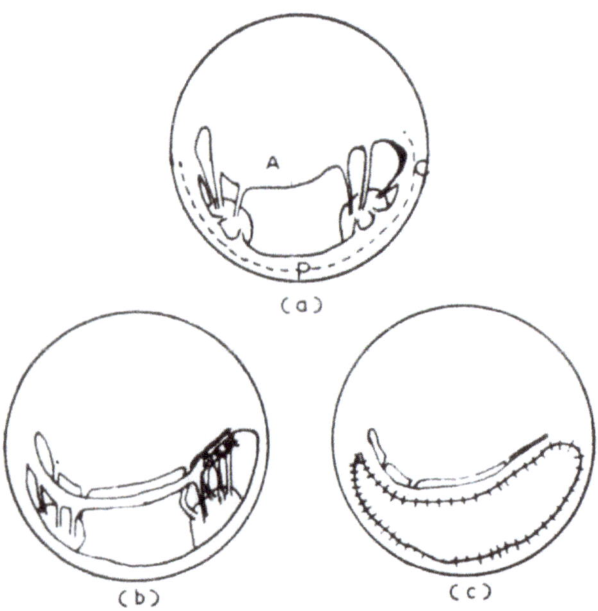

Fig. 8.8. Repair of a rheumatic case in the early 1960s. Combination of chordal transposition and pericardial posterior leaflet enlargement. See text for details ([2]; © Thorax)

8.5 Beginnings of chordal replacement

Chordal transposition was our first solution to chordal elongation, but after further contemplation, replacement seemed an obvious choice. Paul Marchand, a surgeon working with John Barlow in Johannesburg, had replaced ruptured chordae with polyester sutures [7]. They thought they were dealing with rupture of normal chordae but I suspect these were cases of fibroelastic deficiency. There was no follow-up or further work from Johannesburg. We and others (including Edwards in Arizona) started using strips of, at first, autogenous pericardium and later in the 1970s tanned bovine pericardium. In order to obtain the right length, we used understanding that had been gained from studying normal valve function [8].

Given the basic facts that if the free edge of a posterior leaflet with normal chordae, opposite an anterior leaflet with a ruptured cord, is placed under tension so as to straighten the posterior cord, then that level of the free edge is where the anterior leaflet free edge must be fixed. The pericardial strip is stitched to the papillary muscle. It is placed under gentle tension to obtain a straight line and the anterior leaflet is stitched to it so that the anterior and posterior free edges are level. Once this is established, the remaining requirement is that the systolic annular dimension must be sufficiently less than the combined areas of the anterior and posterior leaflets to ensure a good area of coaptation.

In the 1970s and 1980s, many different materials, both inorganic and organic, were tried. Polyurethane was more suited for leaflets than for cords. Organic material had to start as a flat strip or tape rather than a string to have enough strength. Glycerol-treated bovine pericardium initially looked very promising. After 3 months of implantation, it remodeled into a round cord. However, the histology of the collagen looked bad: it was poorly stained and further testing showed a significant immunologic response to the glycerol-treated pericardium. Host healing response to the collagen seemed slower in humans than in sheep or dogs, and we were afraid that ruptures might result in humans that could not be predicted by animal studies. Glycerol-treated tissue was also difficult to sterilize and the search for the right material continued. We made a list of desirable properties. We wanted the host to heal to the implant with a fibrosa and an intima. We wanted thickness, flexibility, and strength–strain properties to approximate those of normal cords. Whatever material we chose needed to be easy to use and suitable for placing multiple chordae in one patient.

8.6 Origin and development of the ePTFE idea

At that time, we were studying the healing of synthetic and biologic vascular grafts. Although Gore-Tex® vascular grafts did not acquire an inner host covering and remained bare along almost all their length, the first 1–2 mm from the anastamotic suture line was different: a fibrosa and intima were visible. The structure of the Gore-Tex® used in grafts and sutures had »internodal spaces«. Fibroblasts from the host at the anastomotic line appeared to attach themselves to this surface. This did not happen in tightly woven Teflon™ fabric grafts or Gore-Tex® formulations with a completely uninterrupted smooth surface. Therefore, the question was raised whether Gore-Tex® sutures, used to replace natural chordae and immersed on all sides in blood, might acquire a host fibrosa and intima by growth from the leaflet and papillary attachment points. This possibility was tested by implantation of Gore-Tex® sutures between the anterior leaflet and the appropriate papillary muscle in sheep. Dr. Herbert Vetter performed the first operation and 5 months later, on 5 March 1985, he called me to the lab to see the autopsy on this first sheep. He had inserted two CV-2 sutures between the left papillary muscle and the anterior leaflet (Fig. 8.9). This was one of those very rare moments in research when the hoped for result is achieved at the first experiment. The sheep had grown a new chorda over the template that we had provided. More chordal replacements were performed in sheep and dogs and the results were always the same: a new chorda invariably grew over the template provided by the Gore-Tex® suture. Fig. 8.10 shows the host tissue advancing along a Gore-Tex® suture at 2 months. Our first goal had clearly been met; we had succeeded in growing new chordae. Later, Karyn Kunzelman compared different sutures with porcine chordae. She showed that ePTFE sutures exhibited viscoelastic properties similar (although not identical) to natural chordae, but, nevertheless, appeared to be the best available synthetic material [9].

It was found that the chordae grown over CV2 Gore-Tex® sutures did not have the flexibility of normal chordae. Since main chordae were generally in a straight line throughout both systole and diastole, it was not clear whether this would interfere with normal opening and closing. They were in fact similar in stiffness to many rheumatic chordae in their flexion response to gravity. Claudio Zussa implanted CV5 sutures in dogs in the laboratory. At explan-

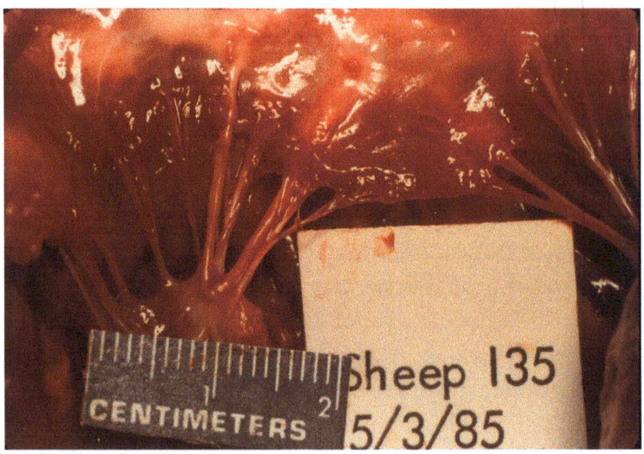

Fig. 8.9. The first sheep sacrificed 5 months after insertion of Gore-Tex® chordae by Dr. Vetter. The two completely covered Gore-Tex® sutures are attached to the papillary muscle just above the 1 cm mark on the ruler and separate by 30° on the way to their attachment to the leaflet

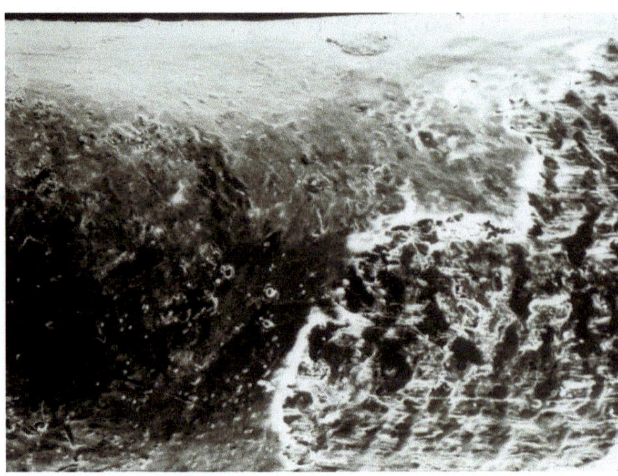

Fig. 8.10. At 2 months, host tissue coming from upper left, is growing over extruded ePTFE. Internodal spaces of the Gore-Tex® are not yet covered on the lower right. Scanning electron microscopy

tation, these were clearly closer to normal chordae in their flexion response to gravity. Guangfu Gong tested the breaking strength of unimplanted CV5 Gore-Tex® sutures and found it to be 1,000 grams. If the suture was crushed in a hemostat or a hemostatic clip, it would break at the point of clamping at 500 grams. The breaking strength of a main chorda of 1 mm diameter is around 400 grams. In 1963, Peter Salisbury [9] published a study on the tension in canine main cords in vivo. Under normal conditions, the tension was between 50 and 60 grams. With adjacent chordae cut and the aorta partially clamped, the tension rose to 150–200 grams. The uncovered strength of CV5 Gore-Tex® seemed to provide a substantial margin of safety. It appeared that we had sufficient information to proceed with human use. There were, in fact, no guidelines, let alone regulations, of any kind regarding replacement of chordae, and we could have used Gore-Tex® sutures for replacing chordae without any preliminary research.

The first presentation of the new chordal replacement technique was made at a meeting in London in 1985 by Dr. Herbert Vetter [10, 11]. There was an interested response from the audience. In the discussion we revealed that, shortly before the meeting, on a visit to the unit of Dr. Garcia-Rinaldi in Houston we had met Jose Revuelta from Santander, Spain, who had started a project with the same goal as ours. In the discussion, we acknowledged Dr. Revuelta's work. On the evening after the presentation, Dr. Tyrone David and I had dinner together. Dr. David told me that he would start using Gore-Tex® sutures in Canada the following week; thus, he became the first surgeon to develop a series of cases [12]. It took us nearly a year to start using the technique in our own institution (Weiler Hospital of Montefiore Medical Center, Albert Einstein College of Medicine, The Bronx, NY).

8.7 Gore-Tex® chordae: a tool in the hands of surgeons

The subsequent history of the use of Gore-Tex® for chordal replacement followed an unusual course for a surgical replacement technique. There was no sponsorship of any kind. There were no formal workshops, no advertising, no promotion. No patents were taken out. Before large numbers of publications appeared, surgeons interested in mitral repair exchanged information and started trying its use around the world. The use of Gore-Tex® as a chordal substitute has been a monument to the ingenuity and enterprise of individual cardiac surgeons. Dr. Zussa began to build a clinical series soon after returning to Italy and produced the definitive textbook on the subject in 1994 [13]. The Gore-Tex® company, observing this spontaneous off-label use of its product, organized a 10th anniversary conference on Gore-Tex® cords in 1996 and obtained FDA 510k approval for the use of its suture for chordal replacement [14–16].

Since the 10th anniversary, in the hands of a steadily increasing number of surgeons around the world, the application of Gore-Tex® chordae has become an essential technique in the armamentarium of valve repair surgeons. Because of the spontaneous nature of this development, many variations have been developed. There have been consistent requirements common to all:

- The length of a new chorda must be such that the free edges of the opposing anterior and posterior leaflets are parallel when the chorae are placed under enough tension to hold them in a straight line.
- Chordal length can be determined preoperatively by echocardiography with a view that cuts through the prolapsing leaflet and the normal leaflet opposite it and, intraoperatively, most often in the arrested heart, by gentle traction on the prolapsing and nonprolapsing

opposing leaflets. In the less common situation in which opposing anterior and posterior leaflets are both prolapsing, a »normal« relationship of the free edge to the annular plane needs to be defined.

- With the free edges parallel, the base to free edge lengths of the opposing leaflets through the contact points must be at least 1 cm more than the systolic annular radius through the contact point. Expressed differently, if the anteroposterior dimension is fixed by annuloplasty at more than 1 cm less than the combined lengths of the anterior leaflet and the central scallop, this will achieve at least 0.5 cm of coaptation.

The details of how many different surgeons have achieved these goals in numerous different ways exceed the scope of this paper. Mohr's use of echocardiography to determine the proper neocordal length in a full beating heart makes eminent sense. Calipers have been used to add precision to length determination and premade lengths of loops of Gore-Tex® have been useful [17]. The use of Gore-Tex® sutures to re-establish annular–papillary continuity after total excision of severely diseased valves was described by Sintek and Khonsari [18].

The question arises as to how to judge the correct length between the papillary muscle and the annulus. Going back to basics, we know that the load-bearing chordae are always under some tension throughout the cycle. Assuming an arrested heart to be in a state somewhat equivalent to diastole, it is reasonable to secure them in a straight line with minimal tension avoiding either pulling the papillary muscle towards the annulus or allowing the suture to be floppy. Komeda [19] studied ventricular function in an animal model of replacement with varying amounts of chordal tension and found 10 grams allowed preserved function, whereas being taut or loose affected it adversely.

I had an opportunity to see the late result of this procedure. A patient, who had a calcified mitral valve replaced with annular–papillary connection preserved with Gore-Tex® sutures placed with sufficient tension to maintain a straight line in the arrested heart, was murdered by her husband in the Bronx. I was allowed to inspect the heart at the autopsy by the Manhattan coroner but, because this was a murder case, I was not allowed to take specimens. The neochordae were thin and flexible and covered with host tissue. I had the impression that the papillary muscle had atrophied, suggesting that I may not have got the tension right.

Gore-Tex® is slippery and surgeons starting to use it have found that tying the knot down resulted in a free edge being pulled down deeper than its correct position with inevitable loss of competence. Various forms of lock stitch have been used to allow the surgeon to tie the knot firmly so as to compress the thread sufficiently to prevent slippage. Four throws with sufficient cinching to compress the suture will not unravel. The alternative of tying multiple relatively loose knots is aesthetically unappealing, looks as though it could be a site for mini-clot formation, and is definitely unnecessary. Tying the knot with the competent valve closed under pressure was introduced by Zussa and has been adopted by many [13, 15].

Recently there has been further interest in using clips to help in achieving correct length [20]. We have avoided hemostatic clips because of the reduction of the breaking strength that they can produce [12]. This prohibition extended to avoidance of temporary clamping of the suture with an arterial hemostat. In recent years, other forms of clips have been used with success particularly during minimally invasive or robotic surgery [20–22]. Our experience with conventional arterial clips has been confirmed in a carefully performed study by Krane et al. [23]. It is possible that the use of conventional arterial clips may not reduce the strength to a level below the forces encountered in a given patient. Nevertheless, they should be avoided. In Krane's study, the use of a Pean clamp to secure the suture while tying a knot did not reduce the breaking strength of the suture. Nor did a knotpusher affect suture strength. Strength testing of knots using nitinol clips would be useful.

With length determination and knot tying techniques established, Gore-Tex® chordal use has become the preferred method of correcting incompetent mitral valves. Artificial chordae were originally introduced for anterior leaflet prolapse or flail, and it is fair to say that their use for this indication has steadily supplanted techniques using other parts of the natural valve. It has also increasingly been used for posterior flail or prolapse, with the notion of resecting less tissue and thereby maintaining a pliable functional posterior leaflet. The slogan »respect instead of resect« was invented by Patrick Perier [24]. Pediatric use is also well established [25–27]. The reason for this steady growth can be attributed to the perception of surgeons that the technique is easy to use and has predictably reproducible results.

Papers have compared the original undoubtedly ingenious and inventive techniques of Alain Carpentier with Gore-Tex® chordal replacement and demonstrated that in their hands the early and late results are better [28, 29]. Others have shown that the previous difference between anterior and posterior repairs has disappeared [31]. The adaptability of chordal replacement to minimally invasive and even robotic approaches has been clearly demonstrated. Indications have included cases of infective endocarditis. The series started by Zussa and continued by Salvador and colleagues [32] has now been in progress for over 20 years and over 700 patients have been followed. It is notable that the only technique used on anterior leaflet pathology was, from the beginning, chordal replacement. Early and late mortality were exceptionally low and follow-up freedom from endocarditis, thromboembolism, reoperation, and recurrent insufficiency all very high. Neither failure nor calcification of the Gore-Tex® material was observed. In 25 reoperations for progression of disease or various causes, the CV4 or CV5 sutures were covered with host fibrosa and endothelium and remained thin and pliable.

There have been two reports in the literature of failure of Gore-Tex® chordae. Butany [33] described rupture of a calcified artificial chorda after 14 years, while Coutinho [34] reported two cases of rupture at 6 and 11 years. These were from an institution that had used Gore-Tex® chordae in more than 500 cases. Although calcification was not grossly evident, the authors speculated that a reaction originating in the host covering had infiltrated and damaged the polytetrafluoroethylene leading to microscopic calcification in the material. Information on the long-term appearance of artificial chordae is for obvious reasons very scarce. Previous pathologic studies of artificial chordae implanted for similar lengths of time [35, 36] have shown no calcium, no damage to the Gore-Tex® sutures, and a continued maintenance of the benign process originally observed in short-term animal studies.

8.8 Conclusion

The ingenious and inventive techniques of mitral valve evaluation and repair which were developed by Alain Carpentier were the subject of intensive teaching programs in North America and Europe. These courses were responsible for a slow but steady change in the proportion of patients with mitral insufficiency receiving repair rather than replacement. The story of chordal replacement has been different: from the beginning, it was driven by the notion of growing new chordae. Once this was achieved experimentally, it was taken up by surgeons in Canada, Italy, Japan, Germany, the USA, and many other countries. Its initial growth was entirely without promotion, sponsorship, or marketing, driven by the desire of individual surgeons to use a technique that they recognized would allow them to achieve the fundamental goals of restoring the parallel free edges and the appropriate coaptation that makes the valve competent. The additional challenge was to master the difficulty of tying a secure knot with a slippery suture. Surgeons developed and used their own chordal replacement methods as they reached for the goal of repairing almost all incompetent valves. I cannot acknowledge all these many individuals. I thank them all for turning an idea into the modern reality of mitral valve repair.

References

1. Tandler J (1913) Anatomie des Herzens. Gustav Fischer Verlag, Jena, Germany, pp 87–90
2. Frater RWM (1964) Anatomical rules for plastic repair of the diseased mitral valve. Thorax 19:458–464
3. Frater RWM (1961) Mitral valve prostheses. Thesis accepted by the University of Minnesota in partial fulfillment of the Degree of Master of Science in Surgery, December 1961
4. Frater RWM, Ellis FH Jr (1961) The anatomy of the canine mitral valve. J Surg Res I:171–178
5. Bellhouse BJ (1970) Fluid mechanics of a model mitral valve and left ventricle. Cardiovasc Res 1970;6:199–210
6. Yellin EL, Laniado S, Peskin C, Frater RWM (1975) Analysis and Interpretation of the normal mitral valve flow curve. In: Kalmanson D (ed) The mitral valve: a pluridisciplinary approach. Publishing Sciences Group Inc., Acton, MA, pp 163–172, 174–176
7. Marchand P, Barlow JB (1966) Mitral regurgitation with rupture of normal chordae. British Heart J 28:7
8. Frater RWM, Gabbay, Shore D, Factor S, Strom J (1983) Reproducible replacement of elongated or ruptured mitral valve chordae. Ann of Thor Surg 35:1
9. Salisbury PF, Cross CE, Rieben PA (1963) Chorda tendinea tension. Am J Physiol 205: 385–392
10. Vetter H, Burack J, Factor S, Macaluso F, Frater RWM (1986) Replacement of chordae tendineae of the mitral valve using the new expanded PTFE suture in sheep. In: Bodnar E, Yacoub M (eds) Biologic bioprosthetic valves. Yorke Medical Books, New York, pp 772–784
11. Cochran RP, Kunzelman KS (1991) Comparison of viscoelastic properties of suture versus porcine mitral valve chordae tendineae. J Cardia Surg 6:508–513
12. David T (1989) Replacement of chordae tendineae with expanded polytertrafluorethylene sutures. J Cardiac Surg 4:286–290
13. Zussa C (1994) Artificial chordae in mitral valve surgery. RG Landes Co, Austin, TX
14. Frater RWM (1996) 10th Goretex chorda anniversary. J Heart Valve Dis 5:348–351
15. Zussa C (1996) Different applications of ePTFE valve chordae: surgical technique. J Heart Valve Dis 5:356–361
16. David TE, Armstrong S, Sun Z (1996) Replacement of chordae tendineae with Goretex sutures: a ten year experience. J Heart Valve Dis 5:352–355
17. von Oppel UO, Mohr FW (2000) Chordal replacement for both minimally invasive and conventional mitral valve surgery using premeasured Gore-Tex loops. Ann Thorac Surg 70:2166–2168
18. Sintek CF, Khonsari S (1996) Use of three extended polytetrafluoroethylene (ePTFE) chordae to re-establish annular-papillary connection after mitral valve excision. J Heart Valve Dis 5:362–364
19. Komeda M, Deanda A, Glasson JR, Bolgert AF, Nikolic SD, Ingels NB, Miller DC (1996) Improving methods of chordal-sparing MVR? Part (I): a novel isovolumic balloon preparation for left ventricle with intact mitral subvalvular apparatus. J Heart Valve Dis 5:376–382
20. Chan DTL, Chin CSW, Chang LL, An TWK (2008) Artificial chordae: a simple clip and tie technique. J Thorac Cardiovasc Surg 136:1597–1599
21. Smith JM, Stein H (2008) Endoscopic placement of multiple artificial chordae with robotic assistance and nitinol clip fixation. *J Thorac Cardiovasc Surg* 135:610–614
22. Rankin J, Alfery D, Orozco R, Binford R, Burrichter C, Brunsting III L (2008) Techniques of artificial chordal replacement for mitral valve repair: Use in multiple pathologies. Op Tech Thorac Cardiovascr Surg 13:74–82
23 Krane M, Braun EU, Mayer H, Knoll A, Bauernschmitt R, Lange R (2007) Mitral valve reconstruction with artificial chordae: how to secure the desired length? Computers in Cardiology 34: 745–748 (http://www.cinc.org/archives/2007/pdf/0745.pdf)
24. Perier P, Hohenberger W, Lakew F, Batz G, Urbanski P, Zacher M, Diegeler A (2008) Toward a new paradigm for the reconstruction of posterior leaflet prolapse: midterm results of the »respect rather than resect« approach. Ann Thorac Surg 2008:86:718–725

25. Murakami T, Yagihara T, Yamamoto F, Uemara H, Yamashita K, Izizaka T (1998) Artificial chordae for mitral valve reconstruction in children. Ann Thorac Surg 65:1377–1380
26. Boon R, Hazekamp G, Hoohenkerk M, Rijlaarsdam M, Schoof P, Koolbergen D, Heredia L, Dion R (2007) Artificial chordae for pediatric mitral and tricuspid valve repair. Eur J Cardiothorac Surg 32:143–148
27. Aganostopoulos PV, Alphonso N, Hornberger L, Raff GW, Azakie A, Tom R (2007) Neonatal mitral and tricuspid valve repair for in utero papillary muscle rupture. Ann Thorac Surg 83:1458–1462
28. Phillips MR, Daly RC, Schaff HV, Dearani JA, Mullany CJ, Orszulak TA (2000) Repair of anterior leaflet mitral prolapse:chordal replacement versus chordal shortening. Ann Thorac Surg 69:25–29
29. Seeburger J, Falk V, Borger A, Passage J, Walther T, Doll N, Mohr FW (2009) Chordae replacement versus resection for repair of isolated posterior mitral leaflet prolapse: an egalite. Ann Thorac Surg 87:1715–1720
30. Chiappini B, Sanchez C, Noirhomme P, Verheist R, Rubay J, Poncelet A, Funken JC, El Khoury G (2006) Replacement of chordae tendineae with polyfluoroethylene (PTFE) sutures in mitral valve repair: early and long-term results. J Heart Valve Dis 15:557–563
31. Rankin JS, Orfosco RE, Rodgers TL, Alfery DD, Glower DD (2006) »Adjustable« artificial chordal replacement for repair of mitral valve prolapse. Ann Thorac Surg 81:1526–1528
32. Lawrie GM, Earle EA, Earle NR (2006) Feasibility and intermediate term outcome of repair of prolapsing anterior mitral leaflets with artificial chordal replacement in152 patients. Ann Thorac Surg 81:849–856
33. Salvador L, Mirone S, Patelli F, Salvatore M, Minetti G, Madat M, Cavaretta E, Valfre C (2008) A 20 year experience with mitral valve repair with artificial chordae in 608 patients. J Thorac Cardiovasc Surg 135:1280–1287
34. Butany J, Collins MJ, David TE (2004) Ruptured synthetic expanded polytetrafluoroethylene chordae tendineae. Cardiovasc Pathol 82:819–826
35. Coutinho GF, Carvalho L, Antunes MJ (2007) Acute mitral regurgitation due to ruptured ePTFE neochordae. J Heart Valve Dis 16:278–281
36. Privitera S, Butany J, David TE (2005) Artificial chordae tendineae: long-term changes. J Card Surg 20:90–92
37. Minatoya K, Kobayashi J, Sesako Y, Ishibashi-Ueda H, Yutani C, Kitamura S (2001) Long-term pathological changes of expanded polytetrafluoroethylene (ePTFE) suture in the human heart. J Heart Valve Dis 10:139–142

Is chordal insertion the procedure of choice in mitral valve repair?

J. Seeburger, F.W. Mohr

9.1 Introduction

Degenerative mitral valve disease is frequently represented by elongated and/or ruptured chordae tendineae which leads to prolapse of the mitral valve (MV) and, thus, to mitral regurgitation (MR). In such cases, MV surgery provides a curative treatment. A simple surgical procedure to address MV prolapse is to replace the diseased chordae tendineae by polytetrafluoroethylene (PTFE) sutures. This idea of chordae replacement was introduced by Frater and colleagues [1]. They followed the attempt of completely replacing diseased chordae with PTFE sutures, a material very similar to native chordae in terms of biomechanical characteristics. Until today, several different techniques for implantation of neochordae in MV repair have been described with a very high rate of success and good long-term durability [2–5]. Despite these promising results, the question remains whether chordal insertion is the procedure of choice in mitral valve repair?

9.2 Methods and results

The surgical technique of chordal replacement follows a very simple principle: the elongated and/or ruptured chordae tendineae of the MV are simply replaced with PTFE sutures. This can be achieved by replacing one chordae at a time or several chordae at once. Until today a large diversity of different techniques for implantation neochordae has been described.

Frater and colleagues assessed biomechanical properties of the PTFE material ex vivo and in vitro. Then introducing this repair technique into clinical practice, they suggested a simple one suture technique to repair the MV. In the area of prolapse, the PTFE suture should be placed in order to re-establish the continuity between the papillary muscles and the mitral leaflet edge [1]. This was accomplished by fixing the PTFE to the body of the papillary muscle, adjusting for the desired length of the sutures, and finally fixing the suture to the prolapsing segment of the MV leaflet.

The group of David and colleagues adopted this technique in the late 1980s and since then has acquired experience [2]. They were able to confirm that the technique is highly applicable for correction of MV prolapse and stabilization of MV leaflets. It also has proven to be a durable repair technique with excellent long-term clinical results regarding the high freedom from reoperation and high survival after MV repair [3]. David, however, modified the technique by using one suture to create something like a »woven net«: by fixing the suture to the papillary muscle and then leading it to the prolapsing leaflet edge and back to the papillary muscle, and now repeating this process as many times as the width of the prolapsing segments requires.

Most recently, another modification has been reported for the repair of isolated posterior leaflet prolapse by Perrier and colleagues [6]. This group uses the »original« technique, however, with modification regarding the fixation of the PTFE suture to the leaflet. They use one suture at a time, but then the fixation on the leaflet edge is performed by initially tying the PTFE on the atrial side three times, then tying it on the ventricular side and finally again on the atrial side. This is very time consuming but highly effective.

Another similar technique is used by Rankin and colleagues [7]. However, this group mostly uses a limited number of sutures irrespective of the width of the prolapse. Even for repair of extensively prolapsing segments, they were able to achieve excellent results with »only« two sutures. They have nicely demonstrated this and made the operative procedure accessible for the public as a video presentation on the Internet [8]. Rankin also proposed to use the implantation of neochordae as a repair alternative to leaflet extension in patients with systolic anterior motion and hypertrophic obstructive cardiomyopathy and demonstrated the feasibility in a patient with very good postoperative results.

All three techniques, however, »lack« the possibility to assess the correct length in advance. The technique introduced by von Oppel in 2000 allows for preimplantation measurement of the correct size of the neochordae using a caliper and followed by implantation of a premade bundle of sutures representing four independent loops, the so-called loop technique [9]. This technique has shown to contribute to the reparability of the historically more difficult anterior leaflet prolapse and bileaflet prolapse [4, 5,10]. Regarding isolated posterior mitral leaflet (PML) prolapse, the loop technique has proven to reach a higher freedom from reoperation rate than the classical resection technique, introduced by Carpentier [11, 12]. The loop technique aims to imitate native valve anatomy which allows for physiological leaflet motion, creation of a large mitral orifice area, and for creation of a long surface of coaptation [13]–which is supposed to be associated with a long durability [12,14].

9.3 Conclusion

The implantation of neochordae represents a highly feasible repair technique for MV prolapse. It provides an excellent intraoperative handling, it allows for re-establishing physiological leaflet function of the MV leaflets and, thus, excellent hemodynamics, it creates a larger mitral orifice area compared to the more classical technique of resection and has proven superior mid-term outcomes. Furthermore, there is a very low risk of systolic anterior motion (SAM) associated with the insertion of neochordae.

The idea of the technique to replace the diseased chordae tendineae is both highly effective and very simple. The PTFE sutures have proven to be of utmost importance and able to provide the best possible biomechanical characteristics. However, it is certainly not the only technique to repair MV prolapse. There are other very successful techniques, such as the widely performed quadrangular triangular resection with or without sliding plasty, chordae transfer, papillary muscle shortening, and the edge-to-edge technique–many of these techniques have shown very good results. In order to answer the initial question as to whether chordal insertion is the procedure of choice in MV repair, these successful repair techniques have to be addressed.

In cases of excessive leaflet tissue, one may be forced to perform a resection, whether quadrangular or triangular with or without sliding plasty, or shorten the height of the leaflet using the »haircut« technique. It may also be necessary to save native chordae from the anterior leaflet and transfer them to the area of prolapse at the posterior leaflet. In highly complex cases, the edge-to-edge technique may represent a final repair technique to achieve a competent valve. In rheumatic disease, leaflet augmentation with a pericardial patch may be adequate.

Compared to these techniques, however, chordal replacement has the advantage of imitating native valve anatomy; thus, it may be best suitable for repair of MV prolapse with restitution of a more physiologic MV. Therefore, the initial idea of Frater and colleagues, modified by many different surgeons, has led and still is leading this simple technique to be a very powerful tool for MV repair.

Chordal insertion is not the only procedure to accomplish a successful MV repair. It also has to be emphasized that the procedure does not apply in all pathologies of the MV. Detailed preoperative planning and imaging of the MV are crucial in combination with a highly individual repair concept for each patient. Chordal insertion is a true alternative to the widely used leaflet resection technique, providing even slightly improved results with regard to a higher freedom from reoperation in the treatment of isolated posterior leaflet prolapse. Furthermore, it allows for successful repair of complex cases, such as bileaflet prolapse. However, until today only a few groups of surgeons have been able to report mid- and long-term results with the chordal replacement technique. In order to refer to this technique as the procedure of choice in MV repair, these results have to be confirmed by other groups. Until then, it remains not the only procedure for successful MV repair, however, a very powerful one.

References

1. Frater RW, Vetter HO, Zussa C, Dahm M (1990) Chordal replacement in mitral valve repair. Circulation 82:IV125–130
2. David TE, Bos J, Rakowski H (1991) Mitral valve repair by replacement of chordae tendineae with polytetrafluoroethylene sutures. J Thorac Cardiovasc Surg 101:495–501
3. David TE (2004) Artificial chordae. Sem Thorac Cardiovasc Surg 16:161–168
4. Seeburger J, Kuntze T, Mohr FW (2007) Gore-tex chordoplasty in degenerative mitral valve repair. Sem Thorac Cardiovasc Surg 19:111–115
5. Kuntze T, Borger MA, Falk V, Seeburger J, Girdauskas E, Doll N, Walther T, Mohr FW (2008) Early and mid-term results of mitral valve repair using premeasured Gore-tex loops ('loop technique'). Eur J Cardiothorac Surg 33:566–572
6. Perier P, Hohenberger W, Lakew F, Batz G, Urbanski P, Zacher M, Diegeler A (2008) Toward a new paradigm for the reconstruction of posterior leaflet prolapse: midterm results of the »respect rather than resect« approach. Ann Thorac Surg 86:718–725
7. Rankin JS, Binford RS, Johnston TS, Matthews JT, Alfery DD, McRae AT, Brunsting LA 3rd (2008) A new mitral valve repair strategy for hypertrophic obstructive cardiomyopathy. J Heart Valve Dis 17:642–647
8. Rankin CTS Net Video at www.ctsnet.org/sections/clinicalresources/videos/vg2010_RankinS_ACR_Barlows.html
9. Oppell UO, Mohr FW (2000) Chordal replacement for both minimally invasive and conventional mitral valve surgery using premeasured Gore-tex loops. Ann Thorac Surg 70:2166–2168
10. Seeburger J, Borger MA, Doll N, Walther T, Passage J, Falk V, Mohr FW (2009) Comparison of outcomes of minimally invasive mitral valve surgery for posterior, anterior, and bileaflet prolapse. Eur J Cardiothorac Surg 36(3):532–538
11. Seeburger J, Falk V, Borger MA, Passage J, Walther T, Doll N, Mohr FW (2009) Chordae replacement versus resection for repair of isolated posterior mitral leaflet prolapse: a egalité. Ann Thorac Surg 87:1715–1720
12. Carpentier A (1983) Cardiac valve surgery – the »French correction«. J Thorac Cardiovasc Surg 86:323–337
13. Falk V, Seeburger J, Czesla M, Borger MA, Willige J, Kuntze T, Doll N, Borger F, Perrier P, Mohr FW (2008) How does the use of polytetrafluoroethylene neochordae for posterior mitral valve prolapse (loop technique) compare with leaflet resection? A prospective randomized trial. J Thorac Cardiovasc Surg 136:1205; discussion 1205–1206
14. Braunberger E, Deloche A, Berrei A, Abdallah F, Celestin JA, Meimoun P, Chatellier G, Chauvaud S, Fabiani JN, Carpentier A (2001) Very long-term results (more than 20 years) of valve repair with Carpentier's techniques in nonrheumatic mitral valve insufficiency. Circulation 104:I8–11

Artificial chordal replacement for complex mitral valve repair*

J.S. Rankin, D.D. Alfery, R. Orozco, R.S. Binford, C.A. Burrichter, L.A. Brunsting III

* The video presentation associated with this paper is published at CTSNet.org and can be downloaded from: http://www.jsrmd.com/ftp/24_ACR_in_Complex_MVR.m4v

10.1 Introduction

The development of mitral valve repair is one of the all-time success stories in medicine. In the 1960s and 1970s, mitral valve replacement was the highest risk adult cardiac procedure in most centers, with operative mortalities approaching 20–30% in many categories [1]. Based on innovation from many sources [2], reparative methods were refined and developed, and Carpentier's lecture before the American Association for Thoracic Surgery in 1983 brought together the techniques of ring annuloplasty, leaflet reconstruction, and chordal shortening/transfer into a unified approach [3]. Carpentier's contributions stimulated great interest in repair, and progress continued on many fronts.

10.2 Basic chordal replacement technique

The use of polytetrafluoroethylene (ePTFE) suture as a chordal replacement subsequently was described by Vetter and Frater in 1986 [4, 5]. Dr. Frater's choice of ePTFE, or Gore-Tex®, suture as a chordal substitute was based on many years of research [6], going back to the first days of cardiac surgery at the Mayo Clinic in the 1950s, when Frater was a fellow with Dr. F. Henry Ellis [7]. Frater realized the advantages of valve repair early on and stated in a 1962 editorial [8] to *The Lancet* »...the patient with a mitral prosthesis is a patient for life. There is a need for satisfactory techniques of repair for the valves that fall between those suitable for

annuloplasty procedures and those for which replacement is mandatory. Procedures using pericardial autografts are promising in this regard«. After 24 additional years of investigation, Frater and his research colleagues developed Gore-Tex® artificial chordal replacement (ACR).

Our group tried ACR early-on, but had difficulty getting chordal lengths right, until 1995, when we learned to adjust neochordal length with a slip knot at the end of the procedure–after annuloplasty ring placement [9, 10]. As shown in ▫ Fig. 10.1, a pledgeted anchor suture is placed in the posterior papillary muscle, oriented longitudinally, and a 2-0 Gore-Tex® suture is passed through the pledget and left untied. The Gore-Tex® chord is stuffed into the ventricle, and after ring placement, it is retrieved and woven into the prolapsing segment in three full-thickness bites: free edge, surface of coaptation, and line of coaptation, emerging onto the atrial surface. This forms a loop that stabilizes the lateral aspects of the segment, with the two arms automatically assuming proper length. The Gore-Tex® chord is tied with a slip knot, and an atraumatic clip is placed lightly on the knot. The valve is tested by instillation of cold saline into the left ventricle across the valve, and if the chord to the leaflet is a little tight or too loose, the clip is removed, and the slip knot is lengthened or tightened. This process is continued until, on re-testing, normal anterior–posterior and left-to-right symmetry is established. Then the final knot is tied tightly against the clip. These knots can come untied, so tying against the clip is important. The clip is removed, the suture is cut, and the goal is for the valve to have a large coaptation area and no residual leak. If leak continues, leaflet clefts are closed, or the procedure is repeated as necessary to obtain full competence. One advantage of ACR, however, is that the steps usually proceed in an organized and timely fashion, without the need to »innovate on the spot«.

Another advantage of ACR is that leaflet tissue is not resected, and maintenance of leaflet surface area promotes competence. In cases of mitral prolapse, 95% of patients have no residual leak at the end, independent of which leaflet is involved [10]. Because the prolapsing

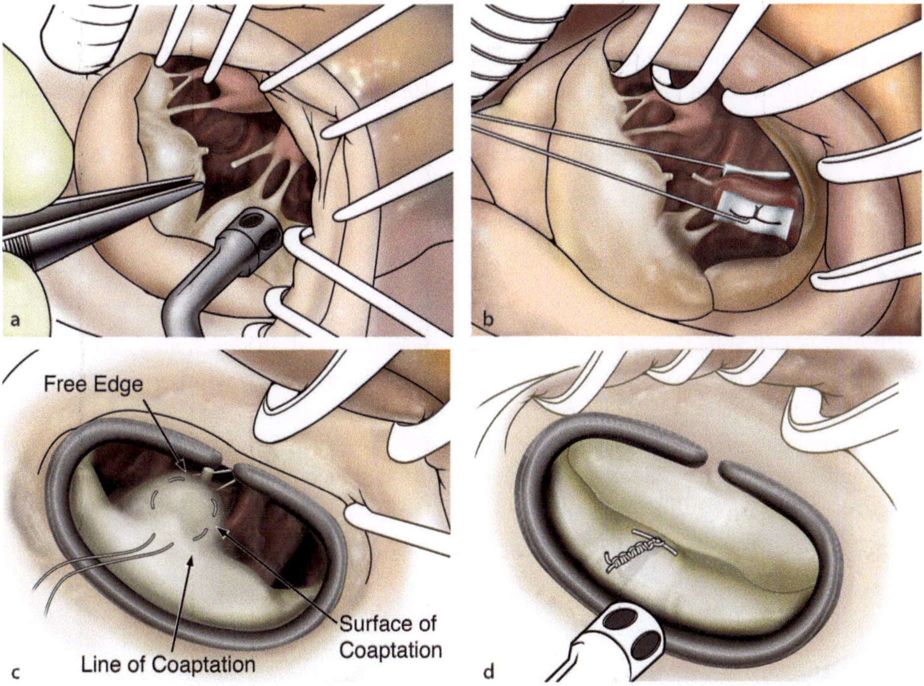

Fig. 10.1. Sequential steps in adjustable artificial chordal replacement. **a** A ruptured chord from the posterior papillary muscle to the posterior leaflet is evident. **b** A pledgetted anchor suture is placed longitudinally in the papillary muscle, and a 2-0 Gore-Tex® artificial chord is passed through the anchor pledget and left untied. **c** After Carpentier ring placement (AnnuloFlow, Sorin Group), the chord is retrieved and woven as a loop into the leaflet in three full-thickness bites: free edge, flaring laterally through the surface of coaptation, and then angled back medially through the line of coaptation, emerging onto the atrial surface of the leaflet. **d** The chordal slip knot is adjusted during valve testing to produce good anterior–posterior and left-to-right leaflet symmetry, and no residual leak

segments are pulled down into the ventricle, mitral systolic anterior motion and outflow tract obstruction do not occur. However, leaving chords to the posterior leaflet too long can cause mild posterior leaflet prolapse, moving the coaptation line proximally on the anterior leaflet and resulting in the distal anterior leaflet flipping into the outflow tract. Conversely, making chords too short can tether the leaflet and prevent proper valve closure. Both of these problems can be prevented by adjusting chordal lengths properly and illustrate how important it is to obtain precise chordal lengths.

10.3 Pure annular dilatation

Patients with pure annular dilatation, by definition, have no chordal abnormalities and do not require chordal procedures [11]. They are comprised of patients with medical disorders, such as hypertension, that cause dilatation of the mitral annulus, although many have leaflet clefts predisposing them to valve leakage with annular enlargement. This group is discussed here for completeness and accounts for only 13% of patients undergoing mitral repair. Patients are predominantly female, have significant comorbidities, and frequently exhibit ventricular dysfunction. Risk-adjusted prognosis after mitral repair is similar to patients with myxomatous prolapse, although raw survival is lower because of the higher incidence of comorbidities [11]. Aggressive mitral full ring annuloplasty is indicated in this group with negligible late failure rates.

10.4 Robotic ACR

ACR also is well-suited to minimally invasive approaches and, in our center, robotic ACR is used primarily for repair of patients with simple prolapse, usually clearly defined isolated posterior leaflet defects [12]. Thus, robotic cases are carefully selected, but even then, evidence may be emerging that complications are higher with minimally invasive procedures. At any rate, more complicated repairs are still performed through median sternotomy incisions in our practice, with the overriding principle that the first priority is achieving an excellent repair.

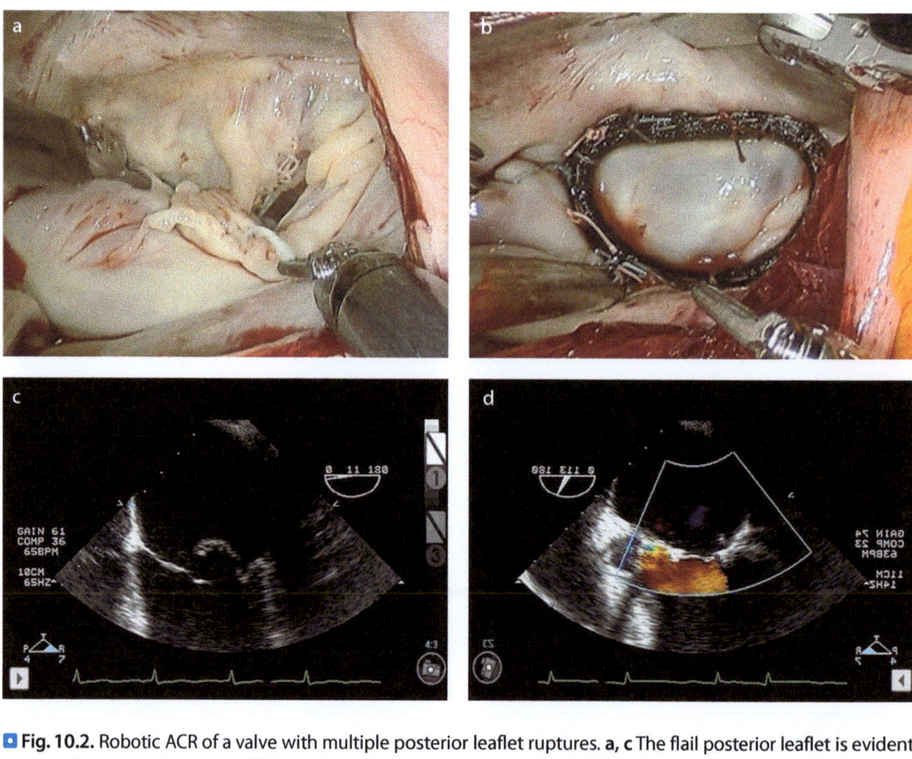

Fig. 10.2. Robotic ACR of a valve with multiple posterior leaflet ruptures. **a, c** The flail posterior leaflet is evident. **b** After placement of a single ACR from the posterior papillary muscle to the posterior leaflet, as shown in Fig. 10.1, the valve is completely competent. **d** After ACR, the prolapsing posterior leaflet is well below the annular plane, with a good surface area of coaptation, and complete recovery of competence. Chordal length adjustment was performed after placement of the full annuloplasty ring (Memo 3D, Sorin group)

In ◘ Fig. 10.2, a valve from a patient with posterior chordal rupture is illustrated before and after robotic ACR. The defect was repaired with a single chord to the posterior papillary muscle and ring annuloplasty. Although techniques for minimally invasive mitral repair are well developed at present, it still remains to be shown (to the authors' satisfaction) that long-term results are as good as with current open methods.

10.5 True commissural prolapse

It is unusual to encounter true commissural prolapse, but in ◘ Fig. 10.3, a patient with severe mitral regurgitation (MR) is shown on echocardiography to have components of posterior leaflet prolapse, normal, and anterior leaflet prolapse. Those findings can indicate true commissural prolapse. On valve testing, the posterior commissure is almost a windsock, with both leaflets involved. Artificial chords were placed to both leaflets, with a good anatomic result and no residual MR.

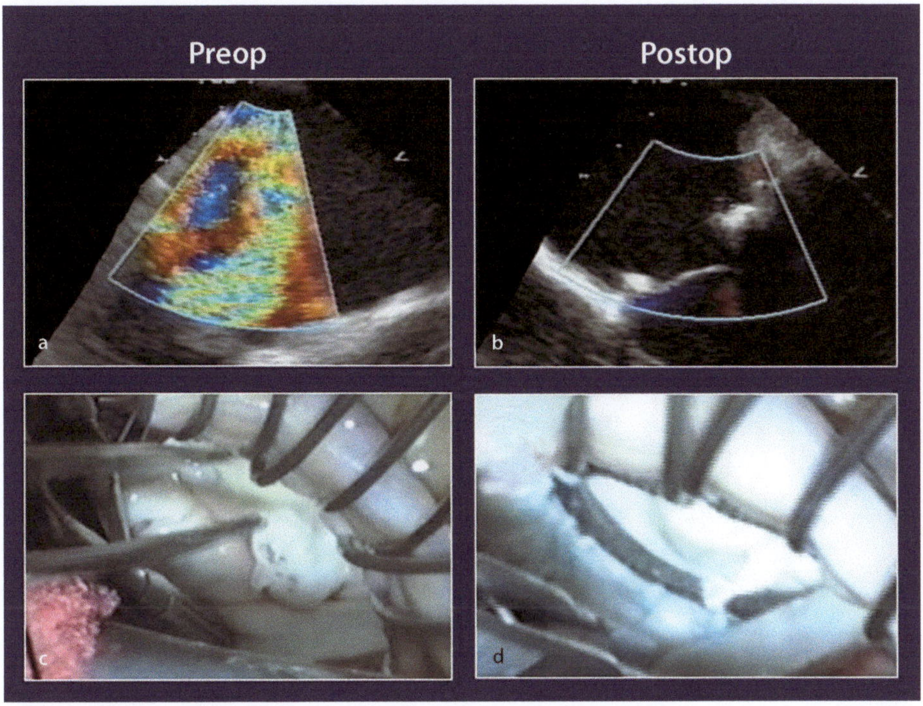

◘ **Fig. 10.3.** Echocardiography and video findings in a patient with true commissural prolapse, before and after ACR repair. **a** Severe MR is evident, and components of anterior, commissural, and posterior leaflet were visualized. **b** After ACR repair, the valve is completely competent with good leaflet position. **c** A »windsock« of true commissural prolapse is present. **d** Valve symmetry and competence are normal after ACR placement to both leaflets and full ring annuloplasty (AnnuloFlow, Sorin Group)

10.6 Barlow's valves

In generalized bileaflet prolapse, or Barlow's valves (Fig. 10.4), two chords are placed to each leaflet [13]. The left chords are anchored to the anterior papillary muscle, and the right to the posterior papillary muscle. Echocardiography shows a typical Barlow's valve with generalized prolapse and a severe central jet. Many Barlow's valves have annular calcification, which is first decalcified. Then multiple segmentations are evident, all of which are prolapsing. After placement of four sets of chords, two are short, and they are independently lengthened. At the end, the valve is nicely symmetrical, with good coaptation area and no residual leak.

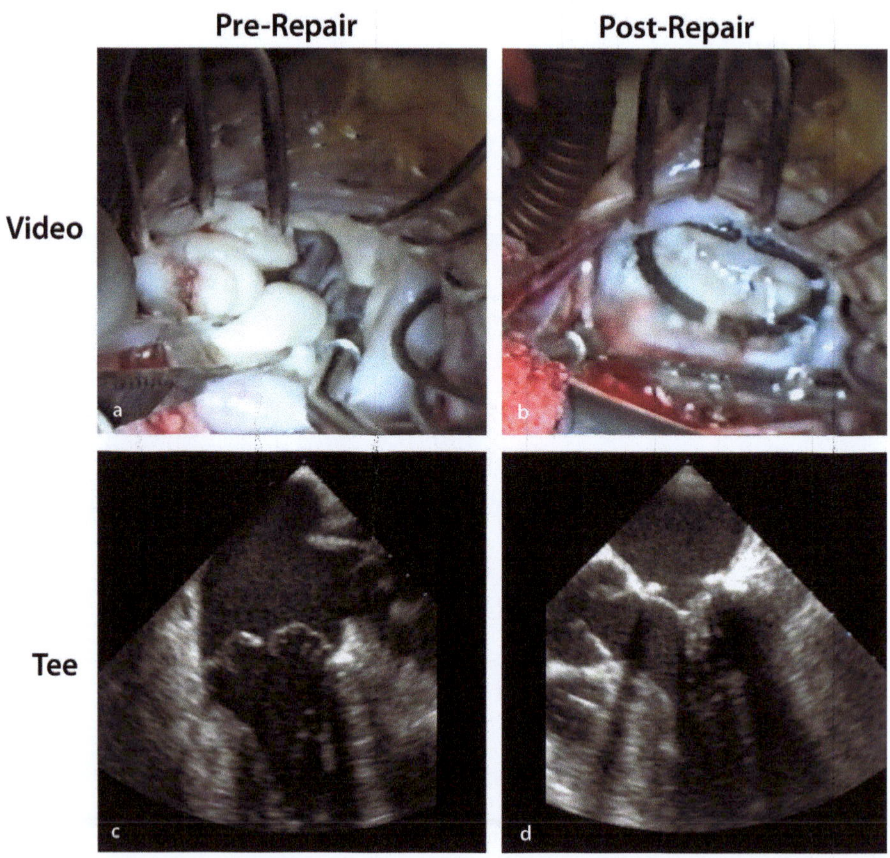

Fig. 10.4. ACR repair of a Barlow's valve with multisegmentation, generalized prolapse, and annular calcification. **a** The repair is begun by limited decalcification of the annulus (enough to allow forward annular positioning with ring placement). Multiple prolapsing segments are evident. **b** After ring annuloplasty (AnnuloFlow, Sorin Group) and placement of four sets of artificial chords (with length adjustment of two), the valve is fully competent. **c** Typical generalized prolapse associated with a Barlow's valve is evident on echocardiography, also with a severe central jet of regurgitation. **d** After ACR repair, leaflet position is excellent with a good surface area of coaptation and no residual leak. The leaflet is never resected, and the authors believe that the concept of »excess leaflet tissue« is not applicable to this situation–the more leaflet surface area, the better the competence

10.7 Endocarditis

Patients with endocarditis represent a difficult group for the cardiac surgeon, and more innovation and development of surgical principles will be required before management of endocarditis is optimized [14]. One candidate for outcome improvement is increasing valve repair, which reduces risk-adjusted mortality in the STS database data set by a third. Obviously, chordal replacement can play a major role in endocarditis repair with disrupted chordal attachments. The timing of intervention is controversial, but the authors suggest that all efforts should be expended to convert each patient from »active« culture positive to »treated« status before undertaking surgery. In the STS database, treated status also is associated with improved results, and in recent practice, it is interesting how many patients can be treated with prolonged antibiotics and be converted to fully culture negative before performing valve repair. As stated by other groups [15], most mitral endocarditis can be successfully repaired with current techniques. A patient with multiple holes in the posterior leaflet and disrupted chordae to both leaflets is illustrated in ◘ Fig. 10.5. After suture closure of the leaflet defects and ACR to both leaflets, the valve is entirely competent. Larger leaflet

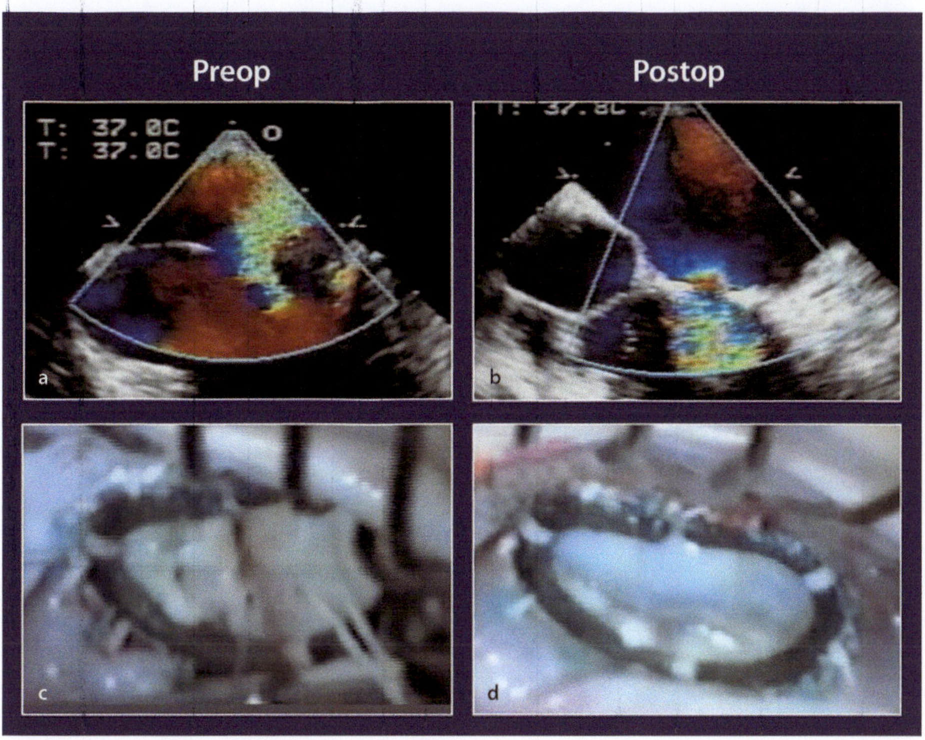

◘ **Fig. 10.5.** ACR repair of a patient with fully treated endocarditis. **a** Echocardiography exhibits severe valve leak. **b** After repair with suture closure of multiple posterior leaflet holes and ACR to both leaflets, the valve is fully competent. **c**The multiple holes in the posterior leaflet are evident; these are suture closed and ACRs are being performed after ring placement (AnnuloFlow, Sorin Group). **d** With valve testing after ACR repair, the symmetry of the competent valve appears normal defects can be managed with patch augmentation using glutaraldehyde-fixed autologous pericardium [16, 17].

10.8 Reoperative mitral repair

The patient in Fig. 10.6 had a failed repair at another hospital 11 months earlier. He continued to deteriorate symptomatically, and on echocardiography, severe MR is evident from two separate jets. There is an inadequate posterior leaflet from overresection and a hole adjacent to an anterior annular suture. The Alfieri stitch is taken down, and the previous ring removed. At that point, a prolapsing commissural cusp is evident. A Gore-Tex® suture is placed into the posterior papillary muscle and stuffed into the ventricle. The anterior leaflet hole is sutured, the posterior leaflet is disconnected from the annulus, and a lightly tanned autologous pericardial patch is inserted into the posterior leaflet. A Carpentier ring (AnnuloFlow, Sorin Group) is true-sized to a ring that is smaller than chosen previously.

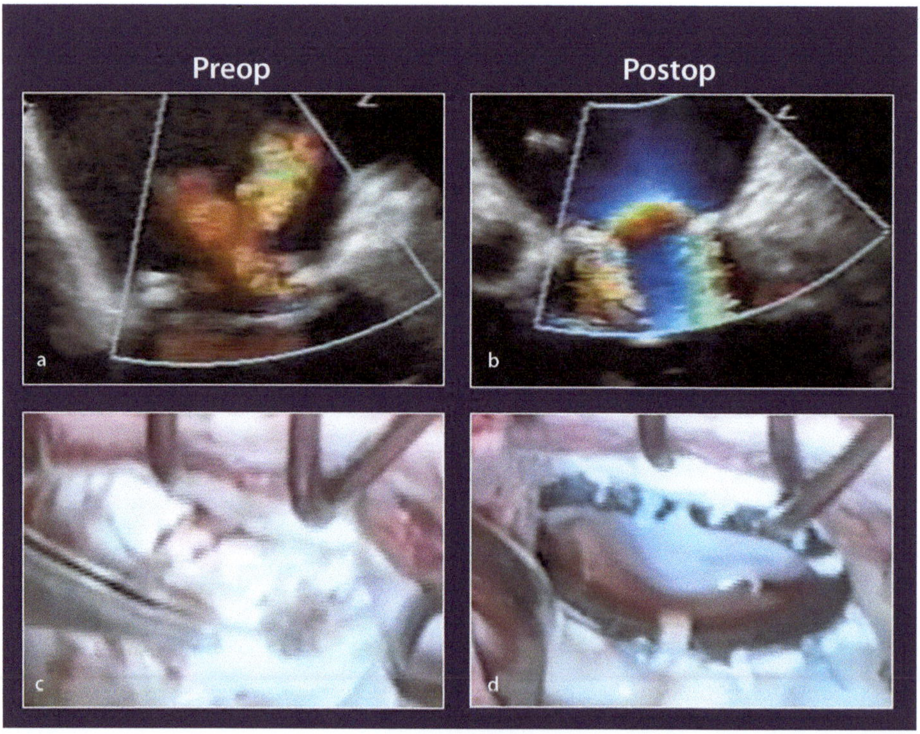

Fig. 10.6. Re-repair of a prolapse valve after failed reconstruction. **a** Two jets of regurgitation are evident–one from a leak through a suture hole in the anterior aspect of the ring sutures and a second from an inadequate posterior leaflet after overresection. The leaflet hole is closed, an Alfieri stitch is taken down, a posterior leaflet autologous pericardial patch is placed to compensate for insufficient leaflet surface area (**c**), and a Gore-Tex® ACR is placed to a prolapsing commissural cusp (that was overlooked during the first procedure). After ring placement (true-sized to a smaller diameter; AnnuloFlow, Sorin Group), the chord is adjusted once, and the valve is fully competent (**b**). The tied ACR and the good leaflet symmetry are shown in **d**

The artificial chord is placed to the commissural cusp and is short on testing. Therefore, the slip knot is lengthened, and then the valve is fully competent, with good coaptation, and no residual leak.

10.9 Rheumatic mitral repair

In previous experience, rheumatic repairs failed because of scarred retracted posterior leaflets or persistent submitral pathology. In our current practice (◘ Fig. 10.7), posterior leaflet pericardial patches are routinely inserted in rheumatic valves, because a retracted or tethered posterior leaflet is such a prominent pathologic feature [18, 19]. If anterior leaflet chords are immobile or tethered, the entire submitral apparatus to the anterior leaflet is resected and reattached by two sets of artificial chords. As in Barlow's valves, the chord to the left front corner of the anterior leaflet is taken to the anterior papillary muscle, and the chord to the right front corner is attached to the posterior papillary muscle. Again, chordal lengths are adjusted at the end of the procedure, after ring placement. Care is taken to perform a complete com-

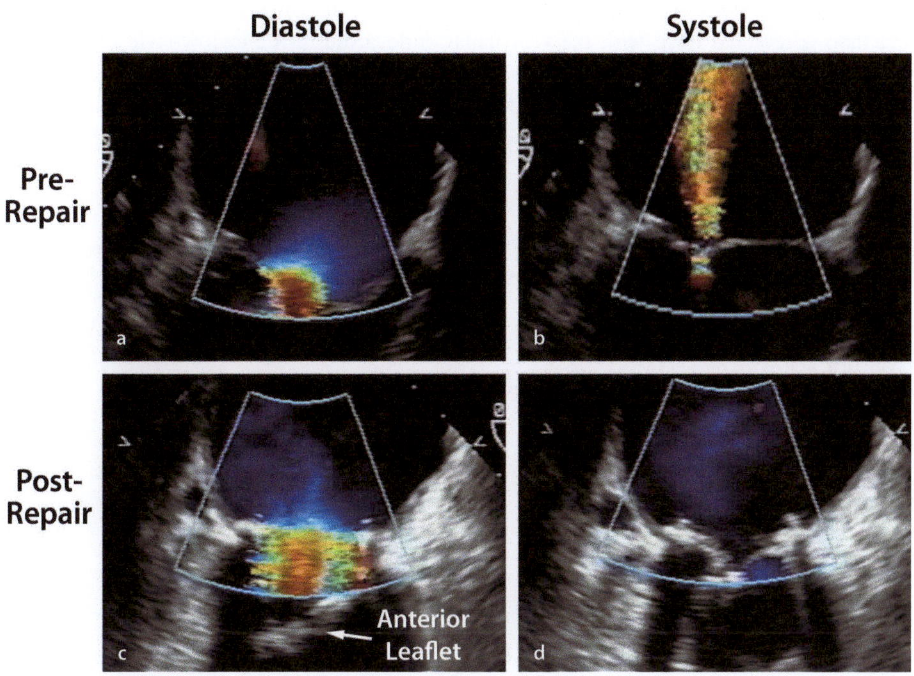

◘ **Fig. 10.7.** A patient with long-standing rheumatic mitral stenosis and regurgitation undergoing a rheumatic repair. **a, b** On pre-bypass echocardiography, the stenotic and insufficient mitral valve is demonstrated. **c, d** After insertion of an autologous pericardial patch into the posterior leaflet, decalcifying commissurotomy, resection of the submitral apparatus to the anterior leaflet, and re-attachment of the mobile anterior leaflet to both papillary muscles with adjustable ACR, the valve is fully competent with insignificant gradient. A full rigid ring also is placed (AnnuloFlow, Sorin Group). These types of more comprehensive ACR repairs for rheumatic valves have been quite stable in the intermediate term missurotomy and to resect all calcium in the subendocardium of the anterior leaflet. Proper valve function is dependent on good anterior leaflet mobility, and thickened fibrous chordal insertions on the underside of the leaflet can be trimmed. In the end, a quite functional anterior leaflet can usually be recovered, even in the most diseased valves, with minimal gradient and residual regurgitation (Fig. 10.7).

10.10 Hypertrophic obstructive cardiomyopathy with mitral anomalies

Hypertrophic obstructive cardiomyopathy is sometimes accompanied by severe mitral anomalies, including papillary muscle prolapse into the outflow tract and severe MR [20, 21]. Recently, a repair approach has been devised for this difficult anomaly, including septal myectomy, anterior papillectomy, and reconstruction of the mitral valve with artificial chords. The patient illustrated in Fig. 10.8 is recovering from HOCM crisis with pulmonary edema, severe MR, and apical LV dysfunction. On echocardiography, severe systolic anterior motion of the mitral valve is evident, and one can see the papillary muscle prolapsing into the outflow tract and butting against the hypertrophied septum. The MR is severe, and on 3D echocardiography, the anterior papillary muscle tip is visualized prolapsing into the outflow tract on multiple views. Through an oblique aortotomy, the anterior papillary muscle is identified in the outflow tract. The entire papillary muscle is disconnected from the mitral valve and then is resected flush with the ventricular endocardium. A Morrow-style myectomy is performed to the left of the ventricular septum, and the aortotomy is closed. The left atrium is opened, and the left aspects of both mitral leaflets are disconnected from chordal support and flail. Three artificial chords are placed into multiple posterior papillary muscle heads, and

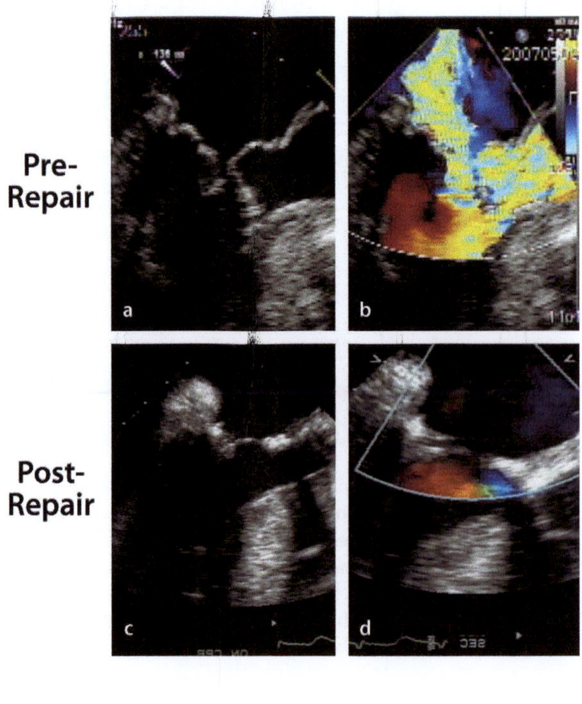

Fig. 10.8. ACR mitral repair in a patient with HOCM crisis and severe mitral anomalies. **a, b** Pronounced systolic anterior motion of the anterior mitral leaflet and anterior papillary muscle prolapse against an asymmetrically hypertrophied septum produces severe outflow tract obstruction and mitral regurgitation. **c, d** After septal myectomy, resection of the obstructing anomalous anterior papillary muscle, and mitral reconstruction with ACR and ring annuloplasty (AnnuloFlow, Sorin Group), the outflow obstruction is relieved, the systolic anterior motion is eliminated, and the valve is fully competent. This type of repair has been quite stable to the intermediate term

after ring placement, they are retrieved and woven into the anterior leaflet, commissure, and posterior leaflet. On testing, the valve is completely competent, with good coaptation, and no residual leak (◘ Fig. 10.8). In addition, outflow gradients with this technique are reduced to physiologic levels and have remained stable in the long term. It may be important to attach the chords to multiple posterior papillary muscle heads, since funneling all of the chords to one point might obstruct mitral outflow.

10.11 Ischemic mitral regurgitation

Ischemic MR (IMR) is usually managed with rigid ring annuloplasty alone [22, 23], but as in George Burch's original drawings [24], IMR can be complicated by leaflet tethering due to infarct expansion, or prolapse from papillary elongation. These complex anatomies are more common in chronic IMR patients and can require additional repair techniques beyond ring annuloplasty to avoid late MR recurrence. The patient in ◘ Fig. 10.9 has severe MR associated with posterior leaflet tethering, but also anterior leaflet prolapse due to elongation of a papillary muscle head. He had a previous coronary bypass, and his ventricle was severely dysfunctional. This exceptional anatomy illustrates two of the more complicated problems that can

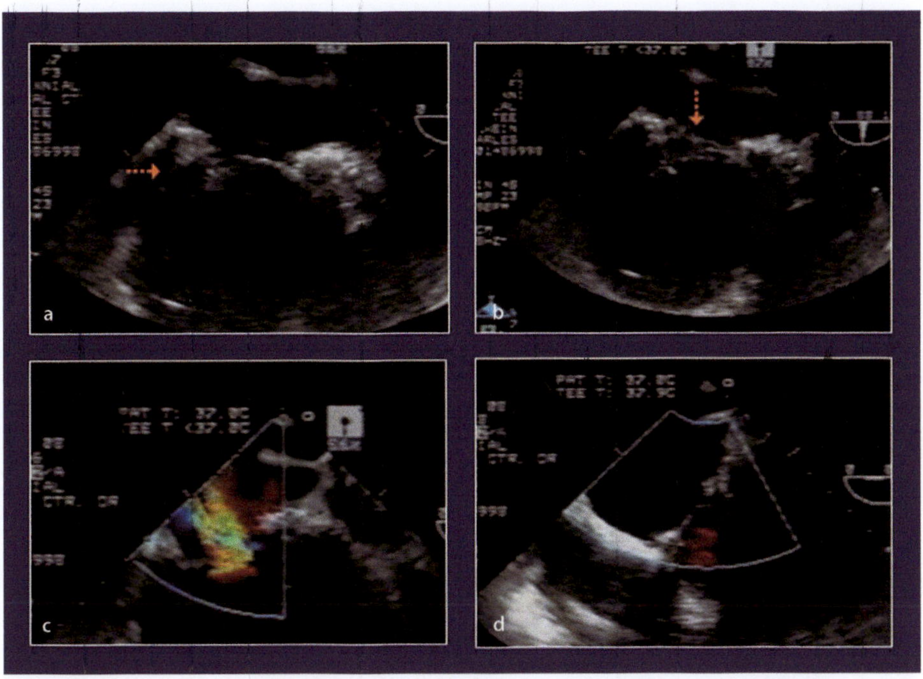

◘ **Fig. 10.9.** ACR repair of complex IMR in a reoperative patient with severe LV dysfunction. **a** The posterior leaflet does not close properly due to tethering (*arrow*) from posterior wall infarct displacement. **b** However, on a different view, a segment of anterior leaflet also is prolapsing (*arrow*) due to papillary muscle elongation. **c** The severe MR from both leaflet abnormalities is evident. **d** After pericardial patch augmentation of the posterior leaflet and ACR to the anterior leaflet, the valve is fully competent. Full ring annuloplasty also was performed (AnnuloFlow, Sorin Group)

be encountered in IMR. In this case, Langer's posterior leaflet pericardial patch [25] was performed to compensate for the posterior leaflet tethering, and the anterior prolapse was corrected with a single chord to an anterior papillary muscle, with full competence (◘ Fig. 10.9). It is important to place artificial chords in IMR to viable papillary muscles to avoid the consequences of late infarct expansion and leaflet tethering. It is a tricky issue to adjust both leaflets just right, but a precise repair usually can be achieved with excellent valve competence long term, even in the most complex cases.

10.12 Tricuspid valve repair

Finally, ACR techniques are equally applicable to the tricuspid valve. The patient in ◘ Fig. 10.10 is undergoing a multiple valve procedure, and the associated tricuspid regurgitation (TR) is thought to be functional. After placement of a Carpentier tricuspid ring, however, the anterior tricuspid leaflet is found to be severely prolapsing. While this is not common, tricuspid prolapse can accompany myxomatous disease of the mitral valve. A single chord is placed from a right ventricular papillary muscle to the anterior tricuspid

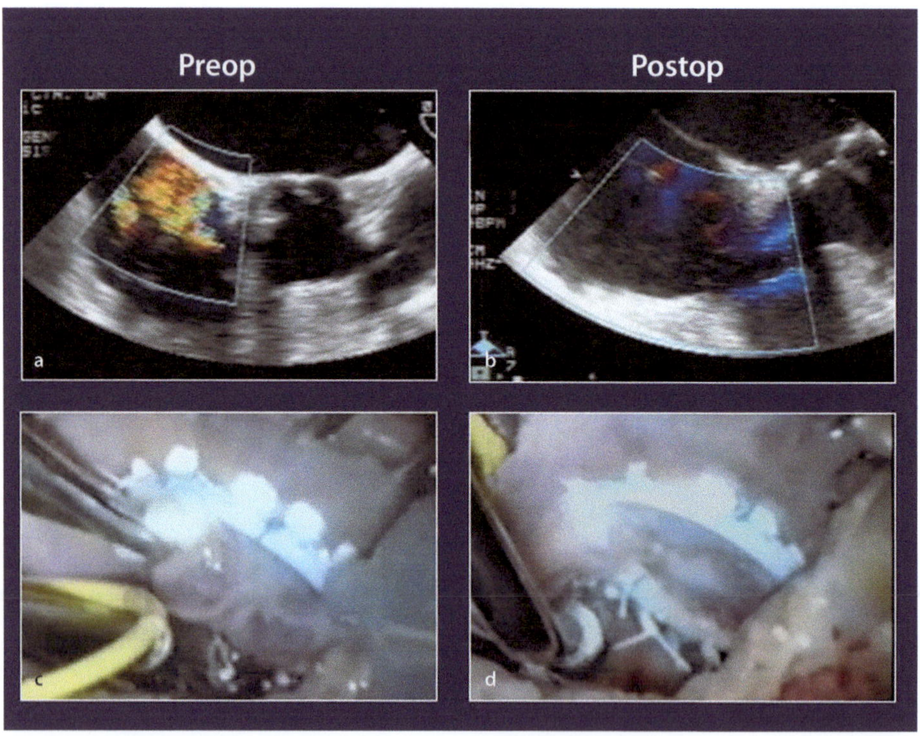

◘ **Fig. 10.10.** A patient undergoing mitral and tricuspid valve repair is thought to have severe TR for functional reasons (**a**). However, after Carpentier tricuspid ring annuloplasty (Edwards Lifesciences), a prominent prolapse of the anterior tricuspid leaflet and persistent valve leak are noted (**c**). ACR is performed from an RV papillary muscle to the anterior leaflet (**d**) with complete recovery of competence (**b**)

leaflet (and length adjustment performed as for the mitral valve), which corrected the defect nicely.

10.13 Clinical outcomes

The perfection of ACR in recent years has probably been a significant factor in increasing application of repair to mitral valve surgery [26]. In many practices, repair rates for all mitral disease are approaching 100% [27], and because operative mortality after mitral repair is lower in sicker subsets [28, 29], early postoperative mortality is approaching 0% (Fig. 10.11). The combination of ACR, autologous pericardial leaflet augmentation, and full ring annuloplasty allows repair of virtually all mitral and tricuspid pathologies. In over 2,000 patients having mitral surgery over the past 20 years [30], risk-adjusted survival across all pathologies is best with mitral repair at all ages (Fig. 10.12). Interestingly, patients receiving mitral bioprostheses have worse risk-adjusted outcomes than either mechanical valves or repair, and at no age do tissue valves equal the other two options. These and other data [31 ,32] support the recent trend toward increasing mitral repair for all ages and for all etiologies of mitral valve disease. Moreover, information is available now from multiple sources that ACR may be associated with lower failure rates and better late outcomes than other techniques [33–40], so the clinical advantages of mitral valve repair are likely to increase further as ACR is adopted more widely.

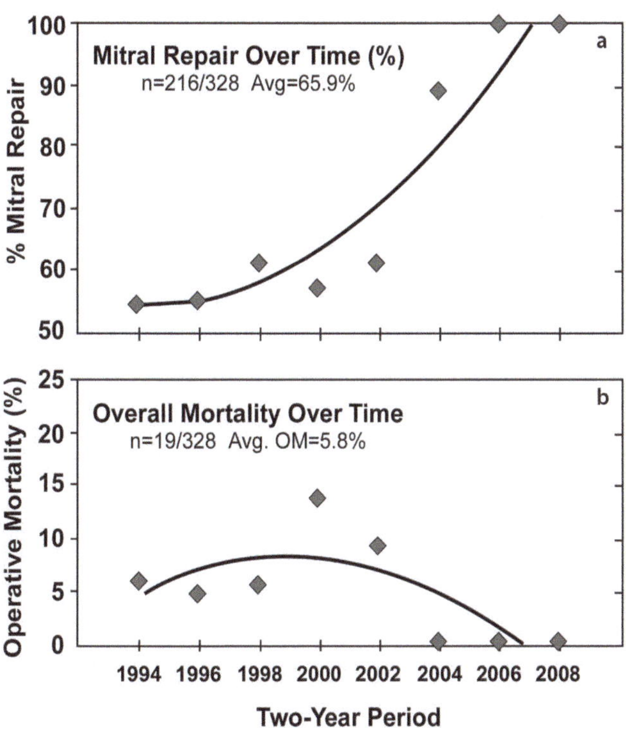

Fig. 10.11. Mitral repair rates and operative mortalities for all mitral procedures (including multiple valves) in the author's practice [27]. The recent increase in repair rates toward 100% has been due to perfection of ACR techniques, together with aggressive use of pericardial patches. With increasing repair (and certainly for other reasons) operative mortality is very close to zero. These data support the increasing use of valve repair across the spectrum of mitral pathologies

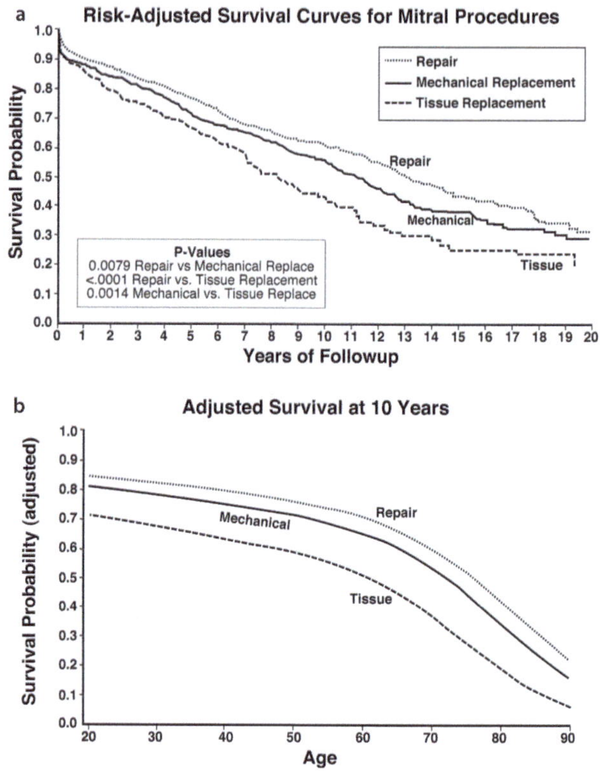

Fig. 10.12. a Long-term survival characteristics after mitral procedures for all pathologies at Duke University over a 20-year period. Mitral repair was associated with a significantly better risk-adjusted survival than valve replacement, and tissue valve replacement was the worst. **b** Risk-adjusted 10-year survival was better with mitral repair for all patient ages at the time of implant. At no patient age did tissue valve replacement achieve equivalent outcomes to either mechanical valves or repair, but repair was clinically and statistically the best [30]

10.14 Conclusions

Gore-Tex® ACR allows a greater percentage of mitral and tricuspid pathologies to be repaired. When combined with autologous pericardial leaflet augmentation and full ring annuloplasty, close to 100% of all patients with mitral and tricuspid valve disease can benefit from repair. Artificial chords also seem to increase stability of repair and reduce late failure rates. Operative mortalities and long-term patient outcomes may be correspondingly improved. Thus, artificial chordal replacement in adult patients is now a key technique in the armamentarium of the cardiac surgeon.

References

This paper is referenced primarily with the authors' manuscripts, but within each work, a full reference list is given.

1. Kouchoukos NT (1973) Problems in mitral valve replacement. In: Kirklin TW (ed) Advances in cardiovascular surgery. Grune & Stratton, New York, pp. 205–216
2. Rankin JS (1986) Mitral and tricuspid valve disease: historical aspects. In: Sabiston DC, Jr. (ed) Textbook of surgery. WB Saunders Company, Philadelphia, p 2345
3. Carpentier A (1983) Cardiac valve surgery - the »French correction«. J Thorac Cardiovasc Surg 86:323–337

4. Vetter HO, Burack JH, Factor SM, et al. (1986) Replacement of chordae tendineae of the mitral valve using the new expanded PTFE suture in sheep. In: Bodnar E, Yacoub M (eds) Biologic bioprosthetic valves. Yorke Medical Books, New York, pp 772–784
5. Frater RWM, Vetter HO, Zussa C, et al. (1990) Chordal replacement in mitral valve repair. Circulation 82 (suppl IV):125–130
6. Frater RWM, Gabbay S, Shore D, et al. (1983) Reproducible replacement of elongated or ruptured mitral valve chordae. Ann Thorac Surg 35:1428–1436
7. Frater RMW (1964) Anatomical rules for the plastic repair of a diseased mitral valve. Thorax 19:458–464
8. Frater RWM (1962) Artificial heart valves. The Lancet 280:1171
9. Rankin JS, Orozco RE, Addai TR, et al. (2004) Several new considerations in mitral valve repair. J Heart Valve Dis 13:399–409
10. Rankin JS, Orozco RE, Rodgers TL, et al. (2006) »Adjustable« artificial chordal replacement for repair of mitral valve prolapse. Ann Thorac Surg 81:1526–1528
11. Glower DD, Tuttle RH, Bashore TM, Harrison JK, Wang A, Gehrig T, Rankin JS (2009) Pure annular dilatation as a cause of mitral regurgitation: a clinically distinct entity of female heart disease. J Heart Valve Dis 18:284–288
12. Brunsting LA, Orozco RE, Rankin JS, Binford RS (2009) Robotic artificial chordal replacement for repair of mitral valve prolapse. Innovations 4:229–232
13. Rankin JS, Alfery DD, Orozco RE, et al. (2008) Techniques of artificial chordal replacement for mitral valve repair: use in multiple pathologies. Op Tech Thorac Cardiovasc Surg 13:74–82
14. Gaca JG, Sheng S, Rankin JS, et al. (2010) Outcomes for endocarditis surgery in North America: a simplified risk scoring system and need for clinical innovationJ Thorac Cardiovasc Surg (in press)
15. Shang E, Forrest GN, Chizmar T, et al. (2009) Mitral valve infective endocarditis: Benefit of early operation and aggressive use of repair. Ann Thorac Surg 87:1728–1734
16. 35. Chauvaud S, Jebara V, Chachques JC, et al. (1991) Valve extension with glutaraldehyde-preserved autologous pericardium. Results in mitral valve repair. J Thorac Cardiovasc Surg 102:171–177
17. Ng CK, Nesser J, Punzengruber C, et al. (2001) Valvuloplasty with glutaraldehyde-treated autologous pericardium in patients with complex mitral valve pathology. Ann Thorac Surg 71:78–85
18. Rankin JS, Sharma MK, Teague SM, et al. (2008) A new method of mitral valve repair for rheumatic disease: Preliminary study. J Heart Valve Dis 17:614–619
19. Rankin JS, Orozco RE, McRae AT (2009) Mitral valve repair for rheumatic disease. Surgical video presented at the Southern Thoracic Surgical Association meeting, November, 2009, to be published at CTSNet.org. Video downloadable from: http://www.ctsnet.org/sections/clinicalresources/videos/vg2010_RankinS_MVR_Rheumatic.html
20. Rankin JS, Binford RS, Johnston TS, Matthews JT, Alfery DD, McRae AT, Brunsting LA III (2008) A new mitral valve repair strategy for hypertrophic obstructive cardiomyopathy. J Heart Valve Dis17:642–647
21. Rankin JS (2010) Mitral valve repair for HOCM with severe mitral anomalies. Presented at the STS meeting and published at http://www.theheart.org/article/1138915.do
22. Glower DD, Tuttle RH, Shaw LK, Orozco RE, Rankin JS (2005) Patient survival characteristics after routine mitral valve repair for ischemic mitral regurgitation. J Thorac Cardiovasc Surg 129:860–868
23. Milano CA, Danishmand MA, Rankin JS, et al. (2008) Survival prognosis and surgical management of ischemic mitral regurgitation. Ann Thorac Surg 86:735–744
24. Burch G, DePasquale N, Phillips J (1968) The syndrome of papillary muscle dysfunction. Am Heart J 75:399–412
25. Langer F, Rodriguez F, Cheng A, et al. (2006) Posterior mitral leaflet extension: an adjunctive repair option for ischemic mitral regurgitation? J Thorac Cardiovasc Surg 131:868–877
26. Gammie JS, Sheng S, Griffith BP, Peterson ED, Rankin JS, O'Brien SM, Brown JM (2009) Trends in mitral valve surgery in the United States: results from the Society of Thoracic Surgeons adult cardiac database. Ann Thorac Surg 87:1431–1439
27. Rankin JS, Burrichter CA, Walton-Shirley MK, et al. (2009) Trends in mitral valve surgery: a single practice experience. J Heart Valve Dis 18:359–366
28. Rankin JS, Livesey SA, Smith LR, et al. (1989) Trends in the surgical treatment of ischemic mitral regurgitation: effects of mitral valve repair on hospital mortality. Semin Thorac Cardiovasc Surg 1:149–163
29. Rankin JS, Feneley MP, Hickey MSJ, et al. (1988) A clinical comparison of mitral valve repair versus valve replacement in ischemic mitral regurgitation. J Thorac Cardiovasc Surg 95:165–177
30. Daneshmand MA, Milano CA, Rankin JS, et al. (2010) Influence of patient age on procedural selection in mitral valve surgery. Ann Thorac Surg 90:1479–1486
31. Daneshmand MA, Milano CA, Rankin JS, et al. (2009) The surgical treatment of mitral valve prolapse: a 20-year perspective. Ann Thorac Surg 88:1828–1837

32. Daneshmand MA, Gaca JC, Rankin JS, Milano CA, Glower DD, Wolfe WG, Smith PK. Effects of valve repair on long-term patient outcomes after mitral valve surgery. In: Hetzer, Rankin,Yankah (eds) Mitral Valve Repair. Springer Verlag, Berlin, pp 195–209
33. Salvador L, Mirone S, Bianchini R, et al. (2008) Twenty-year experience of mitral valve repair with artificial chordae in 608 Patients. J Thorac Cardiovasc Surg 135:1280–1287
34. Chiappini B, Sanchez A, Noirhomme P, et al. (2006) Replacement of chordae tendineae with polytetrafluoroethylene (PTFE) sutures in mitral valve repair: early and long-term results. J Heart Valve Dis 15:657–663
35. Lawrie GM, Earle EA, Earle NR. (2006) Feasibility and intermediate term outcome of repair of prolapsing anterior mitral leaflets with artificial chordal replacement in 152 patients. Ann Thorac Surg 81:849–856
36. von Oppell UO, Mohr FW (2000) Chordal replacement for both minimally invasive and conventional mitral valve surgery using premeasured Gore-Tex loops. Ann Thorac Surg 70:2166–2168
37. David TE, Omran A, Armstrong S, et al. (1998) Long-term results of mitral valve repair for myxomatous disease with and without chordal replacement with expanded polytetrafluoroethylene sutures. J Thorac Cardiovasc Surg 115:1279–1285
38. Nigro JJ, Schwartz DS, Bart RD, et al. (2004) Neochordal repair of the posterior mitral leaflet. J Thorac Cardiovasc Surg 127:440–447
39. Duebener LF, Wendler O, Nikoloudakis N, et al.(2000) Mitral-valve repair without annuloplasty rings: results after repair of anterior leaflet versus posterior-leaflet defects using ePTFE sutures for chordal replacement. Eur J Cardiothorac Surg 17:206–212
40. Tesler UF, Cerin G, Novelli E, Popa A, Diena M (2009) Evolution of surgical techniques for mitral valve repair. Tex Heart Inst J 36:438–440

Twenty-year results of artificial chordae replacement in mitral valve repair

L. Salvador, E. Cavarretta, C. Valfrè

11.1 Introduction

Mitral valve repair (MVR) is the treatment of choice in cases of degenerative mitral valve (MV) regurgitation, with superior results compared to MV replacement. The feasibility of the procedure is up to 95% and it should be considered in all patients. Different techniques have been described, comprising procedures on valve leaflets, the subvalvular apparatus, and annulus. Posterior leaflet prolapse is traditionally corrected by Carpentier's quadrangular resection with or without sliding plasty. Anterior leaflet prolapse is still more technically demanding and various types of reconstructive techniques have been described, not always leading to satisfactory overall results. Efforts to find a substitute for elongated or ruptured chordae date back to the 1960s. In 1962, January et al. [1] described the case of a patient operated on by placing two 00 sutures through the base of the papillary muscles and through the margins of the unsupported portion of the mural leaflet. In 1965, Frater and coworkers published their experimental studies of glutaraldehyde-tanned xenograft pericardium and autologous pericardium as a chordal substitute. In 1984, Vetter began animal experiments with CV 2-0 and 3-0 Gore-Tex® chordae, and 1 year later, Frater introduced experimentally chordal replacement with expanded polytetrafluoroethylene (e-PTFE) sutures (Gore-Tex® sutures, W. L. Gore & Associated Inc., Flagstaff, AZ). Clinical use started in 1985, mainly in three centers (Albert Einstein College of Medicine, The Bronx, New York, USA; Toronto General Hospital, Toronto, Canada; Hospital Nacional Marquès de Valdecilla, Santander, Spain), where e-PTFE chordae were evaluated in clinical practice [2]. The performance of this material, applied to neochordae, was very interesting as it permits infiltration of tissue cells into its porous microstructure, creating a firm adherence of the growing tissue, which was found to be a self-limiting process [3]. In 1986, the clinical use of e-PTFE chordae was introduced in our center, and over the years it has become the preferred technique, in addition to annuloplasty with/without quadrangular resection and sliding. Studies by David et al. [4, 5] confirmed the very good results at intermediate and long-term follow-up. Current use of e-PTFE chordae permits repair of complex mitral regurgitation, and it is now a widely adopted technique. For years, many surgeons remained skeptical and were critical of what they considered a complex repair technique with uncertain follow-up, compared to more diffuse and time-saving technique as, for example, quadrangular resection. We sought to evaluate the very long-term follow-up of mitral valve repair with the use of e-PTFE chordae in a large, homogenous population, referring to a single surgical center.

11.2 Patient population

From 1986–2006, 1,092 consecutive patients underwent MVR for severe degenerative MV regurgitation at the Cardiac Surgery Department, S. Maria dei Battuti Hospital, Treviso. Among these, 608 patients (433 men, 71.2%; mean age 55.5±11.5 years) had artificial neochordae implanted. Patients' characteristics are shown in ◘ Table 11.1. In 5 patients with mild ascending aorta dilation and 3 patients without significant aortic valve disease, there was no concomitant surgical indication. The cause of valve disease was purely degenerative in 91.3% of patients. A total of 53 patients (8.7%) had degenerative mitral regurgitation (MR) complicated by infective endocarditis. Coronary angiography was performed to rule out coronary artery disease (CAD) in patients older than 45 years and in those with suspected pathology. If the MV exhibited evidence of degenerative disease, associated CAD and the need for associ-

Table 11.1. Clinical characteristics of patients with severe mitral regurgitation

	Total
Number of patients	608
Age, years (mean±SD)	55.5±11.5
Male gender	433 (71.2%)
Electrocardiogram	
Sinus rhythm	491 (80.7%)
Atrial fibrillation	117 (19.3%)
Mitral valve pathology	
Pure degenerative	555 (91.3%)
Degenerative + endocarditis	53 (8.7%)
Prolapsing leaflet	
Anterior	47 (7.7%)
Posterior	308 (50.7%)
Bileaflet	253 (41.6%)
New York Heart Association functional class	
I	155 (26.7%)
II	270 (46.6%)
III	134 (23.1%)
IV	21 (3.6%)
Associated disease	125 (20.5%)
Coronary artery disease	24 (3.9%)
Atrial septal defect/PFO	43 (7.1%)
Aortic valve disease	14 (2.3%)
Tricuspid valve regurgitation	13 (2.1%)
Dilatation of ascending aorta	8 (1.3%)
Previous cardiac surgery	3 (0.5%)
Left ventricular ejection fraction <40%	47 (7.7%)

ated coronary artery by-pass graft was not considered an exclusion criteria, nor were other associated procedures, e.g., tricuspid valve repair.

Demographic, morphologic, echocardiographic, and surgical data were obtained from hospital records. Patients were followed up at annual intervals with telephone interviews and echocardiographic studies. The median follow-up was 5.2 years (interquartile range

(IQR) 1.8–9.0 years). Complete follow-up information was available for 602 survivors of the initial hospital stay (100%). The median follow-up was 5.7 years (IQR 2.2–9.8 years, range 0–19.4 years).

11.3 Operative technique

Until April 2006, all patients were operated using a midsternotomy. Since then, most operations have been performed using a videoscopic port-access approach through a right minithoracotomy. MVR was performed under moderate hypothermia with cardiopulmonary bypass (CPB). Myocardial protection was achieved by both intermittent cold blood cardioplegia and topical cooling in case of sternotomy, whereas in minimally invasive surgery cold crystalloid solution infusion was preferred. The MV was approached through a standard left atrium (LA) incision, just behind the interatrial groove. The entire MV apparatus was carefully inspected to identify the prolapsing leaflet and its scallops, comparing the free margin levels.

The main indications of neochordae implantation were the following: (1) MV prolapse, regardless whether the anterior leaflet, posterior leaflet, or bileaflet; (2) chordal rupture or elongation; (3) after a large posterior mitral leaflet (PML) resection in the presence of extensive flail; (4) to avoid a PML resection; (5) as a sentinel chordae, to prevent progression of the degenerative disease; (6) endocarditis etiology, and (7) rarely, rheumatic etiology.

Since 1991, intraoperative transesophageal echocardiography (TEE) has routinely been used to confirm the pathological mechanism in the preoperative setting and to assess the MVR outcome after CPB weaning.

In addition to chordae implantation, 99% of patients had annuloplasty, mostly (80.1%) with a pericardial ring [7]. In 5 cases, no pericardial or prosthetic ring annuloplasty was performed: 3 patients underwent simple suture annuloplasty and 2 had the annulus stabilized by calcification or fibrosis. In 351 (57.7%) patients, quadrangular posterior leaflet resection, according to Carpentier's technique [6], was performed; however, this was more common in the older cases of this series. At the present, we prefer to resect only excess PML excess tissue, parallel to the free margin, in order to align the P2 height to the P1 height, when this scallop appears to be of normal size and to spare as much tissue as possible.

The neochordae implantation technique has been described previously [2]. Briefly, an ePTFE double-armed suture (Gore-Tex® CV-5) is passed through the papillary muscle with a mattress technique and is reinforced with autologous pericardial pledgets (or, rarely, with Gore-Tex® pledgets) on both sides of the muscle. Each end of the suture is then fixed to the prolapsed leaflet free margin and is reinforced with a small autologous pericardial pledget (or, less frequently, a small Gore-Tex® pledget). The length of the artificial chordae is adjusted to maintain the corresponding free margin of the leaflets at the desired level in the ventricular cavity. To determine the correct length of the artificial chordae so that an adequate coaptation area is obtained and all significant prolapses are reduced, the neochordae are tied at the end of all other repair procedures, after the ventricular cavity is filled with saline solution. In 48 (7.9%) selected cases, if thin or fragile natural chordae tendineae were identified after the leaflet repair was accomplished, even if not elongated or ruptured, a couple of artificial chordae were implanted as a protective function (»sentinel« neochordae) to prevent the effects of disease progression. None of the patients received only sentinel neochordae. These were placed as an extra support to ensure better stability. According to the Cox regression analysis, no differences were found in terms of durability of the repair, presence of significant MR, or mortality [8]. Their precise role and, eventually, possible protective factors should be the subject of more in-depth analyses with a larger series of patients.

In all cases, warfarin sodium for anticoagulation was administrated during the first 3 months after surgery and was discontinued if sinus rhythm was established. Operative data are summarized in ◻ Table 11.2.

◻ Table 11.2. Operative data

	Total
Operations performed	
Chordal replacement with e-PTFE	608 (100%)
Mean	6 (4, 8)
Anterior chordal replacement	325 (53.5%)
Posterior chordal replacement	544 (89.5%)
Sentinel neochordae	48 (7.9%)
Mean	3 (2, 6)
Resection of posterior leaflet	351 (57.7%)
Mitral annuloplasty	606 (99.7%)
None	2 (0.3%)
Suture annuloplasty	3 (0.5%)
Pericardial ring	487 (80.1%)
Artificial ring	116 (19.1%)
Additional procedures	214 (35.2%)
AF surgical treatment	44 (7.2%)
TV repair	13 (2.1%)
Coronary artery bypass graft	24 (3.9%)
AV replacement	6 (1%)
AV repair	5 (0.8%)
Repair of congenital ASD	43 (7.1%)
LA appendage closure	146 (24%)
AAR	3 (0.5%)
CPB time, min	135.2 (34.5%)
Cross-clamp time, min	109.1 (31.3%)

AF atrial fibrillation, *TV* tricuspid valve, *AV* aortic valve, *ASD* atrial septal defect, *LA* left atrium, *AAR* ascending aorta replacement, *CPB* cardiopulmonary bypass

11.4 Statistical analysis

The STATA software (version 9.2; StataCorp LP, College Station, TX, USA) was used for all statistical analyses. Continuous values are expressed as mean±SD or median and IQR. Comparisons between groups were made with analysis of variance for continuous variables and χ^2 test or Fisher exact test as appropriate for categorical variables. Late survival and freedom from adverse events were estimated with the nonparametric Kaplan–Meier method. Cox regression analysis with backward selection was used to identify the multivariable and independent predictors of late outcomes. Variable retention in the models was set at a p value of 0.05.

11.5 Results

11.5.1 Mortality and morbidity

The 30-day mortality was <1% (6 deaths), all related to low cardiac output syndrome. Among these, 3 patients were reoperated for MV replacement because of severe MR, only 1 due to a medically untreatable systolic anterior motion (SAM). During follow-up, 34 deaths occurred (24 cardiac-related deaths and 10 noncardiac-related deaths). The causes of cardiac-related death were heart failure (n=10), sudden cardiac death (n=9), myocardial infarction (n=3), and stroke (n=2). Cumulative survival at 15 years was 84% (95% confidence interval (CI) 75–90%; Fig. 11.1). According to prolapse localization, survival at 15 years was 82% (95% CI 58–93), 86% (95% CI 75–92), and 89% (95% CI 81–94) for the anterior leaflet (AL), posterior leaflet (PL), and bileaflet (BL), respectively (Fig. 11.2). Perioperative complications occurred in 94 patients (15.5%) and are listed in Table 11.3. Three cases of SAM, requiring a second

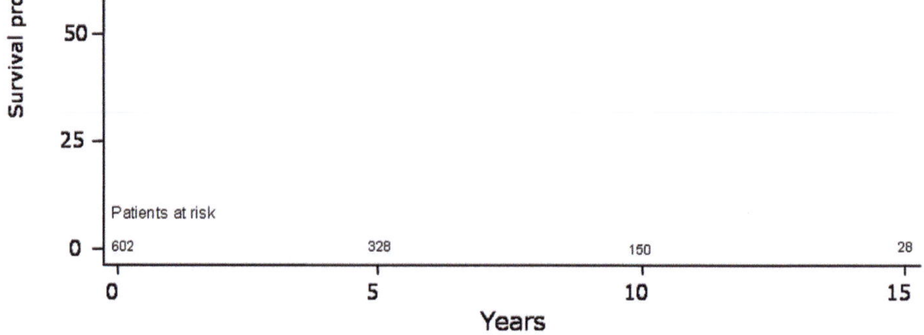

Fig. 11.1. Long-term survival of patients with mitral valve repair with CV-5 e-PTFE suture

CPB run, occurred and were successfully treated by the Alfieri edge-to-edge technique. Two other cases were medically treated with β-blockers and volume adjustment. Causes of SAM were an undersized ring associated with quadrangular resection in 2 cases and ineffective reduction of posterior mitral leaflet length in 4 cases with Barlow disease.

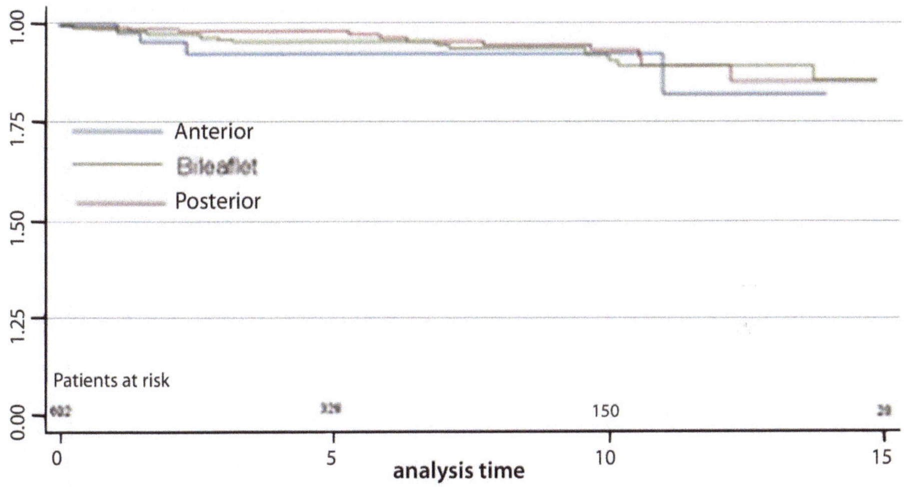

Fig. 11.2. Long-term survival after mitral valve repair, based on prolapse localization. No significant differences are observed, demonstrating that this technique is suitable in all cases of degenerative mitral regurgitation

Table 11.3. Inhospital morbidity and mortality

	Total *n* (%)
Hospital mortality	6 (1.0)
Perioperative morbidity	94 (15.5)
Myocardial infarction	1 (1.1)
Low cardiac output syndrome requiring IABP ± VAD	5 (5.3)
Heart failure	24 (25.6)
Renal failure	9 (9.6)
Respiratory insufficiency	13 (13.8)
Stroke and TIA	10 (10.6)
Postoperative bleeding requiring surgical exploration	32 (34)
MR>2+	2 (0.3)
MR=2+	10 (1.6)

IABP intraortic balloon pump, *TIA* transient ischemic attack, *MR* mitral regurgitation, *VAD* ventricular assist device

11.5.2 Reoperation

A total of 25 patients required MV reoperation: 22 for progression of the degenerative disease and 3 for infective endocarditis. Overall freedom from MV reoperation was 92% at 15 years (95% CI 88–95; Fig. 11.3) with no significant differences between the AL, PL, and BL. Based on the Cox regression, prolapse localization was not identified as an independent risk factor for long-term survival, freedom from reoperation, or recurrent MR. No repair failures arising from spontaneous malfunction of Gore-Tex® chordae were reported in our series.

11.5.3 Infective endocarditis

Seven cases (1.1%) of infective endocarditis were reported; 3 patients underwent a surgical MV procedure: 2 replacements and 1 re-repair. Four cases were successfully treated with antibiotic therapy. All patients survived. In one case, a pair of artificial chordae were involved in a large destruction of the corresponding posterior leaflet and appeared ruptured. Freedom from endocarditis at 15 years was 97% (95% CI 93–99) for all patients.

11.5.4 Recurrent MR

11 Immediately after surgery, 12 (2%) patients had more than mild-to-moderate (≥2+) MR (Table 11.3). Only 2 patients had a 3+ MR on leaving the operating room, which was the result of the lack of transesophageal echocardiography. They were reoperated on a few days later. At the beginning of our experience, we accepted even suboptimal repair, considering

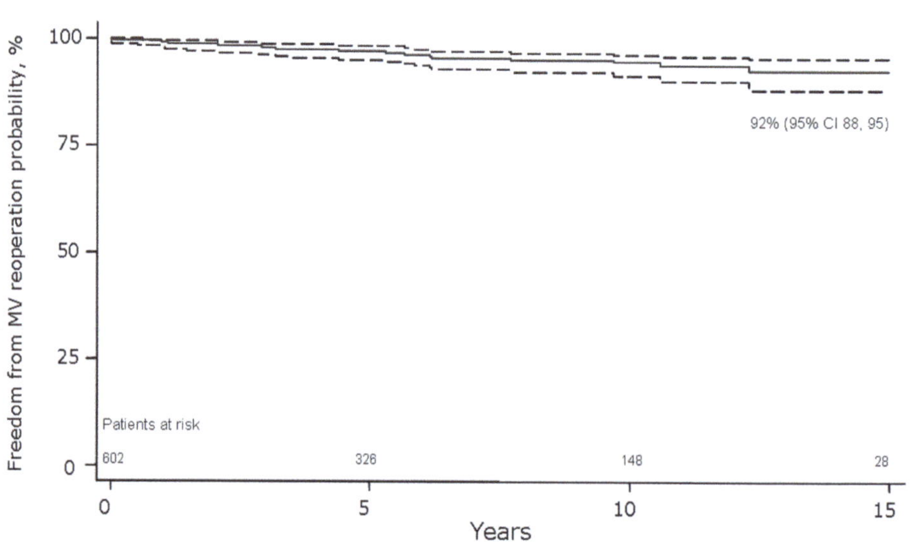

Fig. 11.3. Freedom from reoperation in all patients who underwent mitral valve repair

that in some patients exposure to a second run of CPB would be more life threatening than a 2+ MR. Among these patients, only 3 underwent reoperation, and 1 died of sudden cardiac death. At follow-up, significant MR (more than moderate) was found in 35 patients (5.8%) and 25 underwent reoperation. Overall freedom from significant MR at 15 years was 85% (95% CI 78–91; ▫ Fig. 11.4). Cox regression analysis identified the presence of more than mild MR at discharge as an independent risk factor for significant recurrent MR at follow-up (hazard ratio 12.57, 95% CI 4.14–38.14; ▫ Table 11.4).

11.5.5 Thromboembolic events and anticoagulation-related hemorrhage

Thromboembolic events (stroke and transient ischemic attack) were recorded in 21 patients (3.5%); among these, 4 patients (19%) had atrial fibrillation. Freedom from thromboembolism at 15 years was 92% (95% CI 87–95) for all patients. Since 1999, we have prophylactically closed the left atrial appendage by direct suture in all patients, regardless of sinus rhythm or left atrial dimensions. There were nine major bleeding episodes among those patients receiving anticoagulation therapy. Freedom from major bleeding at 15 years was 96.5% (95% CI 87.6–98.3).

11.5.6 Atrial fibrillation and functional status

At follow-up, 76 patients (12.5%) had permanent AF. Since 2000, a surgical procedure for AF treatment has been performed in 44 selected patients (7.2%). At follow-up, sinus rhythm was restored in 33 patients (75%). New onset of AF was observed in 40 patients (8.2% of 486) who were recorded as having sinus rhythm prior to surgery.

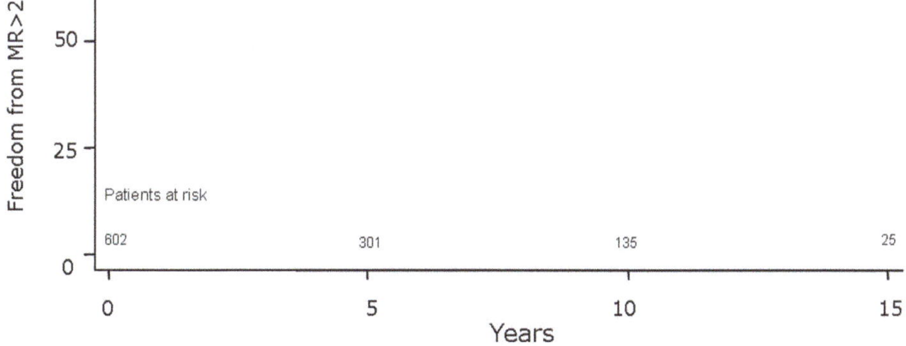

▫ **Fig. 11.4.** Freedom from recurrent moderate to severe mitral regurgitation in all patients

Table 11.4. Cox regression analysis

Outcome	HR (95% CI)	p value
Late mortality (*n*=34)		
Age, 5-year increase	1.35 (1.12, 1.62)	0.002
Segmental resection of posterior leaflet	0.45 (0.22, 0.92)	0.028
Associated CABG	2.85 (1.66, 15.24)	0.004
Perioperative stroke	8.90 (1.81, 43.77)	0.007
Perioperative myocardial infarction	4.96 (1.42, 17.28)	0.012
Perioperative respiratory insufficiency	5.39 (1.52, 19.13)	0.009
Cardiac related mortality (*n*=24)		
Associated CABG	12.25 (3.07, 48.8)	<0.001
Perioperative respiratory insufficiency	9.17 (2.76, 30.50)	<0.001
Reoperation on the MV (*n*=25)		
Age, 5-year increase	1.21 (1.01, 1.44)	0.042
Perioperative MR>2	12.97 (3.58, 44.82)	<0.001
Moderate/severe MR (*n*=35)		
Perioperative MR>2	12.57 (4.14, 38.14)	<0.001
Segmental resection of posterior leaflet	0.39 (0.19, 0.81)	0.012
Thromboembolic cerebral event (*n*=21)		
Perioperative stroke	9.67 (1.21, 77.15)	0.032

CABG coronary artery bypass graft, *MV* mitral valve, *MR* mitral regurgitation, *HR* hazard ratio, *CI* confidence interval

At the latest follow-up, 543 patients were alive and free from reoperation, and 80.8% were in New York Heart Association (NYHA) functional class I, 17.2% in class II, and 2.1% in class III.

11.6 Discussion

Degenerative MR affect about 1–2% of the general population and it has been extensively treated by MVR, which has become the procedure of choice. Compared to MV replacement, MVR shows a better outcome in terms of operative mortality, quality of life, and long-term survival. Symptom-free patients have a survival expectancy identical to that of the general population [9]. A plethora of reconstructive techniques, including triangular resection, chordal transfer, chordal shortening, the edge-to-edge technique, and papillary muscle repositioning, have been described, but long-term results are not always completely satisfactory, and some of these procedures are considered technically demanding and time consuming.

Over the years, many efforts have been made to overcome the differences in the outcome based on the prolapse localization, with anterior leaflet prolapse always being considered a negative prognostic factor. With the introduction of standardized techniques for MVR by Carpentier, technical improvements have been made in order to obtain the most durable repair, particularly in cases of anterior or bileaflet prolapse [10]. While chordal shortening showed significant limitations at intermediate and long-term follow-up [11], chordal transposition proved to have superior results, but it is not always possible in the absence of normal healthy chordae at the site opposite of the prolapsing leaflet. The risk of implanting degenerative chordae can be avoided by using e-PTFE neochordae. In the literature, previous studies [12–14] have already demonstrated good performance at intermediate and long-term follow-up, but to our knowledge, the series from our hospital is the largest series of consecutive homogenous patients who underwent MVR with artificial e-PTFE chordae, for whom the very long-term follow-up can be analyzed.

11.6.1 The role of quadrangular resection

Neochordae implantation has never been performed as the unique repair procedure, but it has always been associated with classic techniques, such as posterior annuloplasty in almost 100% of cases and quadrangular resection with or without sliding in half of the cases. In our series, the need for resection has constantly decreased over the years without an increase in MVR failure and homogenous outcome. This led to a time-saving procedure that preserves leaflet tissue and may result in a wider coaptation. Moreover, it may avoid the implantation of a small ring size annuloplasty, thus, resulting in a low gradient and larger orifice. The possibility to preserve leaflet tissue is particularly appealing in case of re-repair, because a number of other repair procedures can be applied. Our treatment of choice in the vast majority of cases of degenerative MR is e-PTFE neochordae implantation in combination with posterior annuloplasty. When prolapse occurs in the fibroelastic deficiency setting, leaflet tissue is sometimes very thin; thus, it is mandatory to preserve the posterior mitral leaflet, avoiding quadrangular resection to prevent tissue laceration. Usually the free edge is thicker so that neochordae can be safely anchored at this level. Even if Cox regression analysis showed that quadrangular resection is a protective factor associated with neochordae implantation, our change in the operative strategy was motivated by making the simplest, most effective, and physiologic MVR.

11.6.2 e-PTFE properties

Gore-Tex® sutures appeared to be the ideal material for synthetic chordal replacement, because of their biomechanical properties, which ensure long-term durability and allow surface endothelialization with normal fibrosa and intima [15]. The 2-0 or 3-0 Gore-Tex® sutures seem to lose flexibility over time and tissue growth can result in stiffness, which was observed in animal experiments [16]. Kobayashi et al. [17] reported thickening and stiffness of 4-0 artificial chordae at reoperation and they shifted to 5-0 sutures. At our institution, Zussa [16] proved in 1990 that Gore-Tex® CV 5-0 sutures are slightly thicker at explantation from human subjects, maintaining length, flexibility, and resistance. Although a few cases of neochordal rupture or calcification have been reported in the literature, in the series reported here spontaneous rupture or degeneration of implanted Gore-Tex® chordae was never responsible of

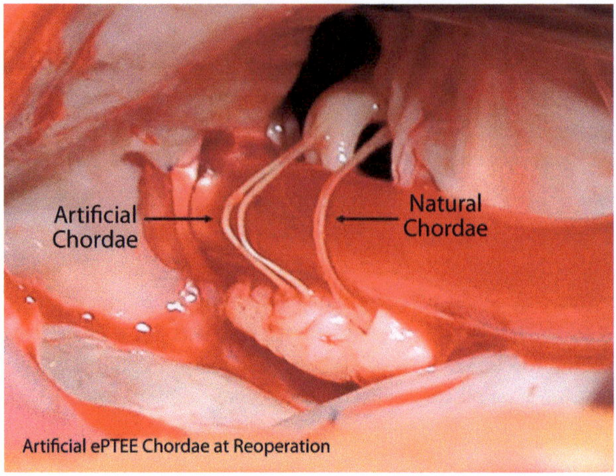

Fig. 11.5. Comparison of artificial and native chordae, seen at reoperation 12 years after mitral valve repair

MVR failure. We can hypothesize that the isolated cases reported in the literature could be related to e-PTFE chordae stretching or pinching by forceps or clips at the time of implantation, which could have created a weakness site.

On the other hand, the rupture could have been consequence of inflammation, like in a subclinical endocarditis setting. In 25 reoperations performed at our center, only in 1 case of acute endocarditis was a pair of ruptured neochordae detected, after being involved in a large erosion of the mural leaflet, caused by a severe and destructive infective process. According to the reports of all the reoperations performed at our center, the artificial chordae explanted were still as pliable, flexible, and resistant as the native chordae (Fig. 11.5). Calcifications have never been found in explanted neochordae at different time intervals or documented at follow-up echocardiograms. Minatoya et al. [18] reported the absence of calcification of e-PTFE sutures 9 years after the implant. Ischemia or rupture of the papillary muscle at the site of implantation was never observed.

11.6.3 Localization of the prolapsing leaflet

According to the Cox regression analysis, anterior leaflet prolapse was not observed as an independent risk factor for MVR failure in terms of reoperation, recurrent MR, or mortality. Based on prolapse localization, no significant differences were found in cumulative survival, freedom from MV reoperation, or recurrent MR. The only independent risk factor for reoperation is the presence of more than mild MR after weaning from CPB. Thus, MVR with the use of artificial chordae and annuloplasty is feasible in over 95% of degenerative MR, independent from the prolapse localization whether anterior, posterior, or bileaflet.

11.7 Conclusion

The predictability of the technique and the stability of the results are demonstrated by the low incidence of long-term mortality, the low rates of reoperation, and the high rates of freedom from moderate/severe mitral regurgitation over 15 years. Thus, the artificial chordal technique, alone or in association with classic techniques, is a procedure with very good long-term results and allows MVR to be performed in almost 100% of patients, independent of prolapse localization.

References

1. January LE, Fisher JM, Ehrenhaft JL (1962) Mitral insufficiency resulting from rupture of normal chordae tendineae. Report of a surgically corrected case. Circulation 26:1329–1333
2. Zussa C (1994) In: Zussa C (ed) Artificial chordae in mitral valve surgery. Medical Intelligence Unit, RG Landes Co., Chapter 7, Artificial chordae clinical experience. Medical Intelligence Unit, RG Landes Co., pp 79–112
3. Frater RW, Vetter HO, Zussa C, Dahm M (1990) Chordal replacement in mitral valve repair. Circulation 82(5 Suppl):IV125–130
4. David TE, Bos J, Rakowski H (1991) Mitral valve repair by replacement of chordae tendinae with polytetrafluoroethylene sutures. J Thorac Cardiovasc Surg 101:495–501
5. David TE, Ivanov J, Armstrong S, Christie D, Rakowski H (2005) A comparison of outcomes of mitral valve repair for degenerative disease with posterior, anterior and bileaflet prolapse. J Thorac Cardiovasc Surg 130:1242–1249
6. Carpentier A (1983) Cardiac valve surgery – the »French correction«. J Thorac Cardiovasc Surg 86:323–337
7. Salvador L, Rocco F, Ius P, Tamari W, Masat M, Paccagnella A, et al. (1993) The pericardium reinforced suture annuloplasty: another tool available for mitral annulus repair? J Card Surg 8:79–84
8. Salvador L, Mirone S, Bianchini R, Regesta T, Patelli F, Minniti G, Masat M, Cavarretta E, Valfrè C (2008) A 20-year experience with mitral valve repair with artificial chordae in 608 patients. J Thorac Cardiovasc Surg 135:1280–1287
9. David TE, Ivanov J, Armstrong S, Rakowski H (2003) Late outcomes of mitral valve repair for floppy valves: implications for asymptomatic patients. J Thorac Cardiovasc Surg 125:1143–1152
10. Gillinov AM, Cosgrove DM, Blackstone EH, Diaz R, Arnold JH, Lytle BW et al. (1998) Durability of mitral valve repair for degenerative disease. J Thorac Cardiovasc Surg 116:734–743
11. Smedira NG, Selman R, Cosgrove DM, MeCarthy PM, Lytle BW, Taylor PC, et al. (1996) Repair of anterior leaflet prolapse: chordal transfer is superior to chordal shortening. J Thoracic Cardiovasc Surg 112:287–292
12. Zussa C, Polesel E, Da Col U, Galloni M, Valfrè C (1994) Seven-year experience with chordal replacement with expanded polytetrafluoroethylene in floppy mitral valve. J Thorac Cardiovasc Surg 108:37–41
13. Nakano K, Eishi K, Kobayashi J, Sasako Y, Kosakai Y (1997) Surgical treatment for prolapse of the anterior mitral leaflet. J Heart Valve Dis 6:470–474
14. David TE, Omran A, Armstrong S, Sun Z, Ivanov J (1998) Long-term results of mitral valve repair for myxomatous disease with and without chordal replacement with expanded polytetrafluoroethylene sutures. J Thorac Cardiovasc Surg 115:1279–1286
15. Frater RW, Vetter HO, Zussa C, Dahm M (1990) Chordal replacement in mitral valve repair. Circulation 82(5 Suppl):IV125–130
16. Zussa C, Frater RW, Polesel E, Galloni M, Valfrè C (1990) Artificial mitral valve chordae: experimental and clinical experience. Ann Thorac Surg 50:367–373
17. Kobayashi J, Sasako Y, Bando K, Minatoya K, Niwaya K, Kitamura S (2000) Ten-year experience of chordal replacement with expanded polytetrafluoroethylene in mitral valve repair. Circulation 102(19 Suppl.3):III30–34
18. Minatoya K, Kobayashi J, Sasako Y, Ishibashi-Ueda H, Yutani C, Kitamura S (2001) Long-term pathological changes of expanded polytetrafluoroethylene (ePTFE) suture in the human heart. J Heart Valve Dis 10:139–142

Current concepts in Barlow's valve reconstruction

J.G. Castillo, A.C. Anyanwu, D.H. Adams

12.1 Introduction

Degenerative mitral valve diseases constitute a spectrum of lesions, varying from simple chordal rupture involving prolapse of an isolated segment in an otherwise normal valve to multisegmental prolapse involving one or both leaflets in a valve with significant excess tissue and a large annular size. Barlow syndrome is the most advanced and complex entity in this spectrum and is distinguished by the characteristic presence of diffuse and complex redundancy of the valve due to myxomatous degeneration (◘ Fig. 12.1a), producing prolapse of multiple segments in one or both leaflets (◘ Fig. 12.1b). Severe annular dilatation with giant valve size is evident (ring size ≥36 mm). In addition, varying degrees of annular calcification is often observed, as well as subvalvular fibrosis and calcification of the papillary muscles, in particular the anterior papillary muscle (◘ Fig. 12.1c). Therefore, surgical repair of the Barlow valve may present specific challenges. In this chapter, we describe our systematic approach to Barlow valve repair; we have found it to possible to repair essentially all Barlow valves by consistent application of the outlined principals.

12.2 Valve exposure

Our standard incision for Barlow's mitral valve repair is a 4 inch (10 cm) skin incision in the lower midline, followed by a median sternotomy, particularly in the case of calcified annulus or giant bileaflet prolapse. Simpler lesions in younger patients may be addressed via a right anterior minithoracotomy according to the patient's preference. Cardiopulmonary bypass is initiated with aortic and bicaval cannulation; peripheral cannulation is sometimes used in limited incisions. Direct aortic clamping and intermittent antegrade and retrograde cold blood cardioplegia is used in all cases. We expose all mitral valves through a left atriotomy in Sondergaard's groove after its generous dissection to allow closer proximity to the valve. The incision in the atrium is often directed behind the inferior caval junction to maximize valve exposure. Self-retaining atrial retractors are used to fix the exposure during valve reconstruction.

12.3 Valve analysis

The valve analysis starts with the echocardiogram, which usually shows the classic features of Barlow syndrome. Intraoperative valve inspection, performed in a systematic fashion as advocated by Carpentier [1], confirms echocardiographic findings. Sometimes in the presence of large distended leaflets, placement of posterior annular sutures is first undertaken to allow adequate exposure for valve analysis. Specifically in Barlow syndrome, it is important to identify and characterize the lesions of the leaflets, chordae, papillary muscles, and the annulus:

- Leaflets: We first identify and document which segments (A1–3; P1–3, anterior and posterior commissures) are distended and/or prolapsing. This requires a combination of echocardiographic information and findings from the direct valvular inspection. Precise identification of every leaflet segment is crucial in the setting of Barlow disease to obtain a good repair. For example, P2 may be distended with excess leaflet height (>1.5 cm) as well as prolapse, while P3 may have intact chordae with excess leaflet height. Both segments would need all identified lesions to be addressed to obtain a good repair result. We also assess for the presence of leaflet restriction, which may occur in those patients with advanced Barlow syndrome, more typically in the P1 segment. Filling the ventricle with saline may help identify the valve dysfunctions; jet lesions also suggest dysfunction in opposing valve segments. Echocardiography may also identify migration of the posterior leaflet hinge toward the left atrium, and if present we usually correct this during valve reconstruction.

- Chordae: Chordal elongation, rupture, or a combination of both must be identified (◘ Fig. 12.1d), in all segments of the valve, including the commissures. Thickened, fibrosed, fused, or calcified chords should also be noted.
- Papillary muscles: Calcification and/or fusion of the papillary muscles may occur in advanced Barlow's disease. If present, these lesions must be addressed during valve reconstruction.
- Annulus: Annular dilatation is usually severe and addressed during valve reconstruction. Calcification of the annulus requires special consideration during a valve reconstruction when identified.

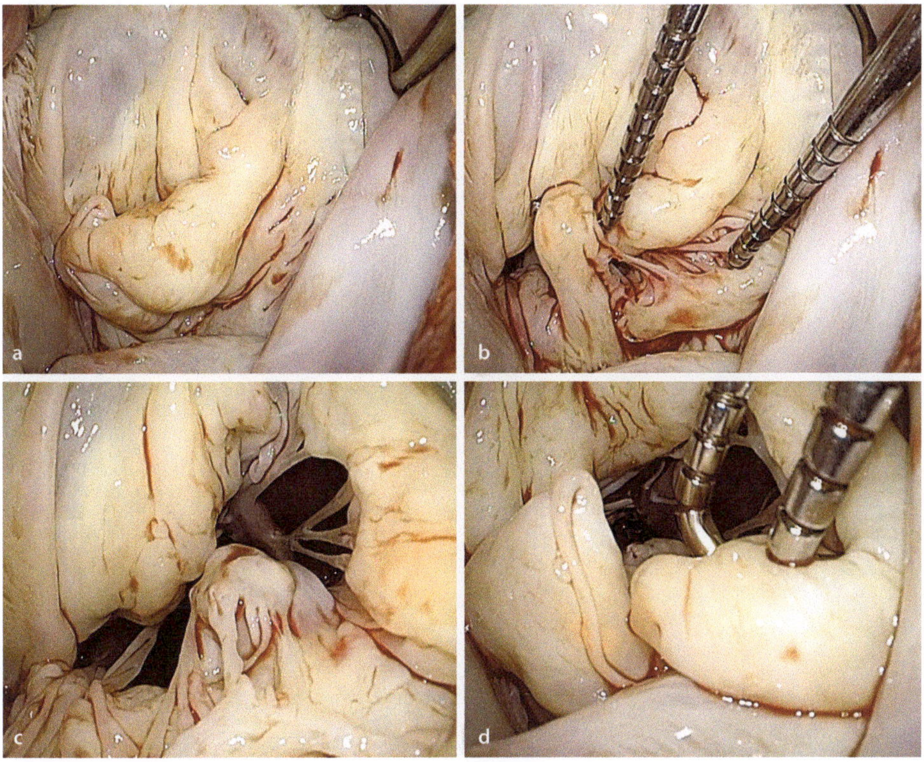

◘ **Fig. 12.1.** Valve analysis shows the variety of lesions encountered in patients with Barlow disease, including a billowing redundant valve with myxomatouos leaflet changes (**a**), deep indentations (**b**), calcification of the anterior papillary muscle (**c**), and chordal elongation and rupture (**d**)

12.4 Posterior leaflet repair

After valve analysis, our first step is the reconstruction of the posterior leaflet. Posterior annular sutures are placed to expose the valve (◘ Fig. 12.2a). The next step is a leaflet quadrangular resection where the prolapse is greatest or leaflet is tallest which may not necessarily be in the center of the valve (◘ Fig. 12.2a). This resection is a narrow rectangle, typically ≤1 cm wide (additional excess tissue can be removed later). If the height is more than 15 mm in any residual leaflet segment, we perform a sliding leaflet plasty to reduce leaflet height to 12–15 mm across the posterior leaflet. In the setting of deep posterior leaflet indentations, these are closed first with a figure-eight suture in order to »treat the segments as one«. Next, starting at the posterior commissure and using a #11 blade, the P3 and remaining P2 segments are detached from the annulus (◘ Fig. 12.2b). We do the same with the left half of the valve with specially angled scissors, starting from the remaining left position of P2 and going to the anterior commissure. At this point, the leaflet segments are suspended by their primary and secondary chordae with the basal chordae remaining on the annular side (◘ Fig. 12.2c). Basal or secondary chordae are

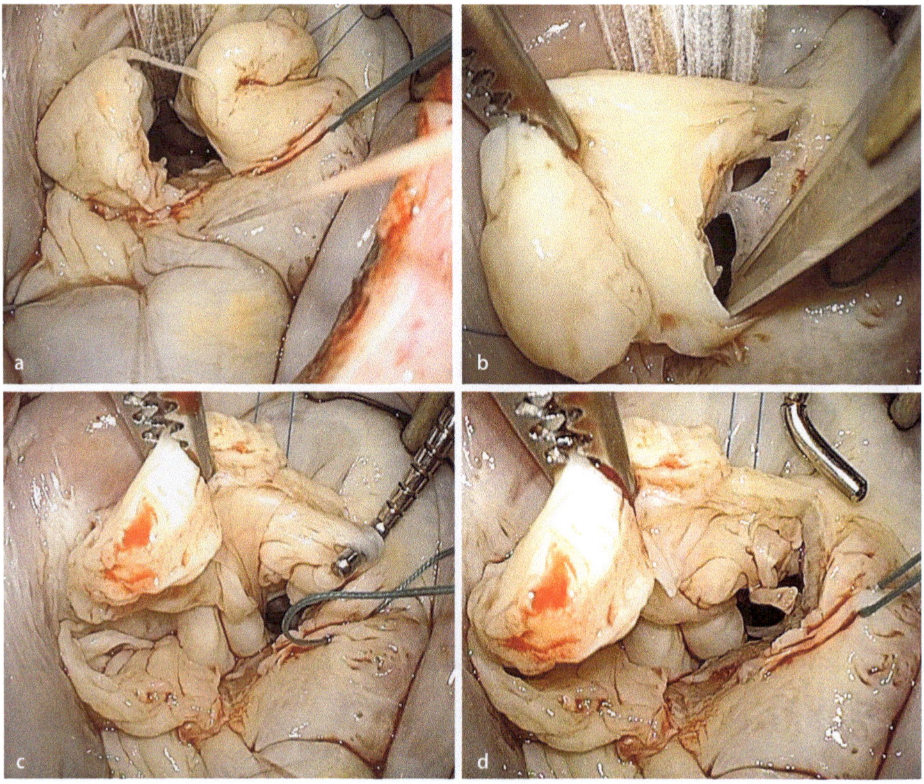

◘ **Fig. 12.2.** After valve analysis, our first step is reconstruction of the posterior leaflet starting by placing posterior annular sutures to expose the valve (**a**). Subsequently, a quadrangular resection (**a**) and detachment of the leaflet from the annulus (**b**) are performed. Secondary chords are then detached to maintain free mobility of the segments after advancement (**c**, **d**)

detached to maintain free mobility of segments after advancement. This prevents secondary chords from restricting the leaflet after leaflet advancement (◘ Fig. 12.2d).

The next steps are critical in leaflet plasty because they determine the final geometry and competency of the valve [2].

- Height reassessment of the left and right portions of the posterior leaflet. As discussed previously, our final target is 10–12 mm. Reattachment of the leaflet to the annulus will reduce the leaflet height several millimeters depending on the depth of suture bites. Therefore, the leaflet height before suturing should ideally be about 15 mm in all segments. If the leaflet is taller than 2 cm, then a horizontal wedge excision is made at the base of the appropriate segment to further reduce its height before reattachment.
- After optimizing the leaflet height, the next step is to assess the residual leaflet volume versus the annular distance that must be covered during leaflet reattachment. Unlike a true sliding plasty that »advances« the position of leaflets along the annulus, in most circumstances, we favor simple »reattachment« of leaflets to the annulus, and this is possible because of the amount of residual tissue. If there is a question about adequacy of residual

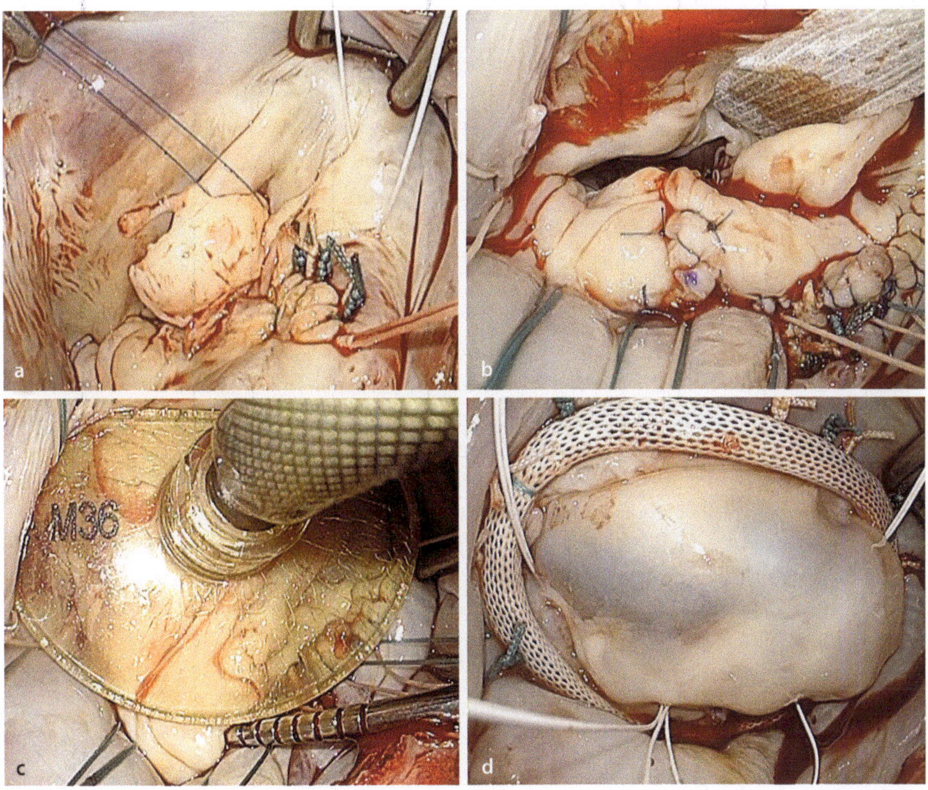

◘ **Fig. 12.3.** Vertical and horizontal placations of the annulus are performed to take tension off the leaflet reconstruction (**a**). The leaflet plasty is completed reattaching the leaflet segments assuring no excess tension on either segment (**b**). Annular sizing is performed by measuring the intercommissural distance and the surface area of the anterior leaflet (**c**). A complete semi-rigid annuloplasty ring is implanted and a saline test shows prolapse of the anterior leaflet (**d**). The areas of prolapse are then marked with ink tissue length, then the circumference of the annulus is decreased with interrupted vertical and/or horizontal plication 2-0 braided polyester sutures (Fig. 12.3a).

- Posterior annuloplasty sutures (2-0 braided polyester) are placed through the annulus and secured on hemostats to be passed through the prosthetic ring at a later stage. If the leaflet was detached, these sutures are placed before leaflet reattachment, as exposure to the annulus is optimal.
- One of two leaflet segments (usually the more robust one) is reattached to the annulus with a single or double layer of 4-0 polypropylene running suture. While running this suture, we continually assess the height of the reconstructed leaflet. Excess height is compensated for by taking sutures up to 5 mm deep into the leaflet, whereas in areas of adequate height, sutures are taken just 1–2 mm from the leaflet edge. The other leaflet segment is reattached to the annulus in a similar fashion assuring no excess tension on either segment (Fig. 12.3b). Saline testing undertaken at this stage confirms appropriate height of the posterior leaflet with a closure line displaced toward the posterior annulus.
- The two leaflet margins are then joined using either running or interrupted 5-0 Prolene sutures. The latter are preferred if the margins are hard to expose, or if there is a height discrepancy, as they allow »fine tuning« of the leaflet repair. Residual clefts or indentations that are indentified are also usually closed with interrupted sutures, to ensure an even surface of coaptation.
- The margins of the reconstructed posterior leaflet are now examined to ensure all segments are adequately supported. Any gaps in support, or areas supported by thinned out chordate (even in the absence of prolapse), are reinforced by transposition of previously secondary chordate attached to a small piece of residual leaflet tissue, or more commonly implantation of artificial polytetrafluoroethylene chords.

12.5 Annuloplasty

After posterior leaflet repair, we next perform annular remodeling. Annuloplasty sutures are placed round the anterior annulus if not previously done; posterior annular sutures are always placed before leaflet height/prolapse correction. Annular sizing is performed by measuring the intercommissural distance and the surface area of the anterior leaflet (Fig. 12.3c). We use a complete semi-rigid ring for all Barlow repairs (Carpentier–Edwards Physio I or Physio II; Edwards Lifesciences, Irvine, CA) and almost invariably the chosen size will be 36, 38, or 40. Sutures are passed through the annuloplasty ring, and the ring is tied down securely. Sizing disparity, whereby the ring size for the anterior leaflet height is more than that determined by the intercommissural distance assessment, is sometimes observed and can often be accommodated by the longer anteroposterior length of the Physio II ring (Edwards Lifesciences). In selected cases where the ring size is 42 mm or larger, an anterior leaflet incision or resection along the base of the annular attachment will allow for optimal ring sizing.

12.6 Anterior leaflet repair

Correction of anterior leaflet dysfunction, if required, will be our next step. Saline testing is performed with moderate pressurization of the left ventricle. Subsequently, one of the following observations may be noted in a patient with bileaflet Barlow syndrome:

- There is no leakage and the anterior leaflet shows no tendency to prolapse or billow. In this instance, no further repair is required (»tendency to prolapse« has been eliminated by correction of the posterior leaflet and annulus).
- There is no leakage, but there is a tendency for a segment to override its corresponding posterior segment or there is substantial billowing. Alternatively there is leakage and prolapse of the anterior leaflet. Areas of prolapse are noted and then marked with ink (◘ Fig. 12.3d).

After analysis of the saline test, the anterior leaflet prolapse is corrected using either one or a combination of the following techniques:

- Chordal transfer of basal or secondary chords kept from the posterior leaflet or divided strut chords from the anterior leaflet to the margin of the prolapsing segment will correct the leaflet dysfunction.
- Neochordoplasty with simple 5-0 polytetrafluoroethylene sutures as artificial chordal replacement (◘ Fig. 12.4a–d) [3].
- Using a polytetrafluoroethylene loop technique to correct multiple prolapsing segments.
- Undertaking a limited triangular resection of a prolapsing segment.

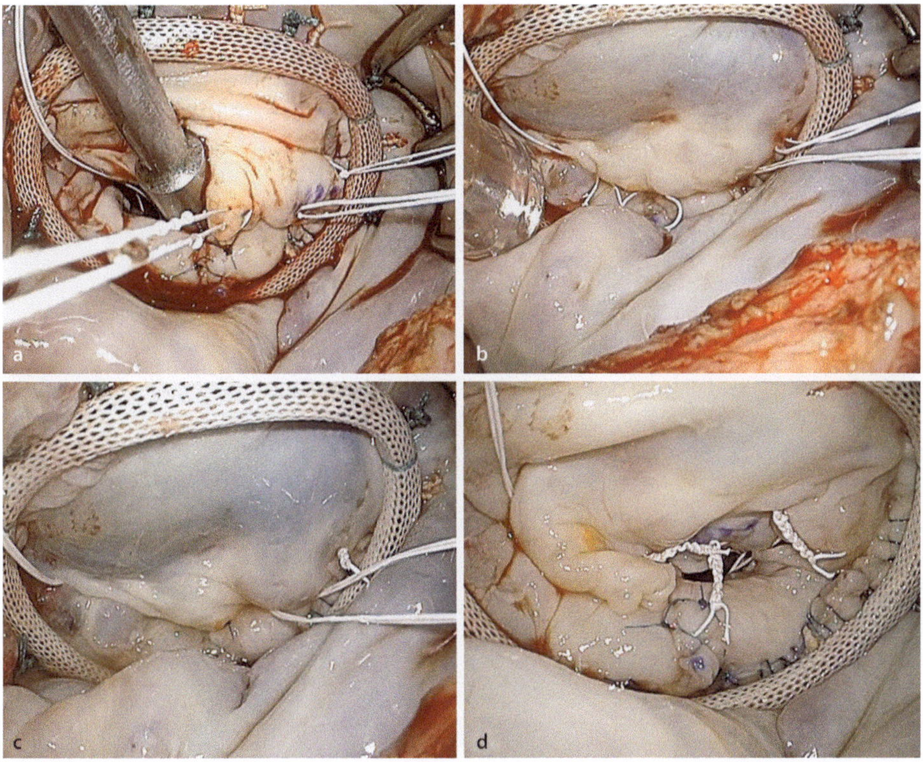

◘ **Fig. 12.4.** Polytetrafluoroethylene (5-0) artificial chords are used to correct the anterior leaflet prolapse. The neochordae are passed through the tip of the papillary muscle head and then the free margin of the leaflet (**a**). Saline testing is used to »functionally adjust« the height of the neochordae (**b**). The final results with three neochordae show a competent valve and symmetric line of coaptation (**c, d**)

12.7 Commissures

In Barlow syndrome, commissural prolapse is usually addressed by placing 1 or 2 vertical mattress sutures (Carpentier's »magic« suture) to fix opposing segments of A1/P1 or A3/P3. Because of the large area of Barlow's valves, there is no risk of stenosis with this maneuver. As a useful alternative, polytetrafluoroethylene chords may be placed to support opposing segments at the commissures, passing one arm of the suture through opposing anterior and posterior leaflet segments.

12.8 Calcification

In the setting of Barlow syndrome, two approaches are typically used to address calcium working around the calcium or resection. Limited calcification and fusion of chords is typically seen in the left side of the valve at P1/A1, where the anterior papillary muscle tip is sometimes fused to the anterior commissure and P1 segments. In this instance, we sometimes simply close off that part of the valve by using 2 or 3 »magic« sutures, thus, excluding the

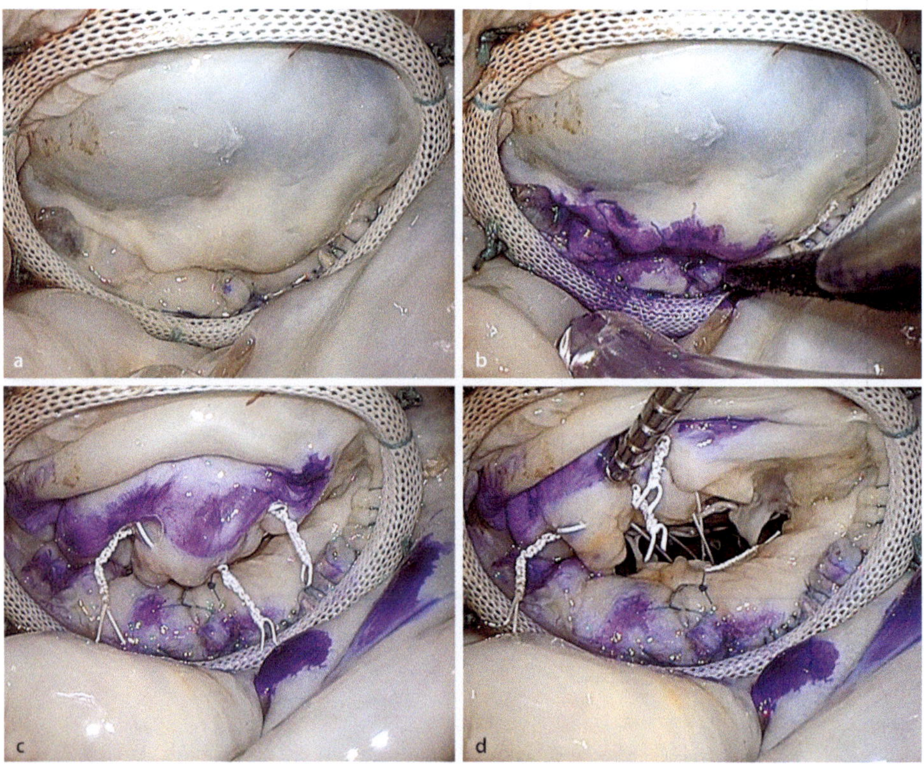

Fig. 12.5. The final saline test confirms no prolapse or billowing, no incompetence, a symmetric closure line, and an anterior leaflet that occupies most of the valve orifice (**a**). The ink test (**b**) reveals a coaptation zone of at least 6 mm and no more than 1 cm of the anterior leaflet beyond the ink (**c, d**)

calcified area from the coaptation zone. If mitral annular calcium is extensive, we often place pledgeted sutures from the ventricle to the atrium around the calcium bar and then oversize the annuloplasty ring. For limited annular calcification, we usually resect it en bloc following leaflet detachment during the posterior leaflet repair.

12.9 Evaluation of repair

The final step of the repair is evaluation of adequacy of repair. An optimal Barlow repair should meet the following criteria: (1) the valve is competent on saline testing, (2) there is good surface of coaptation, (3) there is a symmetric line of closure where the anterior leaflet occupies 80% or more of the valve area, (4) there is no residual billowing, and (5) there is no tendency to systolic anterior motion.

Evaluation for all these points requires two different intraoperative tests: the saline test and the ink test.

- The saline test is performed by filling the ventricle with saline. Examination of the valve confirms no prolapse or billowing, no incompetence, a symmetric closure line, and an anterior leaflet that occupies most of the valve orifice. If neither of these is observed, then necessary adjustments must be made to the repair until these criteria are met (Fig. 12.5a).
- The ink test is performed by drawing a line on the valve closure line during maximum saline insufflation (Fig. 12.5b) [4]. The coaptation zone beyond the ink is examined and should be at least 6 mm in length (this will transform to approximately 10 mm on echocardiography as part of the ink is within the coaptation zone). Also, there should be no more than 1 cm of the anterior leaflet beyond the ink line as this would signify a risk for systolic anterior motion (Fig. 12.5c,d).

12.10 Summary

Barlow valve disease presents special challenges to valve reconstruction. We have found Carpentier's techniques [4] to be allow a near 100% repair rate regardless of lesions or dysfunctions when applied systematically in a fashion outlined above.

References

1. Carpentier A (1983) Cardiac valve surgery–the »French correction«. J Thorac Cardiovasc Surg 86:323–337
2. Anyanwu AC, Adams DH (2007) The intraoperative »ink test«: a novel assessment tool in mitral valve repair. J Thorac Cardiovasc Surg 133:1635–1636
3. Adams DH, Kadner A, Chen RH (2001) Artificial mitral valve chordae replacement made simple. Ann Thorac Surg 71:1377–1378; discussion 1378–1379
4. Carpentier A, Adams DH, Filsoufi F (2010) Carpentier's reconstructive valve surgery. Elsevier Saunders, ISBN: 978-0-7216-9168-8

IV Ischemic mitral regurgitation

Robotic mitral valve surgery

E. Rodriguez, W.R. Chitwood, Jr.

13.1 History

The first robotic mitral valve repair was performed in May 1998 by Dr. Carpentier using an early prototype of the da Vinci® articulated intracardiac »wrist« robotic device [1]. A week later, Dr. Mohr performed the first coronary anastomosis and repaired five mitral valves with the device [2]. Grossi et al. [3] of New York University partially repaired a mitral valve using the Zeus™ system (Computer Motion, Inc.) but no annuloplasty ring was inserted. Four days later, in May 2000, our group performed the first complete da Vinci® mitral repair in North America. Subsequently, we performed 20 other mitral repairs as part of a phase I safety and efficacy Food and Drug Administration (FDA) trial [4]. These initial results were encouraging and prompted a phase II multicenter FDA trial that was completed in 2002 [5]. A total of 112 patients were enrolled at 10 different institutions and all types of repair were performed. The excellent results of these studies prompted FDA approval of the da Vinci® system for mitral valve (MV) surgery in November 2002. Just 8 years later, robotic assisted MV repair surgery became standard at many centers across the world with excellent results. All types of repairs, including complex bileaflet repairs, are currently performed routinely using only ports and a 2- to 4-cm mini-incision. Still further technological developments will eventually lead to better total endoscopic mitral valve repairs. To this end, we are on the cusp of developing a closed-chest operation that can be reproduced by many surgeons.

13.2 Robotic system

The da Vinci® system is the only available robotic system for cardiac surgical procedures. A few upgrades have been made to the system compared to the original that we used in May 2000. The latest version is the da Vinci® S HD (high-definition), which was launched in 2009. This system offers enhanced high-definition three-dimensional (3D) vision and improved digital operating room integration. In addition, this system offers a dual-console capability (◘ Fig. 13.1a, b), which allows for better training and the potential for surgeon collaboration during complex cases. The dynamic left atrial retractor (◘ Fig. 13.2a) provides great exposure of the MV and it is very easy to reposition especially when performing concomitant MAZE procedures for atrial fibrillation. In addition, the robotic EndoWrist (◘ Fig. 13.2b) with seven degrees of freedom allows surgeons great dexterity with both dominant and nondominant hands.

13.3 Anesthesia and patient positioning

The patient is positioned first in the supine position, and double lumen endotracheal intubation and placement of transesophageal echocardiogram (TEE) is performed. Some centers prefer bronchial blockers instead of double lumen endotracheal tubes and the surgeon should select the method that is better for the institution. The anesthesia team then places a 17 Fr thin-walled Bio-Medicus cannula (Medtronic, Minneapolis, MN) into the distal superior vena cava via the right internal jugular vein under TEE guidance. For smaller patients, a 15 Fr cannula is available. This cannula offers further venous drainage during cardiopulmonary bypass. The Swan–Ganz catheter is placed either into the subclavian or internal jugular vein (using a »double-puncture« method) (◘ Fig. 13.3). Oxygen saturation

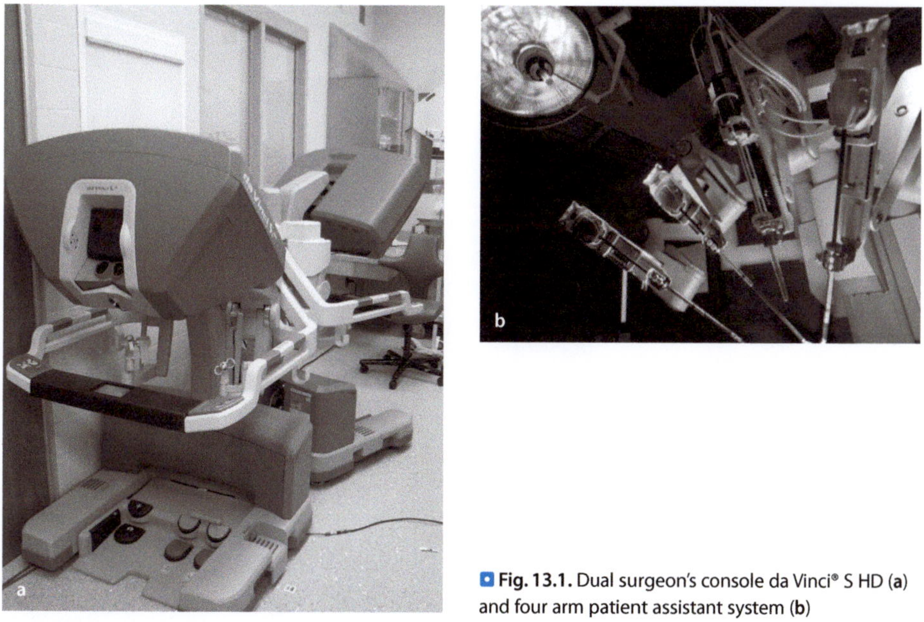

Fig. 13.1. Dual surgeon's console da Vinci® S HD (**a**) and four arm patient assistant system (**b**)

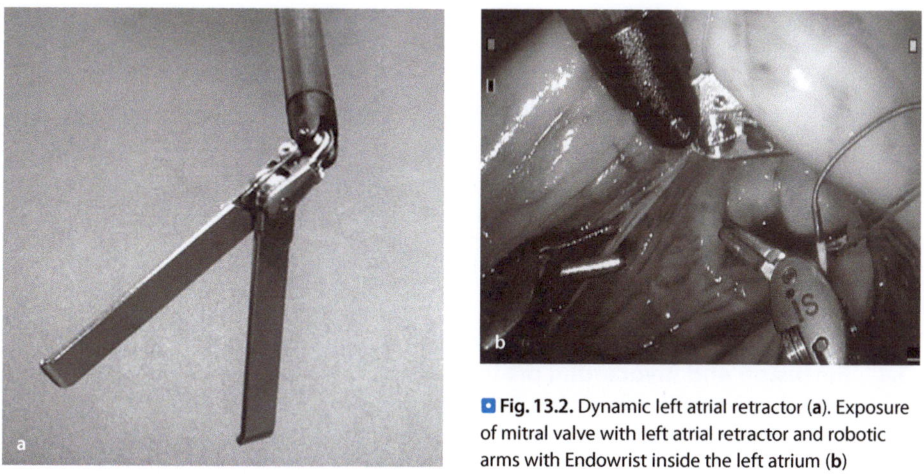

Fig. 13.2. Dynamic left atrial retractor (**a**). Exposure of mitral valve with left atrial retractor and robotic arms with Endowrist inside the left atrium (**b**)

levels are measured in each leg throughout the duration of cardiopulmonary bypass to ensure adequate limb perfusion using the Invos® system (Somanetics Inc., Troy, MI). In the event of inappropriate distal limb perfusion, a 14 Fr angiographic catheter is placed into the distal femoral artery and connected to the arterial perfusion cannula. In our experience, this has reestablished distal limb perfusion as measured by the Invos® system (Fig. 13.4a, b). The patient is then placed in a semi-left lateral decubitus position with the right arm on the side of the patient (Fig. 13.5a, b).

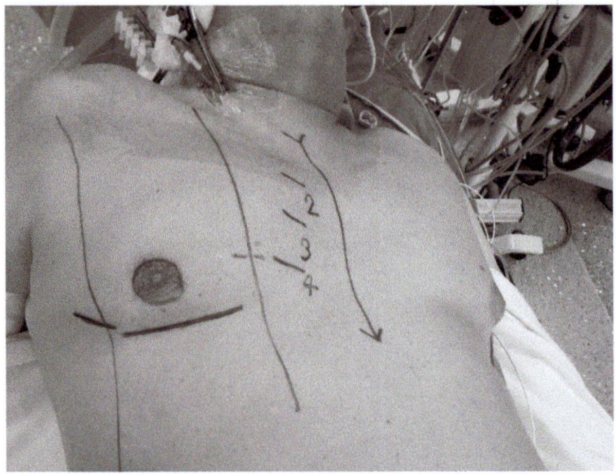

Fig. 13.3. Neck venous cannula in place as well as Swan–Ganz catheter

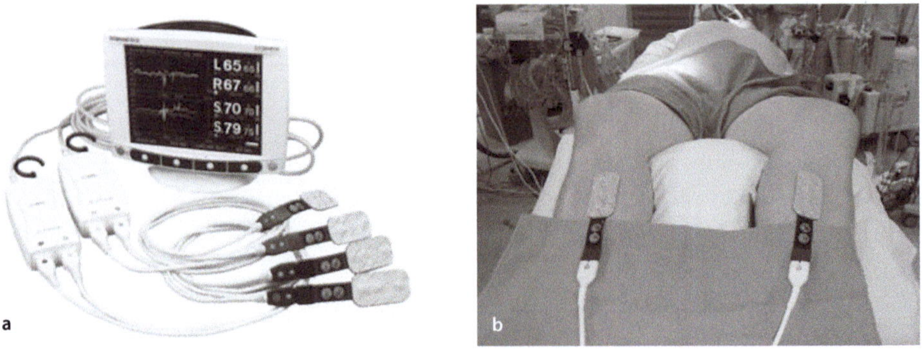

a b

Fig. 13.4. Invos® monitoring system (**a**). Lower extremity monitoring system in order to access proper lower extremity perfusion during cardiopulmonary bypass (**b**)

13.4 Perfusion and myocardial protection

Typically the right femoral artery and vein are used for peripheral cannulation. A small 1-cm incision is made over the femoral vessels, minimal dissection is performed, and only the anterior surface of the vessels is exposed in order to minimize the chance for lymphocele formation. Adventitial purse-string sutures (4-0 Prolene, Johnson & Johnson, Piscataway, NJ) are placed for introduction near the inguinal ligament. After adequate heparinization, arterial (17–19 Fr) and venous (21 Fr) Bio-Medicus cannulae (Medtronic, Minneapolis, MN) are positioned using the Seldinger guidewire technique under TEE guidance. The cannulae could be introduced directly via the groin incision but alternatively, especially in obese patients; a counterincision is made below the surgical incision and the cannulae are tunneled through the subcutaneous tissue of the leg. This is done to allow the cannulae to enter the vessels at a 45° angle, which makes for easier passage. If the angle is too acute, entry is difficult and the potential for vessel disruption or dissection of the posterior wall is increased. After appropri-

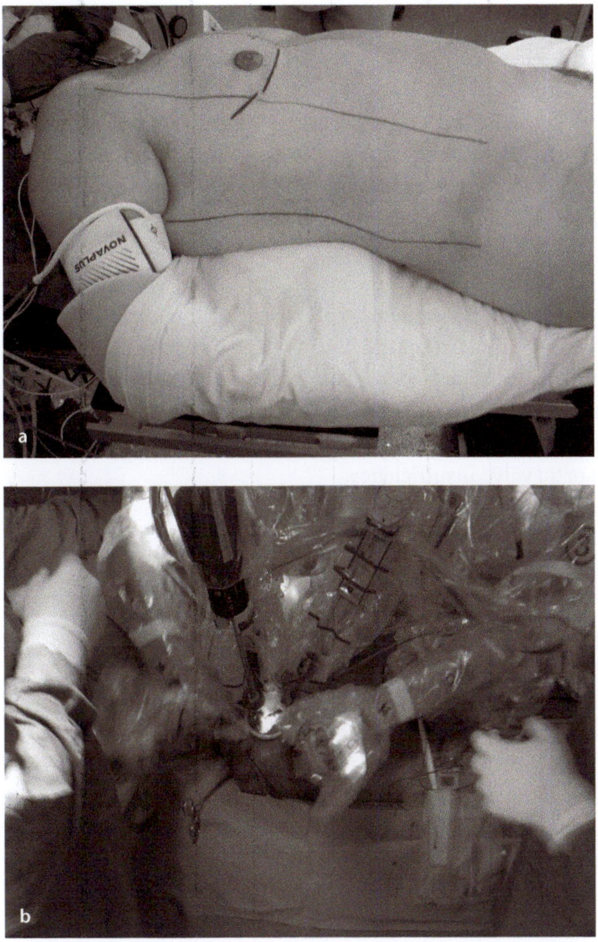

Fig. 13.5. Patient positioning and markings (**a**) in order to plan proper trocar placement (**b**)

ate positioning of the cannulae, cardiopulmonary perfusion can be instituted. In patients with severe peripheral vascular disease, axillary cannulation or direct ascending aortic cannulation through a trocar located in the 2nd intercostal space could be performed. When axillary cannulation is required, we prefer to use an 8 Fr Gelco woven graft, which is anastomosed to the axillary artery using 5-0 Prolene suture. This graft is then connected to the bypass circuit with a 3/8th inch connector.

We routinely use antegrade cold blood cardioplegia administered through the ascending aorta into the aortic root via a long dual cardioplegia/root vent catheter (Medtronic), which is passed through the access incision and secured with a pledgeted 4-0 Gore-Tex® (Gore Medical, Flagstaff, AZ) suture in the proximal ascending aorta. In order to cross clamp the ascending aorta, we most commonly use the Chitwood transthoracic aortic cross clamp (Scanlan International, Minneapolis, MN). This clamp is passed through a stab incision in the 2nd intercostal space at the superior right axillary line into the thoracic cavity. Care must be taken to avoid injury to the right pulmonary artery, the left atrial appendage, and the left main coronary artery.

Alternatively, the Endoclamp system could be utilized (Edwards Lifesciences, Irvine, CA). We also use this system, as it is extremely versatile. It obviates the need for manipulation of the aortic root for placement of the antegrade cardioplegia catheter. In addition, not having the transthoracic aortic cross clamp in the field decreases conflicts with the robotic arms. It is also a good option for reoperations in order to minimize aortic dissection and possible injury to previous grafts. However, it is a more expensive technology and we recommend careful imaging of the vascular tree with CT or MRI on each patient prior to surgery. As is present with any new technology, there is also a learning curve associated with the Endoclamp system, but once over the learning curve it is very reproducible. There is also the Endoplege sinus catheter system (Edwards Lifesciences) which allows placement of a coronary sinus catheter via the jugular system in order to deliver retrograde cardioplegia during the case.

Finally, another approach for myocardial protection is hypothermic (26 °C) fibrillatory arrest. Over 200 procedures have been performed at our hospital using this technique and with excellent results. This approach has become our preferred method for most reoperations unless the patient has significant aortic valve insufficiency.

13.5 Preoperative surgical repair plan

We now rely almost exclusively on intraoperative 3D TEE imaging to plan the MV repair. Each MV segment length is measured using TEE and occasionally also intraoperatively in order to confirm the TEE measurements–thus, we have measurements of the each posterior leaflet segment lengths (P1, P2, and P3) as well as the length of the anterior leaflet. In addition, the location and direction of regurgitant jet(s) are examined in order to determine which areas of the MV are the responsible pathologies. This information allows the potential areas needing resection, cleft closure, and/or chordal support to be determined. It also helps us determine proper postrepair zone of coaptation length.

13

In addition, special attention is paid to the angle between the mitral valve and the aortic annular plane angle. The C–septal distance (distance between the septum at the hinge point of the aortic valve cusp and the coaptation point of the mitral valve leaflets) and thickness of intraventricular septum are also measured. From these parameters, a topographic model is constructed, and the operation and band size are solely planned based on these measurements. The C–septal distance, $\angle\Theta$, anterior leaflet length, and interventricular septum thickness are extensively studied in order to minimize the potential for anterior leaflet systolic anterior motion (SAM) (◘ Fig. 13.6).

Using 3D TEE, it is possible to create preoperative models (◘ Fig. 13.7) or blueprints for a successful repair. A saline test is performed intraoperatively to confirm the echocardiographic findings, but only rarely are any further analyses of the mitral valve pathology performed.

13.6 Robotic mitral valve repair techniques

During our initial experience, simple MV repair patients were selected. Currently we can perform any type of repair using the robotic system. In fact, we believe that the visualization and exposure has improved to the extent that complex repairs are simplified using the da Vinci® system. Also the dexterity of the robotic arms allows the surgeon to precisely place sutures in locations that were routinely difficult to reach (e.g., left trigone) when using sternotomy

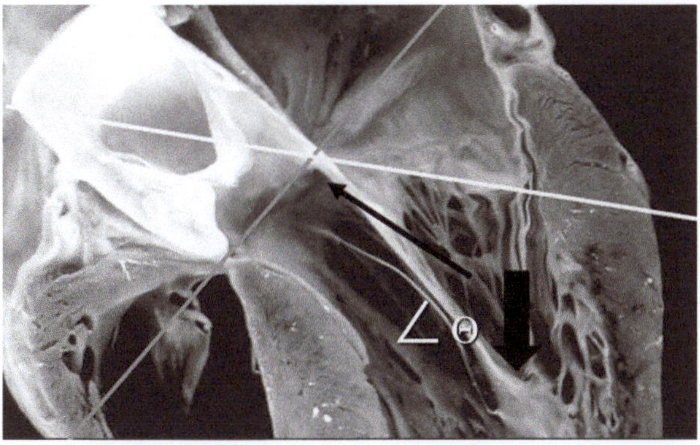

Fig. 13.6. Aortomitral angle and septal thickness are important measurements that determine predisposition for systolic anterior motion (SAM) after mitral valve repair

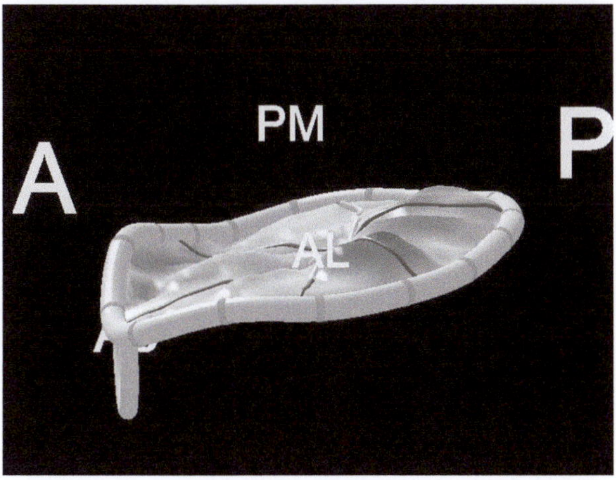

Fig. 13.7. Mitral valve model constructed from 3D TEE imaging, *A* anterior, *P* posterior, *PM* posteriomedial, *AL* anterolateral

or minimally invasive-based approaches. Therefore, the da Vinci® robotic system allows surgeons to perform the same repairs that they are currently doing but with perhaps enhanced visualization and dexterity.

13.7 Robotic mitral valve surgery results

We have performed over 600 robotic MV repairs as a stand-alone or in combination with other cardiac procedures. Between May 2000 and January 2010, 530 patients had undergone isolated robotic MV repair with either 3 or 4+ preoperative mitral insufficiency. Procedures included leaflet resection with an annuloplasty (LRA), LRA plus a sliding plasty and/or chordal procedure (CP), CP with an annuloplasty, LRA with CP, and an annuloplasty alone (n=99, 18.4%; n=130, 24.5%; n=64, 12.1%; n=144, 27.0%, n=58, 11.2%, respectively). Other mitral procedures were performed in 34 (6.6%) patients. Mean age was 57.2±0.9 (mean±SEM) years and 329 (62.1%) were men. Cardiopulmonary bypass, cross-clamp and total robot repair times were 162.0±2.3, 126.0±3.0, and 90.0±2.0 minutes, respectively. All had an annuloplasty band. Group operating room time was 285.5±3.0 minutes. Overall mortality was 1.5% (*n*=8). Length of stay was 4.8±0.2 days. Complex repairs were necessary in 82% of patients and 96.5% had mild or less MR by follow-up TEE. The Cleveland Clinic under the direction of Dr. Mihaljevic has performed over 600 robotic MV repairs without mortality and has reproduced our MV repair results.

Large published robotic MV repair series include:

- Dr. Murphy et al. [6] reported their experience in 127 patients undergoing robotic MV surgery of which 5 were converted to median sternotomy and 1 to thoracotomy; 7 patients had valve replacement and 114 had repair. There was 1 inhospital death, 1 late death, 2 strokes, and 22 patients developed new onset of atrial fibrillation. Blood product transfusion was required in 31% of patients and 2 (1.7%) patients required reoperation. Postdischarge echocardiograms were available in 98 patients at a mean follow-up of 8.4 months with no more than 1+ residual MR in 96.2%.
- Our own institution experience included our initial 300 patients undergoing robotic mitral valve repair between May 2000 and November 2006 having echocardiographic and survival follow-up in 93% and 100% of patients, respectively [7]. There were 2 (0.7%) 30-day mortalities and 6 (2.0%) late mortalities. No sternotomy conversions or mitral valve replacements were required. Immediate postrepair echocardiograms showed the following degrees of mitral regurgitation: none/trivial, 294 (98%); mild, 3 (1.0%); moderate, 3 (1.0%); and severe, 0 (0.0%). Complications included 2 (0.7%) strokes, 2 transient ischemic attacks, 3 (1.0%) myocardial infarctions, and 7 (2.3%) reoperations for bleeding. The mean hospital stay was 5.2±4.2 (standard deviation) days. A total of 16 (5.3%) patients required reoperation. Echocardiographic follow-up demonstrated the following degrees of mitral regurgitation: none/trivial, 192 (68.8%); mild, 66 (23.6%); moderate, 15 (5.4%); and severe, 6 (2.2%).

In addition, most other series have demonstrated low perioperative blood product transfusion rates as well as short hospital length of stays. For example, in a nonrandomized single surgeon experience from the University of Pennsylvania, Woo et al. [8] demonstrated that robotic surgery patients had a significant reduction in blood transfusion and length of stay compared to sternotomy patients. In another series, Folliguet et al. [9] compared patients undergoing robotic assisted mitral valve repair to a matched cohort undergoing sternotomy (*n*=25 each). The robotic group had a shorter hospital stay (7 days vs. 9 days, *p*=0.05) but besides this there were no differences between the two groups.

13.8 Conclusions

Since the first robotic assisted MV repair performed in 1998, there have been great advances and improvements in both the robotic system as well as surgical techniques. Taken together robotic mitral valve surgery is safe and has excellent early- and mid-term results. The introduction of newer robotic instrumentation like the dynamic left atrial retractor and simpler mitral valve repair techniques such as the »Haircut Posterior Leaflet-Plasty« [10] and the »American Correction« [11] will facilitate the use of robotic mitral valve techniques by a larger number of cardiac surgeons. There is no question that there is room for improvement and that further investigation in improved perfusion and myocardial techniques is necessary. Nonetheless, robotic assisted MV repairs have become standard at many institutions with excellent results and these results will continue to improve as experience continues to grow.

References

1. Carpentier A, Loulmet D, Aupecle B, Kieffer JP, Tournay D, Guibourt P, Fiemeyer A, Meleard D, Richomme P, Cardon C (1998) [Computer assisted open heart surgery. First case operated on with success]. C R Acad Sci III 321:437–442
2. Mohr FW, Falk V, Diegeler A, Autschback R (1999) Computer-enhanced coronary artery bypass surgery. J Thorac Cardiovasc Surg 117:1212–1214
3. Grossi EA, Lapietra A, Applebaum RM, Ribakove GH, Galloway AC, Baumann FG, Ursomanno P, Steinberg BM, Colvin SB (2000) Case report of robotic instrument-enhanced mitral valve surgery. J Thorac Cardiovasc Surg 120:1169–1171
4. Nifong LW, Chu VF, Bailey BM, Maziarz DM, Sorrell VL, Holbert D, ChitwoodWR, Jr (2003) Robotic mitral valve repair: experience with the da Vinci system. Ann Thorac Surg 75:438–442;discussion 443
5. Nifong LW, Chitwood WR, Pappas PS, Smith CR, Argenziano M, Starnes VA,, Shah PM (2005) Robotic mitral valve surgery: a United States multicenter trial. J Thorac Cardiovasc Surg 129:1395–1404
6. Murphy DA, Miller JS, Langford DA, Snyder AB (2006) Endoscopic robotic mitral valve surgery. J Thorac Cardiovasc Surg 132: 776–781
7. Chitwood WR, Jr, Rodriguez E, Chu MW, Hassan A, Ferguson TB, Vos PW, Nifong LW (2008) Robotic mitral valve repairs in 300 patients: a single-center experience. J Thorac Cardiovasc Surg 136:436–441
8. Woo YJ, Nacke EA (2006) Robotic minimally invasive mitral valve reconstruction yields less blood product transfusion and shorter length of stay. Surgery 140:263–267
9. Folliguet T, Vanhuyse F, Constantino X, Realli M, Laborde F (2006) Mitral valve repair robotic versus sternotomy. Eur J Cardiothorac Surg 29:362–366
10. Chu MW, Gersch KA, Rodriguez E, Nifong LW, Chitwood WR, Jr (2008) Robotic »haircut« mitral valve repair: posterior leaflet-plasty. Ann Thorac Surg 85:1460–1462
11. Lawrie GM (2006) Mitral valve: toward complete repairability. Surg Technol Int 15:189–197

Ischemic mitral regurgitation: the role of the »edge-to-edge« repair

M. De Bonis, O. Alfieri

14.1 Introduction

Mitral insufficiency is considered to be ischemic in origin when the valve leaflet and chordae are structurally normal and the valve dysfunction is caused by the consequences of myocardial infarction. The main mechanism responsible for ischemic mitral regurgitation (IMR) is tethering of the leaflets which may result either from localized or diffuse left ventricular dysfunction with changes in geometry of the left ventricle (LV) and displacement of one or both papillary muscles. Annular dilatation is often concomitantly present, particularly when the valve insufficiency is severe and long-standing and the LV is remarkably dilated. The diagnosis of IMR is provided by echocardiography, which is able to show the location of the regurgitant jet, the presence of global and regional ventricular wall motion abnormalities, and the severity of MR. Since the mitral valve is structurally normal in the majority of patients with IMR, inspection during the operation is not helpful, and the surgical procedure is guided by the information provided by echocardiography.

14.2 Surgical treatment of IMR

From a surgical point of view, an undersized annuloplasty is the treatment of choice for patients with IMR and dilated cardiomyopathy. The procedure is simple and easily reproducible. In appropriately selected patients, a well-performed restrictive annuloplasty is associated with low operative mortality and is effective in eliminating MR, promoting left ventricular reverse remodeling, reducing symptoms, and improving quality of life. However, patient selection is crucial. Indeed, it has been clearly demonstrated that the ideal candidate for annuloplasty alone is a patient in the early stage of the disease, with a short history of heart failure, and a left ventricle which is not excessively dilated [1, 2]. On the other hand, when the tethering of the leaflets is severe (as typically occurs in patients with a long history of congestive heart failure and advanced left ventricular remodeling), residual/recurrent MR can frequently occur. Such an event has been reported in 20–30% of the patients 1 year after surgery and is strictly related with an unfavorable outcome in terms of heart failure and mortality during follow-up [3, 4]. Therefore, it is extremely important to avoid either residual or recurrent MR. When the preoperative clinical and echocardiographic data suggest that annuloplasty alone is unlikely to be successful and durable, additional surgical procedures should be used to enhance the effectiveness of mitral valve repair. Left ventricular restoration, resection of secondary chordae of the anterior leaflet, external plication or buttressing of the left ventricle, leaflet patch extension, relocation of the tip or the base of the papillary muscles, and the edge-to-edge technique have been proposed.

14.3 The role of the edge-to-edge technique

The edge-to-edge technique was introduced by our group for mitral valve repair in the early 1990s as a simple method to conveniently correct MR in the presence of some complex lesions. The idea behind the edge-to-edge approach is that the competence of a regurgitant mitral valve can be effectively restored with a »functional« rather than an »anatomical« repair. The key point is to identify the location of the regurgitant jet. Exactly at that point, the free edge of one leaflet is sutured to the corresponding edge of the opposing leaflet, thereby, eliminating the incompetence of the mitral valve. When the regurgitant jet is in the central part of the valve, the edge-to-edge repair produces a mitral valve with a double orifice configuration. Depending on the location of the suture, the two orifices can have similar or different sizes. When the regurgitant jet is located in the proximity of a commissure, the edge-to-edge procedure leads to a single orifice mitral valve with a relatively smaller area. The technique is attractive because of its simplicity, reproducibility, and effectiveness even in complex settings and has been adopted by several institutions around the world for selected patients with MR due to different etiologies and mechanisms.

In the setting of functional mitral regurgitation (both ischemic and secondary to idiopathic dilated cardiomyopathy), the edge-to-edge repair has been used with encouraging [5], satisfactory [6], or disappointing results [7]. Most of the unfavorable outcomes, however, have been described when the edge-to-edge technique has been employed without any concomitant annuloplasty [5] or in association with only a posterior flexible band [5, 7], which is unable to prevent the progression of annular dilatation in patients with dilated cardiomyopathy. In particular, the Cleveland Clinic group reported a disappointing 24% recurrence rate of moderate–severe (3+/4+) mitral regurgitation 2 years after edge-to-edge repair for functional mitral regurgitation [7]. However, in that series, the edge-to-edge repair was always employed in association with a posterior flexible band and the patients requiring reoperation almost invariably presented redilatation of the mitral annulus. Moreover the edge-to-edge suture was placed centrally in the great majority of the patients, regardless of the location of the regurgitant jet and there were no restrictions in the use of the technique which was also adopted in the presence of extreme degrees of left ventricular remodeling and tethering.

At our institution, the edge-to-edge technique is added to undersized annuloplasty in functional MR whenever substantial apical tenting was present (coaptation depth >1 cm) with the aim to prevent the recurrence of mitral regurgitation and improve the durability of the repair [8]. The rationale for using the edge-to-edge technique in functional MR is that with this approach the site of the regurgitant jet is specifically addressed, early valve closure is ensured, and the occurrence of the »loitering effect« is abolished. Moreover, by anchoring the leaflets together, the edge-to-edge might exert a kind of »reins« effect on the LV chamber, counteracting the progression of the left ventricular remodeling which can lead to recurrence of mitral regurgitation.

From a technical point of view, the site of the approximating stitch is always guided by the preoperative transesophageal echocardiography which means that it is chosen according to the echocardiographic location of the regurgitant jet. In case of a central jet (between A2 and P2), a central edge-to-edge repair is performed, leading to a double orifice mitral valve configuration. On the other hand, when the regurgitant jet corresponds to the posterior commissure, a commissural edge-to-edge suture is applied. A continuous mattress suture of 4-0 polypropylene is used first, followed by a second over-and-over continuous suture to stabilize the repair. In case of central edge-to-edge repair, care is taken to avoid valve distortion. Moreover, the length of the suture is always kept as short as possible to minimize the risk of postoperative mitral valve stenosis. All patients received (in addition to the edge-to-edge suture) an undersized annuloplasty with a complete ring, rigid or semi-rigid in most cases (usually size 28 or 30 mm). Transesophageal Doppler echocardiographic reassessment of the valve was routinely performed after weaning from cardiopulmonary bypass. Typically, no residual mitral regurgitation was present and two diastolic flows could be visualized through the double orifice mitral valve in case of central edge-to-edge repair (◻ Figs. 14.1 and 14.2).

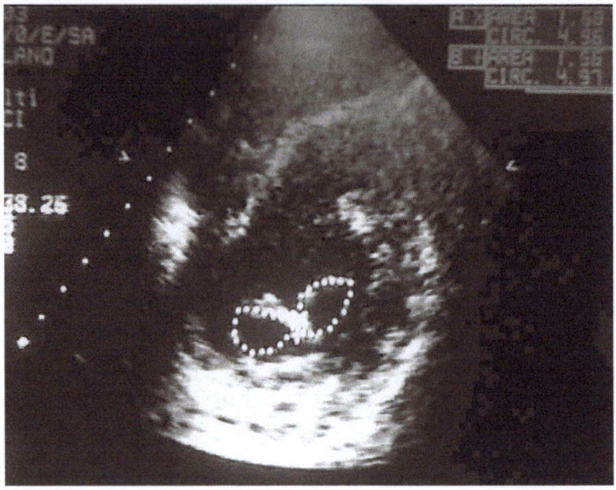

Fig. 14.1. Postoperative echocardiographic view of a central edge-to-edge for ischemic MR. The central suture and the two orifices are shown

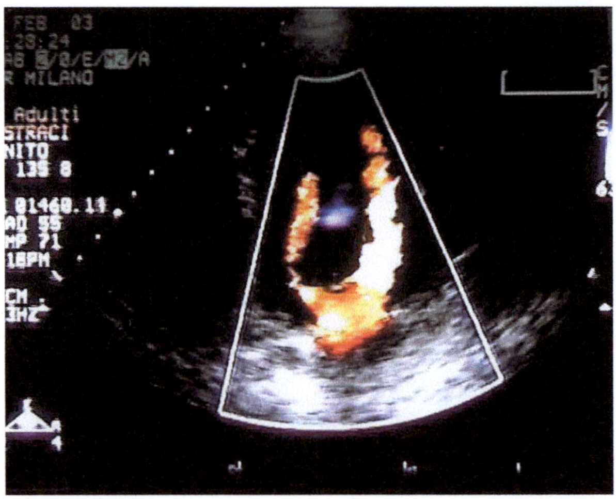

Fig. 14.2. Postoperative echocardiographic view of a central edge-to-edge for ischemic MR showing the two diastolic flows through the two mitral orifices

The valve area was commonly assessed by a planimetric method using the transgastric, short-axis view and no signs of mitral stenosis were ever detected.

In our initial experience, this approach significantly increased the durability of mitral repair with a freedom from recurrence of MR at 1.5 years of 95±3.4% compared to 77±12.1% registered in those patients submitted to isolated undersized annuloplasty in the same time frame (p=0.04). The recurrence rate of MR ≥3+ at follow-up was 3.7%, 6-fold lower compared to those patients registered with the undersized annuloplasty alone (21.7%) despite the edge-to-edge patients having the more advanced degree of leaflet tethering. Moreover, in our series, the use of the edge-to-edge technique was identified as the only significant predictor of durability of the repair [8]. In Tables 14.1–14.3, the preoperative characteristics of the two groups of patients are reported; the recurrence of MR in each group and the predictors of repair failure identified in the initial series were analyzed. Interestingly, the use of the edge-

Table 14.1. Preoperative characteristics of the patients submitted to isolated undersized annuloplasty compared to those who received an undersized annuloplasty + edge-to-edge repair

	Undersized ring only	EE + undersized ring	*p*
Patients (*n*)	23	54	
EF (%)	30±4.3	28±4.2	0.19
LVEDD (mm)	67±8.8	69±6.5	0.5
LVESD (mm)	49±6.8	52±8.4	0.27
LVEDV (ml)	190±68.1	205±62	0.45
LVESV (ml)	132±55.5	145±48.5	0.4
SPAP (mmHg)	50±8.4	50±12.7	0.96
Tenting area (cm^2)	2.2±0.86	2.9±0.99	0.04
Coaptation depth (cm)	0.8±0.11	1.2±0.38	0.006
Ring number	27.3±1.2	28.2±2.3	0.01
Complex jet (*n*, %)	4/23 (17.3%)	17/54 (31.4%)	0.2
Associate CABG (*n*, %)	13/23 (56.5%)	26/54 (48.1%)	0.5

LVEDD left ventricular end-diastolic diameter, *LVESD* left ventricular end-systolic diameter, *LVEDV* left ventricular end-diastolic volume, *LVESV* left ventricular end-systolic volume, *EE* edge-to-edge, *EF* ejection fraction, *SPAP* systolic pulmonary artery pressure, *CABG* coronary artery bypass graft

Table 14.2. Recurrence of MR at follow-up in patients submitted to isolated undersized annuloplasty compared to those who received an undersized annuloplasty + edge-to-edge repair

	Overall	Undersized ring only	EE+undersized ring	*p*
MR 0–1+	61/77 (79.2%)	15/23 (65.2%)	46/54 (85.2%)	0.048
MR 2+	9/77 (11.6%)	3/23 (13%)	6/54 (11.1%)	0.5
MR ≥3+	7/77 (9%)	5/23 (21.7%)	2/54 (3.7%)	0.02

MR mitral regurgitation, *EE* edge-to-edge

to-edge technique showed a trend towards favoring reverse remodeling of the left ventricle compared to isolated annuloplasty. This is extremely important considering that the occurrence of reverse remodeling is associated with longer repair durability and better clinical outcome [2, 4].

In summary, the addition of the edge-to-edge suture to annuloplasty in patients with significant leaflets tethering (coaptation depth greater than 1 cm), significantly improved the durability of the repair and favored reverse remodeling of the left ventricle.

Table 14.3. Univariate analysis of risk factors for MV repair failure (Cox proportional hazards regression)

	Hazard ratio	95% CI	p
Age	0.9	0.9–1	0.8
Ischemic etiology	0.52	0.08–3.1	0.48
Previous AMI	0.3	0.05–1.7	0.19
EF	0.9	0.8–1.1	0.9
SPAP	0.9	0.8–1.0	0.7
LVEDD	1	0.8–1.2	0.8
LVESD	1	0.9–1.1	0.6
LVEDV	0.9	0.9–1	0.9
LVESV	0.9	0.9–1	0.8
Tenting area	1.2	0.3–4.2	0.7
Coaptation depth	2.7	0.1–15.3	0.5
Complex jet	0.8	0.1–4.6	0.8
Absence of edge-to-edge	4.7	1.2–24.1	0.03
Ring number	0.63	0.3–1.1	0.2
Ring type	1.2	0.1–12.1	0.8
Associate CABG	0.6	0.1–1.7	0.5

CI confidence interval, AMI acute myocardial infarction, *LVEDD* left ventricular end-diastolic diameter, *LVESD* left ventricular end-systolic diameter, *LVEDV* left ventricular end-diastolic volume, *LVESV* left ventricular end-systolic volume, *EF* ejection fraction, *SPAP* systolic pulmonary artery pressure, *CABG* coronary artery bypass graft

14.4 Percutaneous edge-to-edge repair

The simplicity and reproducibility of the edge-to-edge repair have recently led to its clinical application by percutaneous methods opening a new age in the fascinating field of reconstructive mitral valve surgery. A dedicated 4-mm wide cobalt/chromium clip (MitraClip, Evalve, Inc., Menlo Park, CA) has been developed for this purpose and is delivered to the mitral valve via percutaneous femoral venous transseptal access. The MitraClip device is made of two arms which can be opened and closed. On the inner portion of the clip are two »grippers« adjacent to each arm to secure the leaflets as they are »captured« during closure of the arms. Each leaflet is independently secured between an arm and a gripper. The clip has a locking mechanism to maintain closure. The clip arms and grippers are covered with polyester fabric to promote tissue ingrowth.

The percutaneous edge-to-edge mitral valve repair for both functional and degenerative mitral regurgitation is performed under general anesthesia, using fluoroscopy and transesophageal echocardiographic guidance. After transseptal puncture, the MitraClip device is advanced into the left atrium, then axially aligned and centered over the origin of the regurgitant jet. The clip is opened to extend the two arms and advanced into the left ventricle below the mitral leaflets. Then, it is retracted until both leaflets are grasped and finally closed to coapt the mitral leaflets. Leaflet insertion into the clip and reduction of mitral regurgitation are assessed by the use of 2-dimensional and Doppler echocardiography. If necessary, the clip can be reopened and the leaflets released and then repositioned. After adequate reduction of MR has been achieved under hemodynamic challenge, the clip is deployed. Despite the fact that the device is manipulated within the mitral orifice in a beating heart, hypotension or significant ventricular arrhythmias are rarely observed.

Recently the clinical results of the percutaneous edge-to-edge repair in a cohort of 107 patients followed for up to 3 years have been reported [9]. Out of 107 patients, 23 patients (21%) had purely functional MR, with a history of coronary artery disease in 74% of the cases and previous bypass surgery in 43%. The remaining 84 patients (79%) had degenerative or combined degenerative and functional disease. Key anatomic inclusion criteria for functional MR included a central regurgitant jet corresponding to segments A2 and P2, a coaptation length of at least 2 mm and a coaptation depth of no more than 11 mm.

Out of 107 patients, 10 (9%) had a major adverse event (MAE), including 1 nonprocedural death. Major adverse events at 30 days were defined as death, myocardial infarction, nonelective cardiac surgery for adverse events, renal failure, transfusion of >2 units of blood, reoperation for failed surgery, stroke, gastrointestinal complications requiring surgery, ventilation for >48 hours, deep wound infection, septicemia, and new onset of permanent atrial fibrillation. Freedom from clip embolization was 100%. Partial clip detachment occurred in 10 (9%) patients. Overall, 79 of 107 (74%) patients achieved acute procedural success defined as a reduction of MR to ≤2+ after clip implantation and 51 patients (64%) were discharged with MR of ≤1+. Mitral valve area (planimetry) was 5.7±1.5 cm² (n=94) at baseline, 3.2±1.2 cm² (n=73) at discharge, and 3.5±1.1 cm² (n=62) at 12 months. The smallest mitral valve area by planimetry was 1.9 cm², and clinically significant stenosis was defined as <1.5 cm². During the 3.2 years after clip procedures, 32 patients (30%) had mitral valve surgery. When repair was planned, 84% (21 of 25) of procedures were successful. Thus, surgical options were preserved. A total of 50 of 76 (66%) successfully treated patients were free from death, mitral valve surgery, or MR >2+ at 12 months. At 3 years, freedom from death was 90.1% and freedom from surgery 76.3%, respectively. Clinical symptoms were improved in 74% of patients, 21% had no change in symptoms, and 6% (3 of 65) had worsened symptoms. The 23 patients with functional mitral regurgitation achieved 83% acute procedural success. Improvement in symptoms was documented in 80% of patients at 12 months, and freedom from surgery was 94.1% at 3 years. These data support the use of this procedure regardless of whether the etiology is functional or degenerative, provided sufficient tissue is available for coaptation.

Certainly, one of the major limitations of the percutaneous edge-to-edge is the lack of annuloplasty, which is very important for the durability of the repair particularly in the setting of functional mitral regurgitation. It is not clear whether any of the percutaneous annuloplasty systems under investigation at the moment will ever be effective and reliable enough to be extensively adopted in conjunction with the MitraClip device. Nevertheless, it is important to emphasize that the septal–lateral annular diameter of the mitral valve remained stable in the patients who had a MitraClip implanted for at least 12 months. In particular, in systole and diastole it was 3.3±0.4 cm and 3.8±0.4 cm, respectively, at baseline and 3.4±0.4 cm and 3.9±0.4 cm at 12 months (p=0.76 and p=0.21, n=35). This is due to the fact that a tissue bridge forms across the clip between the leaflets and that this healing response may help prevent future annular dilation. In addition, continuity created through the tissue bridge between the annulus, the leaflets, the chordae, and the papillary muscles may also help prevent dilation of the LV.

This experience with the MitraClip device demonstrates that the percutaneous edge-to-edge repair can be successfully performed with reduction of mitral regurgitation to less than moderate (2+) in the majority of patients and with low mortality and morbidity. Freedom from death, need for surgery, or recurrent MR >2+ was sustained in a substantial proportion of patients after 1 year. Furthermore, among those patients requiring MV surgery for residual or recurrent MR, surgical options were preserved, with standard repair techniques safely performed in the large majority of patients. A symptomatic improvement was also documented, indicating that clinical benefit was associated with the achieved MR reduction.

Nevertheless, as for the surgical edge-to-edge repair, efficient echocardiographic guidance is essential for this procedure, and a substantial amount of the learning can be attributed to optimizing the use of this modality. Late results are awaited to better define the final role of this new approach in the challenging settings described.

References

1. Bax JJ, Braun J, Somer ST, Klautz R, Holman ER, Versteegh MIM, Boersma E, Schalij MJ, van der Wall EE, Dion RA (2004) Restrictive annuloplasty and coronary revascularization in ischemic mitral regurgitation results in reverse left ventricular remodeling. Circulation 110(Suppl II):II103–II108
2. De Bonis M, Lapenna E, Verzini A, La Canna G, Grimaldi A, Torracca L, Maisano F, Alfieri O (2008) Recurrence of mitral regurgitation parallels the absence of left ventricular reverse remodeling after mitral repair in advanced dilated cardiomyopathy. Ann Thorac Surg 85:932–939
3. McGee EC, Gillinov AM, Blackstone EH, Rajeswaran J, Cohen G, Najam F, Shiota T, Sabik JF, Lytle BW, McCarthy PM, Cosgrove DM (2004) Recurrent mitral regurgitation after annuloplasty for functional ischemic mitral regurgitation. J Thorac Cardiovasc Surg 128: 916–924
4. Hung J, Papakostas L, Tahta SA, Hardy BG, Bollen BA, Duran CM, Levine RA (2004) Mechanism of recurrent ischemic mitral regurgitation after annuloplasty: continued LV remodeling as a moving target. Circulation 110: II85–II90
5. Umana JP, Salehizadeh BS, DeRose JJ, Nahar T, Lotvin A, Homma S, Oz MC (1998) »Bow-tie« mitral valve repair: an adjuvant technique for ischemic mitral regurgitation. Ann Thorac Surg 66:1640–1646
6. Kinnaird TD, Munt BI, Ignaszewski AP, Abel JG, Thompson CR (2003) Edge-to-edge repair for functional mitral regurgitation: an echocardiographic study of the hemodynamic consequences. J Heart Valve Dis 12:280–286
7. Bhudia SK, McCarthy PM, Smedira NG, Lam B, Rajeswaran J, Blackstone EH (2004) Edge-to-edge (Alfieri) mitral repair: results in diverse clinical settings. Ann Thorac Surg 77:1598–1606
8. De Bonis M, Lapenna E, La Canna G, Ficarra E, Pagliaro M, Torracca L, Maisano F, Alfieri O (2005) Mitral valve repair for functional mitral regurgitation in end-stage dilated cardiomyopathy: the role of the »edge-to-edge« technique. Circulation 112(suppl I):I 402–I408
9. Feldman T, Kar S, Rinaldi M, Fail P, Hermiller J, Smalling R, Whitlow PL, Gray W, Low R, Herrmann HC, Lim S, Foster E, Glower D and EVEREST Investigators (2009) Percutaneous mitral repair with the MitraClip system: safety and midterm durability in the initial EVEREST (Endovascular Valve Edge-to-Edge REpair Study) Cohort. J Am Coll Cardiol 54 (8):686–694

14

Mitral valve repair for ischemic mitral incompetence

R. Hetzer, E.M. Delmo Walter

15.1 Background

Ischemic mitral incompetence (IMI) is the most frequent mechanism of mitral regurgitation today and will continue to be so in the future, particularly in developed countries where rheumatic mitral valve disease has been nearly eradicated. It is a complex multifactorial entity related to coronary artery disease that is a frequent complication of myocardial infarction and associated with a poor prognosis. It involves global and regional left ventricular remodeling as well as dysfunction and distortion of the mitral valve (MV), including the chordae, annulus, and leaflets. Mitral regurgitation in the IMI mechanism is characterized by restrictive mitral leaflet mobility due to dyskinesia or even akinesia of the ventricular wall which bears one or both papillary muscles, thus, extending the distance between the ventricular wall and the leaflets, either both or, most frequently, predominantly the posterior leaflet. The posterior papillary muscle and its supporting ventricular wall and the posterior–inferior wall of the left ventricle are most frequently affected.

IMI can be permanent following myocardial infarction, myocardial scarring, or even after the development of an aneurysm; however, IMI can also be transient in ischemia and hibernating myocardium. Both may be marked by fibrotic transformation of the papillary muscles.

IMI has been observed as a frequent and important component of what we have named the »LOCIMAN complex,« which is a combination of left ventricular failure due to hibernating myocardium, left ventricular aneurysm or akinesia, and IMI (Fig. 15.1). This complex rapidly increases in severity in patients who have suffered one or more myocardial infarctions. Eventually, however, these patients will develop chronic heart failure. With increasing life expectancy and the increasingly successful treatment of acute disease episodes, management of this complex will become the most extensive task of cardiology and cardiac surgery.

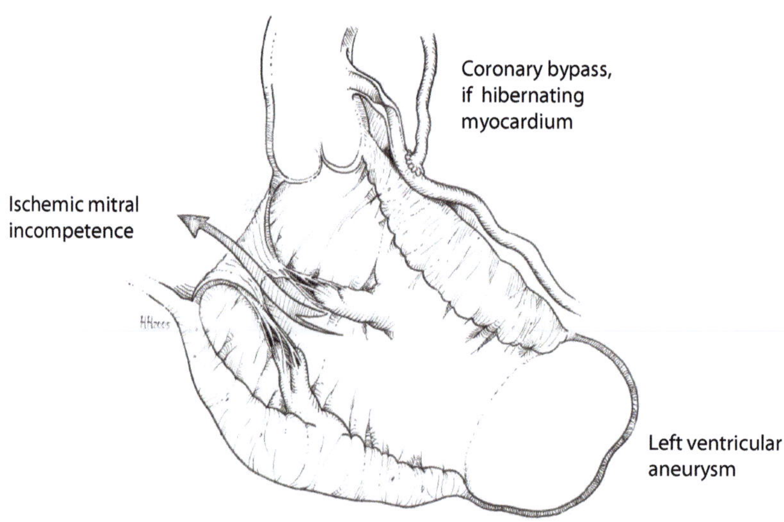

Fig. 15.1. LOCIMAN (Left ventricular failure, Obstruction of the Coronary arteries, Ischemic Mitral incompetence, left ventricular ANeurysm) complex

15.2 Surgical management

Since heart transplantation is beneficial only to a small patient group and since the vast majority of LOCIMAN patients belong to an older age group, eventually many of them will receive a mechanical circulatory support system. However, left ventricular failure can be successfully treated and cardiac performance can be improved by organ-preserving conventional cardiac surgery, including revascularization of hibernating myocardium and improvement of ventricular efficiency by ventricular restoration, either by resection of scar tissue and aneurysms, by repair of the mitral valve, or by both (Fig. 15.1).

In the past, the suboptimal results obtained with the most commonly used surgical strategy, i.e., restrictive annuloplasty combined with coronary artery bypass grafting (CABG), emphasized the need to develop alternative or concomitant surgical techniques that directly target the causal mechanisms of the disease.

Repair of the incompetent mitral valve in the various types of IMI has been a highly debated topic, and there is still no general agreement on the indication, concept, or appropriate techniques to treat IMI. This is mainly due to the fact that in the IMI setting the mitral valve itself, i.e., its leaflets, its annulus and, at least in the cases of transient IMI, the subvalvular apparatus (the chordae and papillary muscles), appears to be normal.

On the other hand, it was observed that even with seemingly perfect repair, mostly with a conventional annuloplasty ring, there was a lasting or at least intermittent recurrence of mitral regurgitation once the ventricle was under load again. Therefore, a number of repair concepts have been introduced, among which are surgical interventions on the afflicted ventricular wall, on the papillary muscles, on the chordal lengths, and, finally, application of specifically bent annuloplasty rings that would compensate for the asymmetric mechanism of IMI mostly affecting the posterior aspect of the mitral valve. This, of course, includes the posterior–inferior wall, the posterior papillary muscle, and the posterior halves of the anterior and posterior leaflets.

Taking into consideration this pathophysiology, we introduced commissuroplasty in the 1980s, whereby the free edges of both leaflets next to the posterior commissure were sewn together, thus, prohibiting valve incompetence in this area (Fig. 15.2). Although this technique was successful in most instances, it was not further pursued since there were a significant number of cases requiring reoperation within the short- and medium-term postoperative period due to residual and/or recurrent mitral valve incompetence.

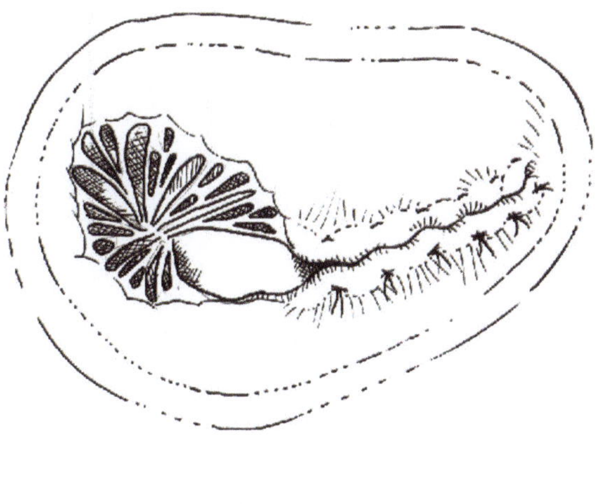

Fig. 15.2. Technique of commissuroplasty: the free edges of both leaflets next to the posterior commissure are sewn together to prohibit valve incompetence in this area

15.2.1 Approaches to mitral valve repair in IMI

We recently published our standard approach for exposure and repair of the mitral valve [1], which can be approached in different ways. In the *conventional* approach, mitral valve repair is performed through a median sternotomy (optimal if coronary revascularization and other intracardiac procedures are to be concomitantly performed). The *optimally invasive* right thoracic approach may be either a *minimally invasive* approach, with a right anterolateral thoracotomy at the 5th intercostal space (a relatively good approach for exposure of the mitral valve, especially when the patient has had previous surgery and a repeat median sternotomy would prove difficult due to scarring and adhesions; in women, it is mainly the patient's choice for cosmetic reasons) or a *semi-invasive approach* through a submammary incision. The comparison of these approaches is shown in Table 15.1.

To approach the mitral valve, we prefer a median sternotomy when additional coronary revascularization and/or even aneurysmectomy is needed and favor a right anterolateral thoracotomy approach in cases of isolated IMI. After cardiac anesthesia, a transesophageal Doppler echocardiographic probe is used to determine the extent and location of the regurgitant jet and degree of mitral valve incompetence. Likewise, the functional anatomy of the mitral leaflets and subvalvular apparatus is assessed. In most cases, the exact prolapsing leaflet, the annular dilatation, and the chordal or papillary muscle rupture can be precisely defined. The decision to treat mild regurgitation caused by ischemic incompetence has been controversial. If during the intraoperative transesophageal echocardiography (TEE), a preoperatively diagnosed mild mitral insufficiency disappears after volume loading, then we would decide to leave the mitral valve alone. However, if it is persistently present, mitral valve repair is performed depending on which component of the mitral valve is causing the insufficiency. Likewise, we proceed with repair of the mildly to moderately incompetent MV in patients with impaired LV function, since it yields better survival and improved LV function. With moderate to severe incompetence, the decision to perform mitral valve repair is unquestioned and straightforward.

In all our mitral valve operations with concomitant coronary revascularization and even with an accompanying left ventricular aneurysmectomy, an individual cannula is placed directly on the caval vein with occluding tapes. Myocardial protection is administered with an intermittent infusion of blood cardioplegia. Distal coronary anastomoses are accomplished before performing the valve repair, except in cases of concomitant left ventricular aneurysm where the aneurysm is resected performed first. In the past, the transventricular approach

Table 15.1. Comparison of optimally invasive mitral valve operations (right thoracic approach)

	Minimal invasive	Semi-invasive
Length of incision	3–5 cm	10–15 cm
Cannulation	indirect	direct
Exposure/overview	limited overview	good overview
Myocardial protection	insecure	controlled
De-airing	insecure	adequate

was used to repair the mitral valve prior to closure of the previously resected aneurysmal ventricular wall; however, because of difficulty in precise evaluation of the valve anatomy, we now reserve this approach for special situations.

15.2.2 Functional valve repair techniques

Because in ischemic mitral incompetence the mitral valve structure apparently appears normal, valve repair is ideal for this lesion. In IMI, mitral insufficiency may be caused by dilatation of the annular–ventricular apparatus and left ventricular wall–papillary muscle dysfunction, alone or in combination, with the net result being failure of leaflet coaptation [2]. In our personal experience, the most significant determinants of mitral valve coaptation, leaflet orifice area, and mitral insufficiency are the dimensions of the mitral valve annulus.

In patients with ischemic annular dysfunction, without structural abnormality of the leaflets and their subvalvular apparatus, the repair technique we now apply is a biological repair which is a combination of posterior annulus shortening and a modified Paneth type annuloplasty (◘ Fig. 15.3a) to a degree that reduces the mitral orifice to between 23 and 25 mm in diameter, which reduces the mitral valve opening area to between 3.5 and 4.5 cm^2. This residual size is sufficient for adults and ensures a sufficiently broad coaptation area of the leaflets. The posterior annulus shortening suture is reinforced by adding a strip of untreated autologous pericardium which avoids redilatation (◘ Fig. 15.3b, c). This basic principle has been applied to cases of ring dilatation of any origin both in adults and in children and has since shown a low and quite satisfactory recurrence rate.

It has also been observed that this technique was quite successful in IMI through a mechanism that we previously explained as being due to augmentation of the posterior annulus caused by the pericardial strip tissue. This means that the area which the posterior leaflet offers to the anterior leaflet for coaptation during the valve closure is enlarged and heightened by the strip tissue, thus, making valve closure possible even in cases of advanced leaflet restriction (◘ Fig. 15.4a, b).

Precautions, however, must be observed to avoid the systolic anterior motion (SAM) phenomenon, which must be anticipated when folding of the anterior leaflet is observed during valve testing with saline instillation into the ventricle (◘ Fig. 15.5). The folding appears when

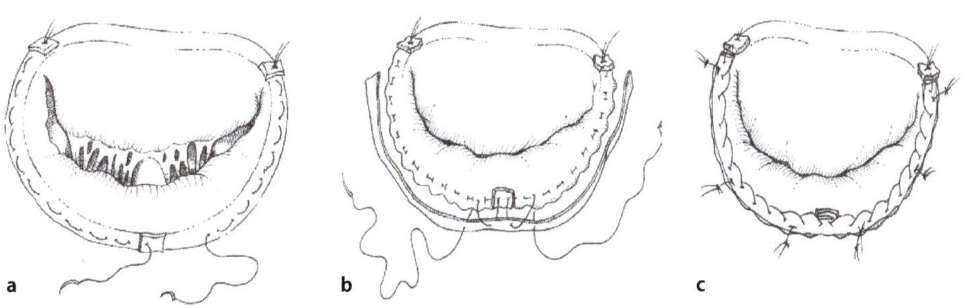
a b c

◘ Fig. 15.3. Modified Paneth–Hetzer technique of posterior annulus shortening plasty (**a**), reinforcement with autologous pericardial strip (**b**), and completed repair (**c**)

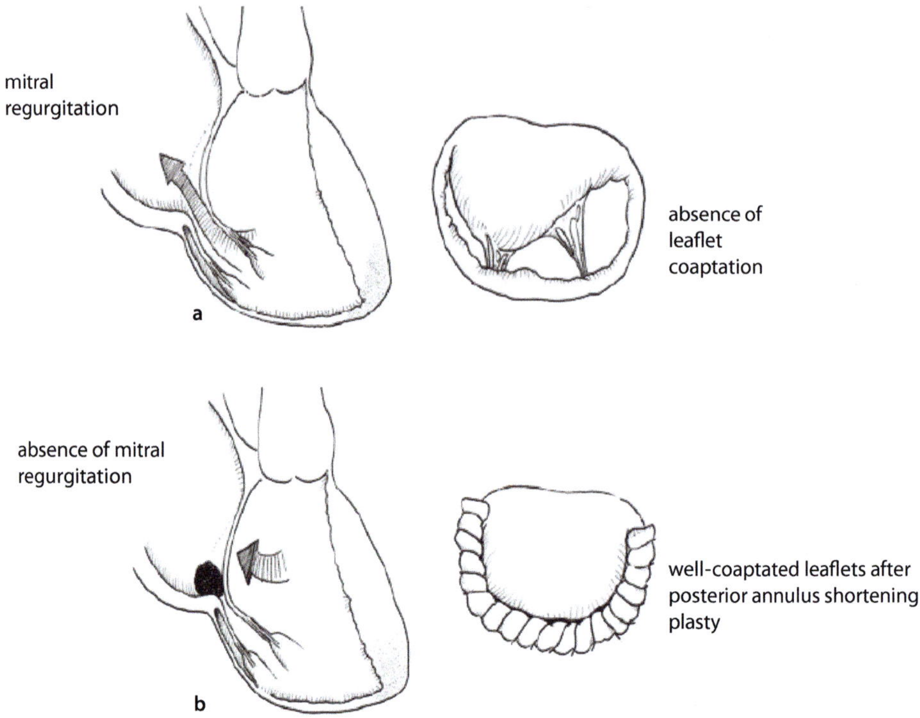

Fig. 15.4. Mitral valve incompetence before repair, showing inability of the leaflets to coapt leading to mitral regurgitation (**a**) and after repair by posterior annulus shortening and augmentation with a pericardial strip showing a broad coaptation of leaflets (**b**)

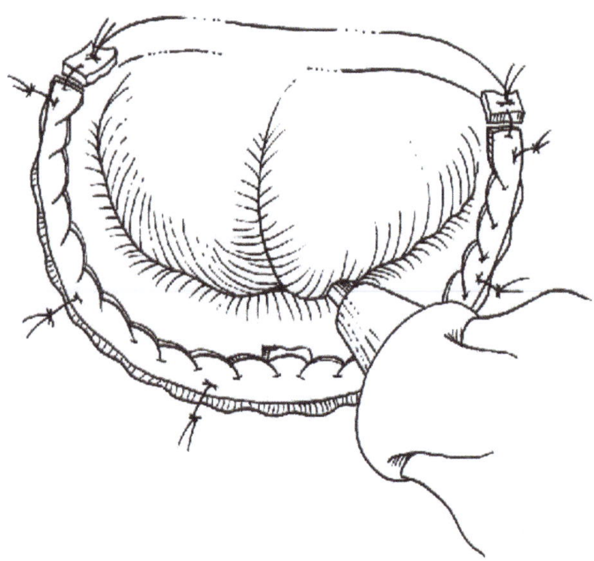

Fig. 15.5. Systolic anterior motion phenomenon observed as an infolding of the leaflet during intravalvular saline testing as a result of overreduction of the posterior annulus

the valve opening is made too narrow by overshortening or overreduction of the posterior annulus, thus, making the anterior leaflet too large relative to the resulting mitral valve opening area.

Mitral regurgitation from IMI may also be caused by chordal rupture, thus, leading to leaflet prolapse (◘ Fig. 15.6a). This is a clinical situation different from ruptured papillary muscle, which may occur following acute myocardial infarction and where surgical management is entirely different [3]. In our personal series, we have seen chordal rupture in patients with a large area of infarcted posterior wall and, interestingly, it was observed in all 18 patients with 90% or complete occlusion of the right coronary artery. It is always accompanied by alterations in papillary–annular geometry, which leads to reduction in the surface area of leaflet coaptation. In this condition, a modified Gerbode–Hetzer plication plasty, where the flail segment is plicated towards the left ventricle by a V-shaped suture line, bringing together the P1 and P3 segments, is employed (◘ Fig. 15.6b). In this manner, the competence of the mitral valve is restored. To avoid further annular narrowing, the annulus is then stabilized with an untreated autologous pericardial strip (◘ Fig. 15.6c).

In patients with a left ventricular aneurysm, both the aforementioned techniques are applied accordingly concomitant with coronary revascularization and resection of the posterior ventricular aneurysm. The mitral valve repair can then be performed by transventricular access. However, this approach is reserved for mitral valve repair in the presence of a small atrium.

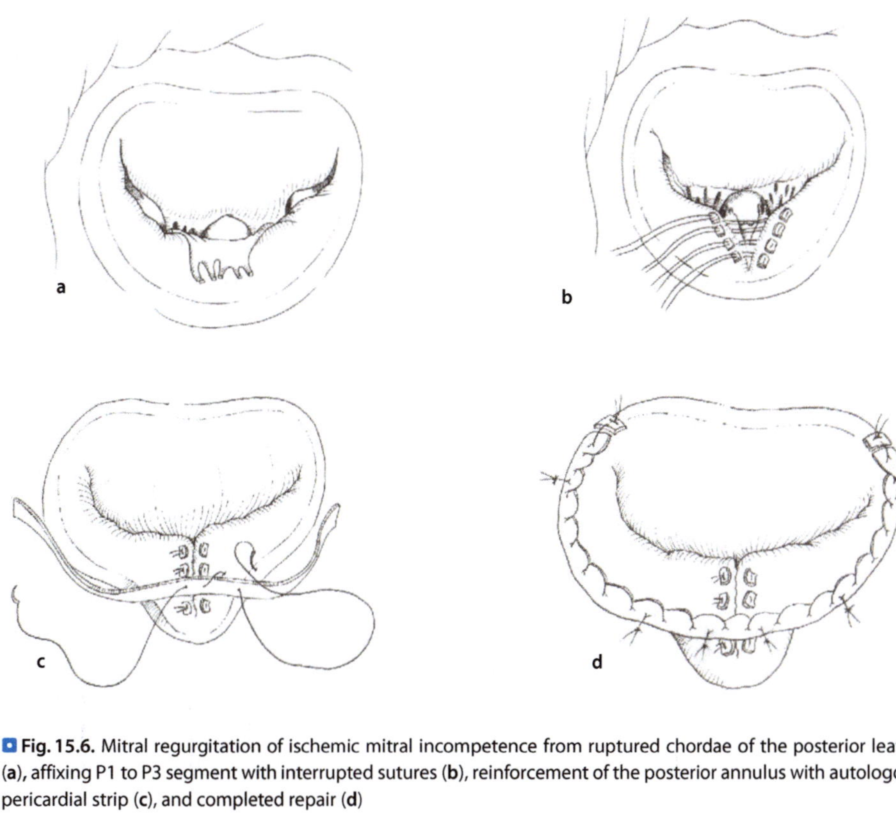

◘ **Fig. 15.6.** Mitral regurgitation of ischemic mitral incompetence from ruptured chordae of the posterior leaflet (**a**), affixing P1 to P3 segment with interrupted sutures (**b**), reinforcement of the posterior annulus with autologous pericardial strip (**c**), and completed repair (**d**)

15.2.3 Evaluation of the adequacy of repair

After repair of the mitral valve, it is obligatory to assess the valve function before closure of the atrium and separation from cardiopulmonary bypass. This is performed by transvalvular saline injection with a bulb syringe under pressure. Any remaining areas contributing to significant incompetence must be attended to before closure of the atrium. Once de-airing has been completed and extracorporeal circulation is discontinued, the repair result must be further evaluated with intraoperative TEE in order to demonstrate mitral opening area, residual incompetence, myocardial ischemia due to coronary kinking, and presence of the SAM phenomenon. Immediate and prompt correction must be made if the repair is shown to be unsatisfactory. Regardless of the underlying pathology and techniques used, no patient should be discharged from the operating room with more than minimal mitral valve incompetence.

15.3 Outcome of mitral valve repair for mitral insufficiency in IMI

In a personal experience series, we have employed these two techniques in 214 patients with mitral regurgitation from ischemic mitral incompetence. The mean age of these patients was 64.05±10.04 years (median 64.02; range 35.1–82.3 years). Most patients (83%) presented with triple-vessel disease and a high prevalence of angina pectoris (70%). Impaired left ventricular function (mean LVEF 0.24) was observed in 80% of patients, which explains the high incidence of patients in NYHA functional class III or IV. Patients had also significant noncardiac comorbidities, e.g., diabetes mellitus, renal insufficiency, hypertension, cerebrovascular events, peripheral arterial disease, and chronic obstructive pulmonary disease. Emergency operations (for cases which are immediately life-threatening and performed within a few hours of admission) were performed in 133 (51.1%) patients, urgent operations (for cases which are potentially life-threatening and must be completed within 24 hours) in 115 (44.2%) patients, and elective surgery was performed in 12 (4.6%) patients; all patients underwent coronary revascularization. Twenty (9.17%) patients had associated resection of ventricular aneurysms. These were the patients with severely impaired left ventricular function (mean ejection fraction (EF) 0.21±0.64, median 0.20, range 0.15–0.35) and 80% were in NYHA functional class IV. Isolated mitral valve repair was performed in 26 (11.9%) patients (mean age 60.6±11.9 years, median 61.07, range 35–82.8 years) underwent. These patients had mild mitral regurgitation upon discharge after previous coronary revascularization, which had progressed to become moderate to severe over time. The basic characteristics of these 260 patients are shown in Table 15.2.

15.3.1 Follow-up

Change in functional class. Postoperatively and at a mean follow-up period of 3.13±3.16 years (median 2.43, range 6 months–13 years), consisting of 1189 patient–years, mean NYHA functional class significantly improved from a preoperative value of 3.4±0.6 (3, range 2–4) to 1.63±0.49 (2, range 1–3) ($p<0.001$). The changes in NYHA functional class are presented in Fig. 15.7a. Improvement in heart failure symptoms occurred significantly within 6 months to 1 year and remained stable at the 5-year follow-up.

Table 15.2. Demographic profile of 214 patients with mitral regurgitation from ischemic mitral incompetence

	Variable	Preoperative	Postoperative follow-up (mean follow-up years)
Mean age at operation (median, range), years	64.2±9.4 (65.4, range 35.1–88.6)		
Sex , male/female	201/39		
Urgency of operation, *n* (%) Emergency Urgent Elective	 133 (51.1) 115 (44.2) 12 (4.6)		
NYHA classification, mean (median, range)		3.4±0.6 (3, range 2–4)	1.63±0.49 (2, range 1–3)
Ejection fraction, mean, (median, range) %		0.37±0.15 (0.35, range 0.13–0.81)	0.57±13.5 (0.55, range 0.30–0.85)
Degree of severity of mitral regurgitation[a], mean		3.27±0.6 (3, range 1–4)	0.72±0.6 (1, range 0–2)
Number of diseased coronary arteries, mean	2.8		
Associated systemic diseases, *n* (%) Diabetes mellitus Renal insufficiency Hypertension Peripheral arterial disease Cerebrovascular accident Chronic obstructive pulmonary disease	 93 (35.7) 72 (28.1) 218 (83.8) 63 (24.2) 42 (16.1) 57 (21.9)		
Surgical procedures, *n* Coronary revascularization + mitral valve repair (annuloplasty with pericardial strip) Coronary revascularization + mitral valve repair (repair of chordal rupture with placation plasty and posterior annuloplasty with pericardial strip) Coronary revascularization + mitral valve repair using various techniques Coronary revascularization + resection of LV aneurysm + mitral valve repair (annuloplasty with pericardial strip) Isolated mitral valve repair after previous coronary revascularization	 64 18 132 20 26		

[a]Echocardiographic grading of mitral valve regurgitation (based on regurgitant fraction)
0 (none) = absence of regurgitant fraction, *1* (mild) = regurgitant fraction of <20%, *2* (moderate) = 20–40% regurgitant fraction, *3* (moderate to severe) = 40–60% regurgitant fraction, *4* (severe) ≥60% regurgitant fraction

Change in left ventricular ejection fraction. Improvement in postoperative left ventricular ejection fraction was observed and is depicted in ◘ Fig. 15.7b. It had increased from a mean of 0.37±0.15 (0.35, range 0.13–0.81) to 0.57±13.5 (0.55, range 0.30–0.85) ($p<0.05$). These patients showed significant improvement at 1 year and remained generally stable during the course of follow-up.

Change in degree of severity of mitral regurgitation. There is a tremendous decrease in the severity of mitral regurgitation, as can be seen in ◘ Fig. 15.7c. The mitral valve regurgitation severity decreased significantly from grade 3.27±0.6 (3, range 1–4) to absent or mild regurgitation of grade 0.72±0.6 (1, range 0–2) at follow-up ($p<0.001$). Significant early (30 days–6 months) postoperative improvement in MR grade was found in almost all patients

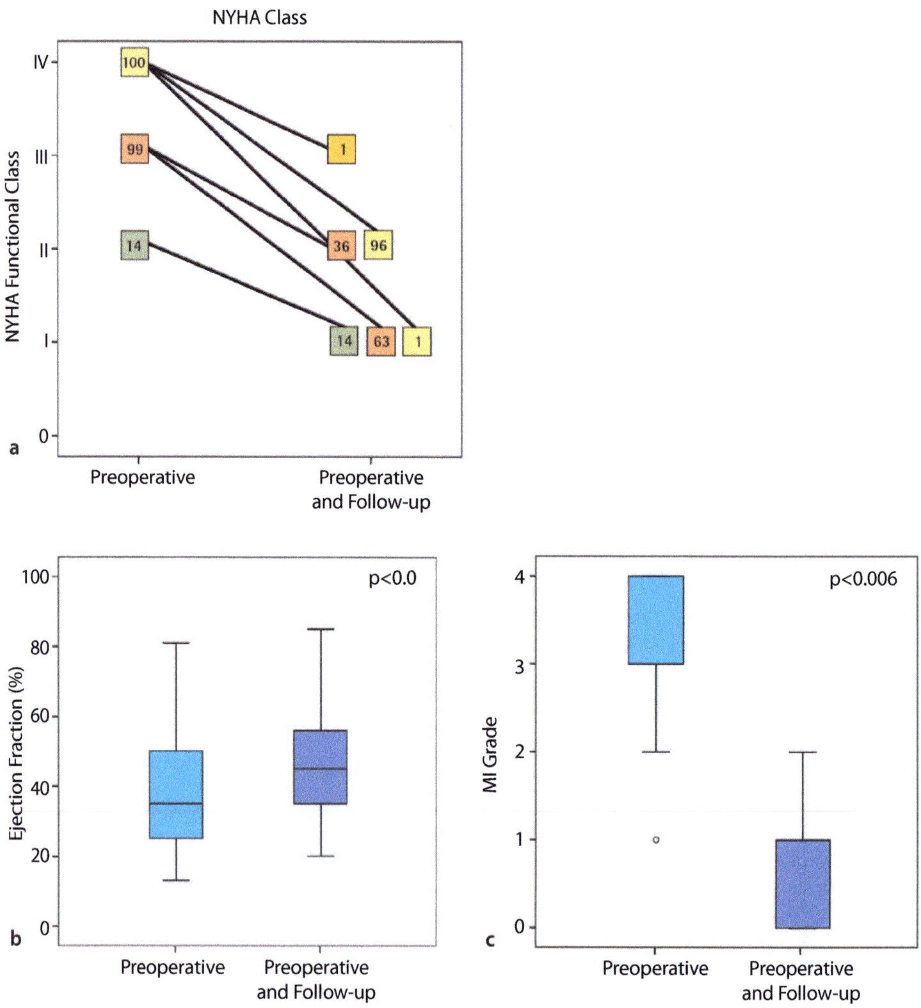

◘ **Fig. 15.7.** Comparison of preoperative and postoperative NYHA classification (**a**), left ventricular ejection fraction (**b**), and degree of mitral regurgitation (**c**)

(96%). There was no worsening of MR observed, except in 3 patients, of whom 1 had suture dehiscence and 2 underwent mitral valve replacement. The increase in severity of their mitral regurgitation, however, did not occur until the late postoperative period.

Freedom from reoperation was 96.5±2.4%, 94.3±3.2%, and 79.1±10.2% at 30 days, 1 year, and both 5 and 10 years, respectively, in patients who received the modified Paneth–Hetzer posterior annulus shortening technique, while freedom from reoperation was 100% at 30 days and 1 year in patients who underwent the modified Gerbode–Hetzer plication plasty (◘ Fig. 15.8a). Reoperation consisted of mitral valve replacement in 2 patients, and 1 patient was reoperated upon due to suture dehiscence in the annulus. Two reoperations unrelated to the mitral valve repair consisted of mechanical circulatory assist device implantation and another 2 patients underwent orthotopic heart transplantation 1 year later. These are the patients who preoperatively had an ejection fraction of 15%, NYHA functional class IV, and MR of grade 4, with associated triple-vessel coronary disease and left ventricular aneurysm.

Freedom from reoperation rates in patients who underwent isolated MV repair for IMI are 96.2±3.8%, 92.0±5.5%, and 80.7±8.9% at 30 days, 1 year, and 5 years, respectively, while freedom from reoperation rates of those who underwent mitral valve repair using various techniques are 96.7±1.4%, 93.8±2.3%, 89.5±3.01%, and 83.0±4.2% at 30 days, 1 year, 5 years, and both 10 and 15 years, respectively. Comparative freedom from reoperation among patients, in whom different techniques of mitral valve repair were used, is shown in ◘ Fig. 15.8a.

Survival rates were 87.7±4.4% 74.5±5.9%, and 72.4±6.1% at 30 days, 1 year, and 5 years, respectively, in patients with the modified Paneth–Hetzer posterior annulus shortening technique, while in those who underwent the modified Gerbode–Hetzer plication plasty, the survival rate was 100% for both at 30 days, 1 year, and 5 years. The patients (n=26) who underwent isolated mitral valve repair for IMI had survival rates of 96.2±3.8%, 92.±5.5%, and 80.7±8.%, at 30 days, 1 year, and 5 years, respectively. Those (mean age 63.9±9.1 years, median 65, range 38–88.6 years) who underwent mitral valve repair with the various techniques used in our first 15 years' experience, as described above, had survival rates of 83.8±3.31, 75.5±3.8%, and 59.7±4.3% at 30 days, 1 year, and 5 years, respectively. Their survival rate decreased at the 10- and 15-year follow-up, because patients who were already >70 years old at the time of operation were very old at the 10- and 15-year follow-up examinations and were dying from other diseases or of old age. Comparative survival rates among patients in whom different techniques of mitral valve repair were used are shown in ◘ Fig. 15.8b.

It might be superfluous to state that our data confirmed the numerous existing data showing that urgency of operation has a significant influence on survival (◘ Fig. 15.9a). Mortality was indeed high when patients were operated upon on an emergency basis. Needless to say, these are the patients who were in NYHA functional class III–IV, with left ventricular ejection fraction of <20%, triple-vessel coronary artery disease, left main coronary stem stenosis, a posterior wall infarction, mitral regurgitation of grade 3–4, and mostly with ventricular aneurysm, aside from associated coexisting noncardiac systemic diseases. Surgical treatment in these patients has been identified as an indicator of poor prognosis [4, 5]. This is primarily due to the ventricular problem that causes MV dysfunction and, despite valve repair, the disease further exists. In these patients, salvage surgery is performed. In the series of other investigators, mortality varies between 2.3% and 19.4% [6–8]. However, the urgency of operation in patients with IMI exerted no influence on the freedom from reoperation (p=0.40) (◘ Fig. 15.9b).

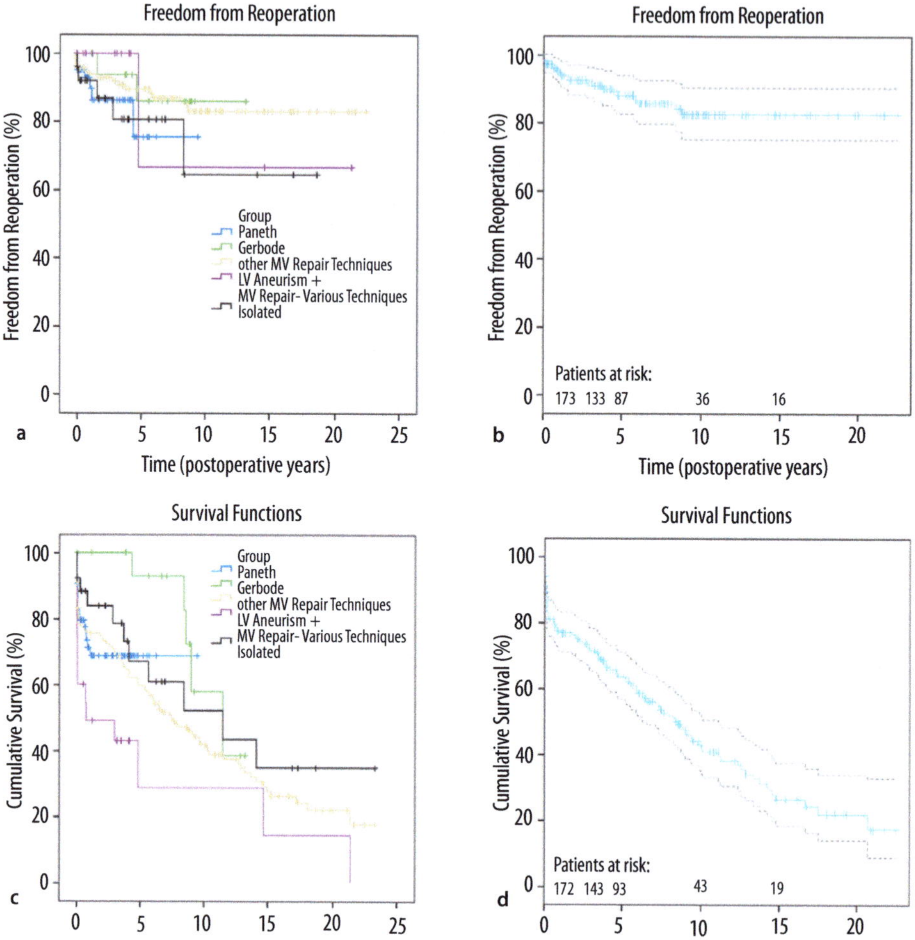

Fig. 15.8. Freedom from reoperation: comparing various mitral valve repair techniques used (**a**) and overall rate with patients at risk at 95% confidence interval (**b**); survival rates comparing various mitral valve repair techniques used (**c**) and overall rate with patients at risk at 95% confidence interval, in mitral regurgitation from ischemic mitral incompetence (**d**)

In 20 patients (mean age 62.63±8.09 years, median 63.2, range 47.7–78.39 years) from our personal series who underwent resection of left ventricular aneurysm along with coronary revascularization and mitral valve repair, 13 (65%) had emergency operations and 5 (25%) were operated upon on an urgent basis. In addition, 80% were in NYHA functional class IV and 15 (75%) had an ejection fraction of <20% and grade 4 mitral regurgitation. They were seriously ill patients whose medical management had been ineffective in improving a severely impaired functional and hemodynamic status. Hence, revascularization of the stenosed coronary arteries and repair of the combined mechanical abnormalities, i.e., mitral regurgitation and ventricular aneurysm, was the best option. Early mortality rate is 39%, while late mortality is 50.9%. Comparing this subset of patients with those who underwent CABG and mitral

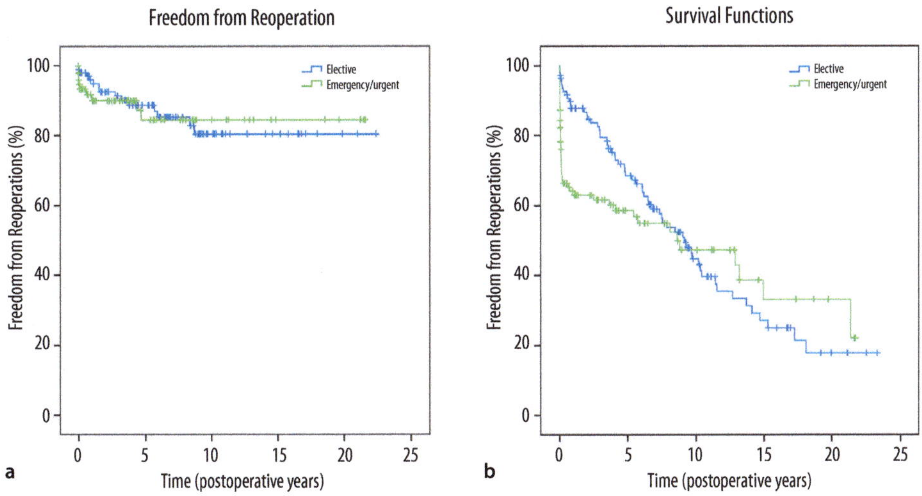

Fig. 15.9. Impact of urgency of operation on freedom from reoperation (**a**) and survival (**b**)

valve repair alone, they did not fare well (Fig. 15.9a, c). Symptomatic improvement of at least two functional classes was noted in the 6 long-term survivors in our series. Needless to say, left ventricular performance after myocardial infarction is directly related to the amount of damaged myocardium and correlates highly with the relative size of an akinetic or dyskinetic segment and congestive heart failure occurs when the length of the abnormally contracting segment exceeds 20% of the total left ventricular end-diastolic circumference. Compensation for the loss of myocardium occurs by augmentation of the contractile state in the residual normal myocardium [9]. Thus, left ventricular aneurysm and mitral regurgitation impose hemodynamic burdens on the left ventricle (i.e., increased LV volume and decreased cardiac output). The superimposition of significant mitral regurgitation on a ventricle with a large ventricular aneurysm would further decrease stroke volume and limit the Frank–Starling compensation [10]. The effects of the two lesions, therefore, are hemodynamically additive; either lesion can limit the ability to compensate for the other [11].

There must be a way to solve this severe condition. If the solution does not lie in our present surgical options, then it would be interesting to know which alternatives can be offered.

The patients in our study, therefore, represented a high predicted mortality among patients with ischemic cardiomyopathy. The surgical mortality in patients with ischemic cardiomyopathy with an age of >60 years has been reported to be between 10% and 48% [9]. A high operative mortality of 21% has been reported among a group of 28 patients undergoing CABG and mitral valve replacement [10].

The operative mortality in patients with IMI is higher than for other forms of regurgitation, especially when the condition is due to restricted leaflet motion [6, 11, 12]. Moderate and severe MR precipitated by myocardial infarction represents the cause of valve pathology in 10% of mitral valve operations [13], but its presence in patients with impaired LV function is a poor prognostic sign [14, 15]. Despite high operative risks, the 30-day mortality in our series was moderate at 6.5%. All patients with early death had ischemic mitral incompetence with previous coronary revascularization and were admitted with severely impaired left ventricular function and operated upon in emergency circumstances.

Mitral valve surgery in patients with LV dysfunction is associated with higher postoperative complication rates. A third of our patients had preoperative atrial fibrillation and/or compensated renal insufficiency and 49.5% of them were older than 70 years. Postoperative morbidity rate was low in this cohort of patients with serious comorbidities. Early complications such as reoperation for bleeding, acute respiratory failure, acute renal failure with dialysis, and ventricular tachycardia developed in 11 (5.04%) patients.

LV function improved significantly in our patients undergoing combined surgery, as a result of the reperfusion of ischemic myocardial areas, stabilization of the mitral annulus, and decreased volume overload secondary to MR correction.

15.4 Comments

The pathophysiology and treatment of ischemic mitral regurgitation has been discussed by Rankin et al. [16] who categorized patients with ischemic mitral regurgitation into those who exhibit posterior papillary–annular dysfunction concomitant with a large posterior wall infarction, those with papillary muscle rupture in which the posterior wall infarction is small and localized, and those with diffuse left ventricular infarctions or anterior aneurysms, in whom the mitral valve incompetence is due to generalized ventricular and annular dilatation and myocardial contraction impairment. In all three categories there is restricted leaflet motion. Valve prolapse results from papillary muscle infarction with elongation, fibrosis, paresis, or rupture of the chordae tendineae. IMI leads then to a cycle of more volume overload, LV remodeling, ventricular enlargement, progressive annular dilatation, loss of contractile forces, congestive heart failure, and more severe regurgitation.

Current surgical options for repair of the mitral valve apparatus, e.g., quadrangular resection of the posterior leaflet with or without sliding annuloplasty, triangular resection of the middle scallop of the anterior leaflet, chordal transfer or transposition, papillary muscle shortening or reimplantation, edge-to-edge leaflet approximation (Alfiere repair), are usually performed in combination with ring annuloplasty using flexible or rigid circular rings and posterior annuloplasty bands or partial rings. We do not employ these methods in ischemic MI. Along with coronary revascularization and left ventricular aneurysmectomy, a simpler repair technique of restoring the ventricular–valvular geometry, such as that we currently employ, also contributes greatly to improving the hemodynamic function and functional status of the patient. We are highly satisfied with our mid- and long-term results of mitral valve repair in ischemic mitral incompetence.

15.4.1 Principles of mitral valve repair for mitral regurgitation in IMI

Our biological mitral valve repair for ischemic mitral incompetence restores valvular–ventricular geometry. This is best achieved by repair techniques applied individually and which avoid any kind of prosthetic material. Repair should be performed using sutures and autologous pericardium only. We use untreated autologous pericardium for posterior annulus reinforcement and as pledget material. There has not been any incidence of calcification, shrinkage, infection, or thrombus formation on the pericardial strip. In a reoperation, the pericardium has been observed to be completely endothelialized, perfectly integrated into the annular tissue, and indistinguishable from the atrial endocardium. When used as an annular reinforcement, the pericardial strip should not lead to further annulus shortening; however, it should stabilize the suture-dependent repair and increase the height of the posterior leaflet coaptation counterpart. Addition of an autologous pericardial strip allows the mitral valve to stabilize its restored geometry.

The primary goal is to achieve complete and rapid closure of the mitral orifice by a well-mobile anterior leaflet and a sufficiently large coaptation area by bringing the posterior leaflet closer to the anterior leaflet. There should be no sutures placed along the anterior leaflet annulus. Depending on the components of the mitral valve contributing to the incompetence, several repair techniques may be required to achieve a competent valve. One must remember that the minimal final mitral valve opening area is 3.5 cm^2. Precautions must be observed to avoid the systolic anterior motion (SAM) phenomenon caused by excessive annulus reduction and too wide a coaptation area, visible by »folding« of the anterior leaflet when the valve is tested with saline instillation into the ventricle (Fig.15.5).

As the left ventricle dilates in functional MR, there is an increase in the regurgitant orifice area and the mitral annulus dilates. Our rationale of shortening the annulus facilitates the return of the zone of coaptation to a normal dimension to correct the insufficiency.

MR of IMI also impacts on coronary flow characteristics. Coronary flow reserve is limited in patients with MR due to an increase in baseline coronary flow and flow velocity, related to LV volume overload, hypertrophy, and preload (LV wall stress). Mitral valve repair, through restoration of LV geometry, improves the baseline coronary flow and flow velocity once the LV preload, work, and mass are reduced,

15.4.2 Trends in the management of IMI

Although ischemic mitral incompetence is in essence »a ventricular and not a valvular disease,« and our repair technique targets the consequence, i.e., mitral regurgitation, our biological »valvular« repair, nonetheless, provides satisfactory results in terms of MR correction and improvement in outcomes. These may seem like simple techniques without elaborate excision, transfers, reimplantation, and imbrication [17] to attempt to remodel the valve to simulate its original morphology; however, they have been proven effective as well as reliable.

Surgical management of IMI has primarily consisted of revascularization with or without the addition of mitral valve repair with a variety of techniques including suture, band, or ring annuloplasty, or even mitral valve replacement. Other surgical interventions to address left ventricular dilatation, e.g., remodeling procedures and passive restraint devices, have been attempted but are not widely used. Most patients with IMI that can be revascularized undergo revascularization to correct any reversible ischemia potentially contributing to left ventricular dysfunction underlying the IMI.

Mitral valve repair for mitral regurgitation of grade 2 or less, in addition to revascularization for IMI, has been advocated by several authors. To date, based on the outcome in our series, a survival benefit has clearly been demonstrated with this combination of surgical therapy over revascularization alone. Other debates concern mitral valve repair versus mitral valve replacement in IMI, and many have argued in favor of repairing the mitral valve with undersized flexible bands or rings or with asymmetrical remodeling rings [18– 23]. However, these still leave 30% of patients with residual or recurrent mitral regurgitation.

Our present surgical technique of biological correction of mitral regurgitation from IMI has shown highly satisfactory outcomes. Use of an autologous pericardial strip to stabilize the shortened posterior annulus not only reinforces the repair but helps maintain the geometry of the mitral valve. This technical strategy offers an incremental benefit over standard annuloplasty or implantation of prosthetic devices in such a way that shortening the posterior annulus reduces the sphericity of the left ventricle as well, thereby improving the ventricular shape and size along with reductions in subvalvular apparatus tethering and interpapillary muscle distance. In effect, this geometrical restoration helps improve the left ventricular function.

In our study, we have shown a hemodynamic advantage in performing posterior annulus shortening plasty. There is a very low incidence of recurrent mitral regurgitation or even residual MR. We believe these results to be due to the restoration of annular shape, with emphasis on anteroposterior to lateral diameter ratio, as well as preservation of the subvalvular apparatus. By increasing the coaptation area, prolapse of the anterior leaflet during systole, which is the common mechanism in recurrent IMI, is thus prevented. Our concern naturally is in patients with diffuse left ventricular dysfunction. In our series, the hemodynamic deterioration is predominantly related to myocardial rather than valvular factors.

There has always been a debate whether to repair the valve or simply replace it in cases of ischemic mitral incompetence. Many favor valve repair. Replacement should be reserved for cases of acute papillary muscle rupture in relation to an acute myocardial infarction, where a large area of the ventricle is infarcted. Intraoperative assessment of the papillary muscle structure and appearance proves to be helpful in surgical judgment, since reimplanting the ruptured papillary muscle to an infarcted area of the ventricle might eventually lead to a repeated rupture; thus, replacing the valve remains the best alternative.

Historically, the surgical approach to patients with functional MR of IMI was to perform mitral valve replacement and little was understood of the consequences that interruption of the annulus–papillary muscle continuity had on LV systolic function. This procedure was associated with prohibitive mortality rates. Techniques of mitral valve replacement, such as prosthesis implantation with preservation of the subvalvular apparatus [24], and prosthesis implantation with preservation of one or both leaflets (usually the posterior leaflet) have evolved to improve the long-term hemodynamic function and clinical status of these patients. However, we avoid replacement of the valve in IMI and we do not advocate this procedure. It has been demonstrated in a number of studies that preservation of the annulus–papillary muscle continuity is of paramount importance to preservation of LV function [25, 26]. It was the excision and disruption of the subvalvular apparatus that accounted for the significant loss of systolic function due to the destruction of the LV that led to the poor outcome in the earlier patients who underwent mitral valve replacement [27]. Preservation of the mitral valve apparatus and LV in mitral valve repair has been demonstrated to enhance and maintain LV function and geometry with an associated decrease in wall stress [28].

Mitral valve replacement is associated with a postoperative loss of LV systolic function because of the interruption of annular–chordal papillary muscle continuity causing a higher operative mortality and poor late survival. It remains unclear whether patients with ischemic mitral incompetence of grade 2–3 and impaired LV function should undergo mitral valve surgery concomitant with coronary revascularization, or simply isolated revascularization. Studies by Hausmann et al. [29, 30] showed that residual MR of grade 1 or above is a strong predictor for poor survival. Prifti et al. [31] demonstrated that grade 2 MR is a strong predictor for poor overall survival in end-stage coronary artery disease patients. Czer et al. [32]

showed that concomitant annuloplasty and CABG significantly reduced regurgitation by re-establishing a more normal relationship between the leaflet and annulus sizes, whereas the reduction in regurgitation grade with revascularization alone was infrequent. Other authors have different opinions on this subject: Christenson et al. [33] reported good survival and morbidity in patients with poor LV function and MVR of grade 2 undergoing CABG alone and demonstrated MVR normalization postoperatively. Likewise, Pinson et al. [34] presented a high estimated 5-year survival with moderate MVR and normal LV function in patients undergoing CABG alone. However, Duarte et al. [8] reported only »acceptable« outcome in his series of 58 patients with moderate ischemic MVR undergoing isolated CABG.

Based on the highly satisfactory outcome of mitral valve repair from our large personal series of 240 patients with MR of IMI, we advocate mitral valve repair for MR of even mild degree in patients with poor left ventricular function, concomitant with coronary revascularization. Operative times are not much increased when using simple repair techniques and exert no great influence on operative outcome in this era of excellent myocardial protection.

15.5 Conclusions

Ischemic mitral incompetence is the most important mitral valve disease of the future. It is a significant complication of myocardial ischemia. This occurs due to progressive dilatation of the annular–ventricular apparatus, altered ventricular geometry, loss of leaflet coaptation, and LV wall–papillary muscle dysfunction, in relation to an increase in preload and a decrease in afterload, which eventually leads to LV dilation and remodeling. Mitral valve reconstruction effectively corrects MR, is a safe procedure in a high-risk population, and has an acceptable mortality rate. Both survival and functional status have improved in these patients.

Our institutional experience has shown that IMI can be excellently corrected by mitral valve repair using our technique of posterior annulus shortening and augmentation of the coaptation area with pericardial strip annuloplasty. The satisfactory outcomes of this procedure in IMI are attributed to the decrease in regurgitant orifice area, better effective forward flow, and an increase in coronary flow reserve, along with revascularization of the affected coronary arteries, and resection of ventricular wall aneurysm, when present and appropriate. All these changes contribute to restoration of the normal valvular–ventricular geometric relationship. We advocate mitral valve repair in mitral regurgitation from IMI of grade 2 and less in patients with impaired left ventricular function, since it yields better survival, enhances patients' hemodynamic status and improves their functional class.

Acknowledgment

We are grateful for the tremendous assistance of Christine Detschades, Anne Gale, Julia Stein, Astrid Benhennour, and Helge Haselbach.

References

1. Hetzer R, Delmo Walter EM (2010) Repair of congenital mitral valve insufficiency. Oper TechThorac Cardiovasc Surg A Comparative Atlas.15(4)260–272
2. Bolling SF (2001) Mitral valve reconstruction in the patient with heart failure. Heart Failure Reviews 6:177–185

3 Gerbode FL, Hetzer R, Krebber HJ (1978) Surgical management of papillary muscle rupture to myocardial infarction. World J Surg 2:791–796
4. Duarte IG, Murphy CO, Kosinski AS, Jnes EL, Craver JM, Gott JP, Guyton RA (1997) Late survival after valve operation in patients with left ventricular dysfunction. Ann Thorac Surg 64:1089–1095
5. Wu AH, Aaronson KD, Bolling SF, Pagani FD, Welch K, Koelling TM (2005) Impact of mitral valve annuloplasty on mortality risk in patients with mitral regurgitation and left ventricular systolic dysfunction. J Am Coll Cardiol 45:388–390
6. Bishay ES, McCarthy PM, Cosgrove DM, et al. (2000) Mitral valve surgery in patients with severe left ventricular dysfunction. Eur J Cardiothorac Surg 17:213–221
7. Rostagno C, Caciolli S, Fradella GF, Stefano PL (2007) Early effects of mitral valve repair in patients with left ventricular dysfunction: an echocardiographic study. Eur J Heart Fail(suppl):26
8. Duarte IG, Shen Y, MacDonald MJ, Jones EL, Craver JM, Guyton RA (1999) Treatment of moderate regurgitation and coronary disease by coronary bypass alone: late results. Ann Thorac Surg 68:426–430
9. Jones EL, Weintraub WS, Craver JM, Guyton RA, Shen Y (1994) Interaction of age and coronary disease after valve replacement: implications for valve selection. Ann Thorac Surgery 58:378–385
10. Ashraff SS, Shaukat N, Odom N, Keenan D, Grotte G (1994) Early and late results following combined coronary bypass surgery and mitral valve replacement. Eur J Cardiothorac Surg 8:57–162
11. Hendren WC, Nemec JJ, Lytle BW, Loop FD, Taylor PC, Stewart RW, Cosgrove DM (1991) Mitral valve repair for ischemic mitral insufficiency. Ann Thorac Surg 52:1246–1252
12. Kay GL, Kay JH, Zubiate P, Yokoyama T, Mendez M (1986) Mitral valve repair for mitral regurgitation secondary to artery disease. Circulation 74(suppl I):88–98
13. Rankin JS, Livesey SA, smith LR, et al. (1989) Trends in the surgical treatment of ischemic mitral regurgitation: effects of mitral valve repair on hospital mortality. Semin Thorac Cardiovasc Surg 1:149–163
14. Von Oppell UO, Stemmet F, Brink J, Commerford PJ, Heijke SA (2000) Ischemic mitral valve surgery. J Heart Valve Dis 9:64–73
15. Lee EM, Shapiro LM, Well FC (1995) Mortality and morbidity after mitral valve repair. The importance of left ventricular function. J Heart Valve Dis 4:460–468
16. Rankin JS, Hickey MSJ, Smith LR, DeBruijn NP, Sheikh KH, Sabiston DC (1991) Current concepts in the pathogenesis and treatment of ischemic mitral regurgitation. In: Vetter, Hetzer, Schmutzler (eds) Ischemic Mitral Incompetence. Springer Verlag, Heidelberg, pp 127–178
17. Menicanti L, Di Donato M, Frigiola A, Buckberg G, Santambrogio C, Ranucci M, Santo D, RESTORE roup (2002) Ischemic mitral regurgitation: intraventricular papillary muscle imbrication without mitral ring during left ventricular restoration. J Cardiothorac Surg123:1041–1050
18. Rothenburger M, Rokusujew A, Hammel D, Dorenkamp A, Scheld HH (2002) Mitral valve surgery in patients with poor left ventricular dysfunction. Thorac Cardiovasc Surg 6:351–354
19. Szalay ZA. Civelek A, Hobe S, Brunner-LaRocca HP, Klovekorn WP, Knez I, Vogt PR, Bauer EP (2003) Mitral annuloplasty in patients with ischemic versus dilated cardiomyopathy. Eur J Cardiothorac Surg 4:567–572
20. Chen F, Adams D, Aranki S, Collins J, Couper G, Rizzo R, Cohn L (1998) Mitral valve repair in cardiomyopathy. Circulation 98:II124–II127
21. Lachmann J, Shirani J, Pletis K, Frater R, Le Jemtel T (2001) Mitral ring annuloplasty: an incomplete correction of functional mitral regurgitation associated with left ventricular remodeling. Curr Cardiol Rep 3:241–246
22. Bolling S (2002) Mitral reconstruction in cardiomyopathy. J Heart Valve Dis 11:S25–S31
23. Silberman S, Klutstein MW, Sabag T, Oren A, Fink D, Merin O, Bitran D (2009) Repair of ischemic mitral regurgitation: comparison between flexible and rigid annuloplasty rings. Ann Thorac Surg 87:1721–1727
24. Hetzer R, Drews T, S iniawski H, Komoda T, Hofmeister J, Weng Y (1995). preservation of papillary muscles and chordae during mitral valve replacement: possibilities and limitations. J Heart Valve Disease 4(Suppl II):S115–S123
25. David TE, Uden DE, Strauss HD (1983) The importance of the mitral apparatus in left ventricular function after correction of mitral regurgitation. Circulation 68(3 pt 2):1176–1182
26. Sarris GE, Cahill PD, Hansen DE, Derby GC, Miller DC (1988) Restoration of left ventricular systolic performance after reattachment of the mitral chordae tendineae. The importance of valvular-ventricular interaction. J Thorac Cardiovasc Surg 95:969–979
27. Huikuri HV (1983) Effect of mitral valve replacement on left ventricular function in mitral regurgitation. Br Heart J 49:328–333
28. Tischler MD, Cooper KA, Rowen M, Le Winter MM (1994) Myocardial function/valvular heart disease/hypertensive heart disease: mitral valve replacement versus mitral valve repair: a Doppler and quantitative stress echocardiographic study. Circulation 89:132–137

29. Hausmann H, Siniawski H, Hotz H, Hofmeister J, Chavez T, Schmidt G, Hetzer R (1997) Mitral valve reconstruction and mitral valve replacement in ischemic mitral insufficiency. J Card Surg 12:8–14
30. Hausmann H, Siniawski H, Hetzer R (1999) Mitral valve reconstruction and replacement for ischemic mitral insufficiency: seven years' follow-up. J Heart Valve Dis 8:536–542
31. Prifti E, Bonacchi M, Frati G, et al. (2000) Early and midterm outcome of coronary artery bypass grafting in end-stage coronary artery disease patients. Cor Europaeum 8:93–99
32. Czer LS, Maurer G, Bolger AF, De Robertis M, Chaux A, Matloff JM (1996) Revascularization alone or in combined with suture annuloplasty for ischemic mitral regurgitation: evaluation by color Doppler echocardiography. Tex heart Inst J 23:270–278
33. Christenson JT, Simonet F, Bloch A, Maurice J, Schmuziger M (1995) Should a mild to moderate mitral valve regurgitation in patients with poor left ventricular function be repaired or not. J Heart Valve Dis 4:484–488
34. Pinson CW Cobanoglu A, Metzdorff MT, Grunkemeier GL, Kay PH, Starr A (1984) Late surgical results for ischemic mitral regurgitation. Role of wall motion score and severity of regurgitation. J Thorac Cardiovasc Surg 88:663–72

Effects of valve repair on long-term patient outcomes after mitral valve surgery

M.A. Daneshmand, J.G. Gaca, J.S. Rankin, C.A. Milano, D.D. Glower, W.G. Wolfe, P.K. Smith

16.1 Introduction

Over the past decade, techniques for mitral valve repair have expanded considerably [1], so that most mitral pathologies now can be repaired routinely [2, 3]. A question still exists, however, whether patients would benefit from more liberal application of repair, and if so, in what disease categories and clinical situations. One way to address this problem, or at least to gain insights, would be to review experiences with previous patient cohorts. Faced with this question 5 years ago, the authors began a systematic analysis of mitral surgery patients receiving care at Duke University over the past 20 years. Because all surgical patients had been entered into a prospective databank over that time, the opportunity existed to examine long-term outcomes, using multivariable analysis methodology. The purpose of this paper is to review those studies, with the goal of summarizing the benefits of mitral valve repair on patient outcomes observed in our clinical experience.

16.2 Methods

All studies of survival after mitral surgery were performed with approval from the Duke Institutional Review Board and under a waiver of informed consent. In the Duke Databank for Cardiovascular Disease, 2,064 consecutive patients with isolated mitral disease who underwent cardiac surgery from January 1, 1986 through December 31, 2006 were reviewed [4]. Patients having concomitant CABG or atrial ablation were included, but other major cardiac procedures were excluded (e.g., aortic valves, tricuspid valves, postinfarct ventricular septal defects, ventricular aneurysm repair). While patients with previous CABG were included, those with previous mitral replacement were excluded, because they potentially were not candidates for either procedure.

Preoperative baseline and intraoperative characteristics for all patients were recorded prospectively over the entire 20 years, with a consistent variable set throughout. Late outcome data were collected prospectively on patients with significant concomitant coronary disease per Duke Databank protocols. A National Death Index (NDI) search was conducted through 2006 to acquire mortality results for remaining patients. Patients were divided into two groups: the first group included patients having mitral repair (n=1,188), and the second group included patients having prosthetic valve replacement (n=876) with mechanical valves (n=680 (78%); predominantly St. Jude valves) or tissue valves (n=196 (22%); predominantly Carpentier Edwards porcine or pericardial bioprostheses). They also were grouped into etiology of mitral disease for each specific study, including elderly patients, degenerative disease, ischemic MR, and rheumatic etiology. Operative notes of all 2,064 patients were audited to ensure proper categorization. Most repairs had full ring annuloplasty (usually Edwards Physio, Carpentier classic, or Seguin rings) along with appropriate leaflet or chordal procedures. Innumerable different repair combinations were used, depending on surgeon preference, anatomy encountered, and evolution of techniques over time, and 18 different surgeons contributed. Partial or total chordal-sparing valve replacement was performed frequently, but this variable was not documented well and was not assessed in the analysis. Follow-up for survival was 92% complete, and only all-cause mortality was consistently available for analysis.

In each study, baseline characteristics and clinical event rates were described using medians with 25th and 75th percentiles for continuous variables and frequencies and proportions for categorical variables. Descriptive data were compared using the Wilcoxon rank-sum test for continuous and ordinal variables, and a Pearson χ^2 or Fisher's exact test for categorical variables. Three propensity models were created to determine the propensity for repair versus mechanical replacement, repair versus tissue replacement, and mechanical versus tissue replacement [5]. A multivariable Cox proportional hazards regression model was employed for each study with an analysis strategy that adjusted for the impact of differences in baseline characteristics on survival [6], allowing assessment of individual procedures for each etiology of valve disease. To develop each risk adjustment model, a pool of all known clinical covariates that have been shown to be important in previous analyses was developed. Variables proving significant by stepwise univariable/multivariable procedures were included in the final Cox model and also used for risk adjustment. Propensity scores were included in most Cox models, as were the valve repair versus replacement variables of interest. Continuous and ordinal variables were tested for linearity over the log hazard and transformed as necessary. Adjusted survival estimates for each group were calculated by applying their baseline hazard functions, along with parameter estimates, to all patients in the entire cohort and then averaging over all patients at each time point. Statistical analyses were performed using SAS version 8.2 (SAS Institute, Cary, NC, USA), and $p \leq 0.05$ was considered significant.

16.3 Results

16.3.1 Overall mitral surgery

Baseline characteristics of the entire population are detailed in ◘ Table 16.1 [4]. Among the groups, tissue replacement patients were significantly older with less elective surgery. Mechanical replacement patients were younger, and repair patients were more predominantly male, had a higher incidence of concurrent 3-vessel disease and CABG, and lower ejection fractions. Procedural incidence over time is shown in ◘ Fig. 16.1 with mitral repair increasing dramatically in

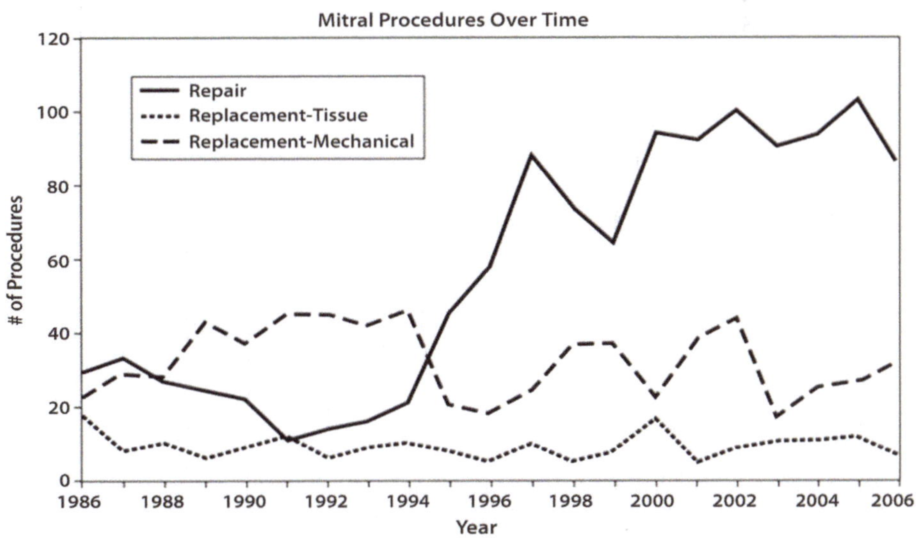

◘ **Fig. 16.1.** Numbers of mitral procedures per year performed at Duke University from 1986 through 2006. Procedures are subdivided into mitral repair (*solid line*), mechanical mitral valve replacement (*dashed line*), and tissue mitral replacement (*dotted line*). Mitral repair increased dramatically over the period

Table 16.1. Baseline characteristics of overall mitral surgery population

	Total (*n*=2,064)	Mitral valve repair (*n*=1,188)	Tissue	Mechanical	Overall p value
			Mitral valve replacement (*n*=196)	Mitral valve replacement (*n*=680)	
Age	64 (53, 72)	64 (53, 72)[*,$]	72 (63, 77)[&,$]	62 (52, 70)[&,*]	<0.0001
Gender					
Male (%)	46%	54%[*,$]	33.7%[&]	36%[&]	<0.0001
Female (%)	54%	46%[*,$]	66%[&]	64%	
Caucasian race	76%	76%	74%	77%	0.6581
History of diabetes	17%	19%[$]	16%	13%[&]	0.0020
Hypertension	50%	55%[$]	49%	44%[&]	<0.0001
Hyperlipidemia	34%	39%[*,$]	28%[&]	28%[&]	<0.0001
BMI	26 (23, 30)	26 (23, 30)[*]	25 (22, 28)[&,$]	26 (23, 30)[*]	0.0024
History of renal failure	4%	4%[*,$]	10%[&,$]	2%[&,*]	<0.0001
NYHA class					
I	32%	33%	29%	29%	0.0428
II	15%	16%	16%	14%	
III	31%	30%	26%	35%	
IV	22%	21%	29%	22%	
Chronic lung disease	10%	10%	9%	10%	0.8542
Infectious endocarditis	3%	2%[*]	7%[&,$]	3%[*]	<0.0001
History of CVA	10%	9%	9%	11%	0.1893
History of MI	24%	30%[*,$]	21%[&]	16%[&]	<0.0001
History of tobacco abuse	42%	41%	39%	44%	0.3539
Ejection fraction	50% (40, 60)	50% (34, 58)[*,$]	55% (45, 64)[&]	55% (45, 63)[&]	<0.0001
3-Vessel disease	22%	29%[*,$]	19%[&,$]	11%[&,*]	<0.0001
Previous CABG	3%	3%	5%	2%	0.1366
Concomitant CABG	39%	46%[$]	39%[$]	29%[&,*]	<0.0001
Clinical status					
Elective	70%	68%[*,$]	59%[&,$]	75%[&,*]	<0.0001
Nonelective	30%	32%[*,$]	41%[&,$]	25%[&,*]	

[*]p<0.05 compared to tissue replacement; [$]p<0.05 compared to mechanical replacement; [&]p<0.05 compared to repair

recent years. Regardless of age and operative procedure, the most common etiology of mitral valve disease was degenerative followed by ischemic (Table 16.2). Rheumatic patients comprised 20% of the population and more frequently underwent mitral replacement (88%), while ischemic and degenerative etiologies usually had repair. Raw *unadjusted* 30-day mortality was 3.5% for mitral repair, 5.9% for mechanical replacement, and 8.2% for tissue replacement. Long-term *unadjusted* Kaplan–Meier survival was not significantly different between mitral valve repair and mechanical mitral valve replacement for the overall population (Fig. 16.2a), and both groups had significantly better raw survival as compared to tissue valve replacement. Final Cox model coefficients are shown in Table 16.3, and after having been adjusted for dif-

Table 16.2. Distribution of valve disease etiology

	Total (*n*=2,064)	Mitral valve repair (*n*=1,188)	Tissue mitral valve replacement (*n*=196)	Mechanical mitral valve replacement (*n*=680)
Degenerative	42%	51%	32%	28%
Ischemic	22%	31%	12%	9%
Rheumatic	20%	4%	26%	47%
Other	11%	11%	12%	11%
Infectious	5%	3%	18%	5%

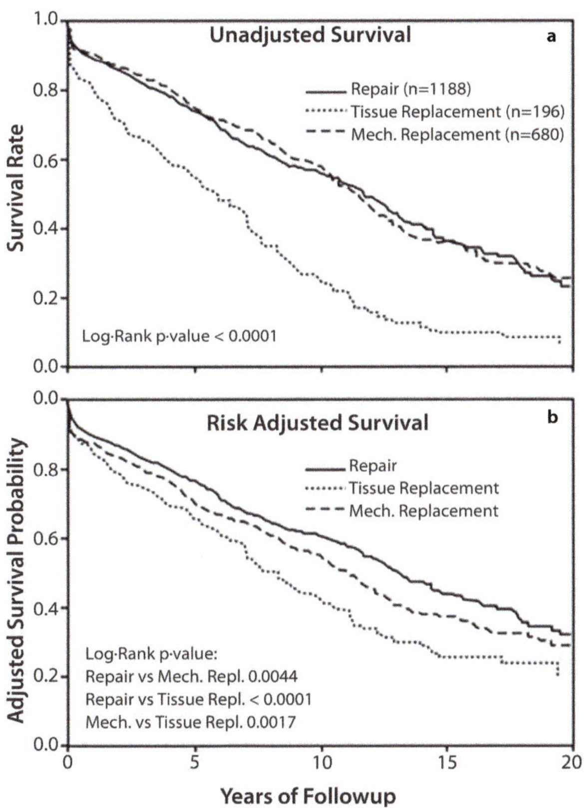

Fig. 16.2. Patient survival in the overall group (*n*=2,064) after mitral repair (*solid line*), mechanical mitral replacement (*dashed line*), and tissue mitral replacement (dotted line). Unadjusted Kaplan–Meier survival data are shown in **a**, and survival adjusted by the Cox model for differences in baseline characteristics are illustrated in **b**. Adjusted survival was significantly better with mitral repair, and worse with tissue mitral replacement

Table 16.3. Overall Cox model parameters

Risk factor	Wald χ^2	HR	95% CI		p value
Dialysis	6.9	2.2	1.2	3.9	0.0088
Tissue valve replacement	28.9	1.8	1.5	2.3	<0.00001
History of peripheral vascular disease	24.5	1.7	1.4	2.1	<0.00001
History of CABG	10.2	1.7	1.2	2.3	0.0014
Full sternotomy	7.3	1.5	1.1	1.9	0.0069
History of cerebrovascular disease	12.4	1.4	1.2	1.8	0.0004
Age (HR per 10 years; truncated low end at 50)	32.7	1.4	1.3	1.6	<0.0001
History of diabetes	12.7	1.4	1.2	1.7	0.0004
Nonelective surgery	10.8	1.4	1.1	1.7	0.0010
Chronic lung disease	5.6	1.3	1.0	1.6	0.0180
Mechanical valve replacement	8.1	1.3	1.1	1.5	0.0044
Ischemic valve etiology	4.8	1.3	1.0	1.5	0.0287
GFR (HR per 5 unit decrease; truncated high end at 100)	27.6	1.2	1.1	1.4	<0.00001
Number of diseased vessels (HR per increase of 1)	2.3	1.1	1.0	1.1	0.1323
Ejection fraction (HR per 5% decrease)	11.2	1.0	1.0	1.1	0.0008
Year of surgery (HR per 1 year increase)	11.3	1.0	1.0	1.0	0.0008
Caucasian race	7.8	0.8	0.7	0.9	0.0052
Mechanical vs. tissue replacement propensity	8.8				0.0031
Repair vs. tissue replacement propensity	7.3				0.0070
Repair vs. mechanical replacement propensity	7.2				0.0072

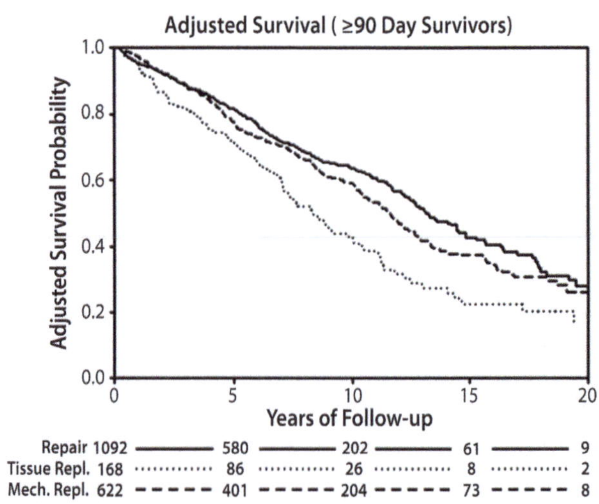

Fig. 16.3. In patients surviving the 90-day operative period, risk-adjusted late survival was still statistically best in patients receiving mitral repair and worse in those having tissue mitral valve replacement

ferences in baseline characteristics, the *risk-adjusted survival estimates* for the overall population are displayed in Fig. 16.2b. Adjusted curves demonstrated better survival with mitral repair than mechanical replacement, and even after adjustment for adverse risk profiles, tissue replacement survival was still inferior to both. In another Cox model, survival curves were generated for patients surviving 90 days after surgery in order to compare relative late mortalities. Conditional adjusted survival estimates demonstrated persistent superiority of repair over mechanical replacement, and both were better than tissue valve replacement (Fig. 16.3).

16.3.2 Elderly patients

In an analysis subset ≥65 years of age (*n*=998), baseline characteristics were more similar between groups, but mitral repair patients (*n*=563) still had more 3-vessel disease, CABG, nonelective presentation, and lower ejection fractions [4]. Elderly mitral replacement patients (mechanical *n*=293; tissue *n*=142) were more predominantly female. The finding of better raw survival after repair was preserved in the *unadjusted* Kaplan–Meier survival comparison of patients ≥65 years (Fig. 16.4). In the Cox model, no treatment interaction was observed between procedural choice and age (p=0.1781). In other words, the hazard associated with each treatment was the same across all ages. Finally, adjusted survival probabilities at 10 years versus age at valve implant are shown in Fig. 16.5. Regardless of patient age, mitral repair was associated with better risk-adjusted 10-year survival compared to either mechanical or tissue valves. At no age did tissue valve replacement achieve equivalent results to either of the other two procedures [4].

16.3.3 Ischemic mitral regurgitation

In a subanalysis of patient having mitral surgery for postinfarction ischemic mitral regurgitation, patients were divided into two groups. Group I (*n*=16,209) consisted of coronary artery disease patients having no evidence of ischemic mitral regurgitation (IMR) based on preop-

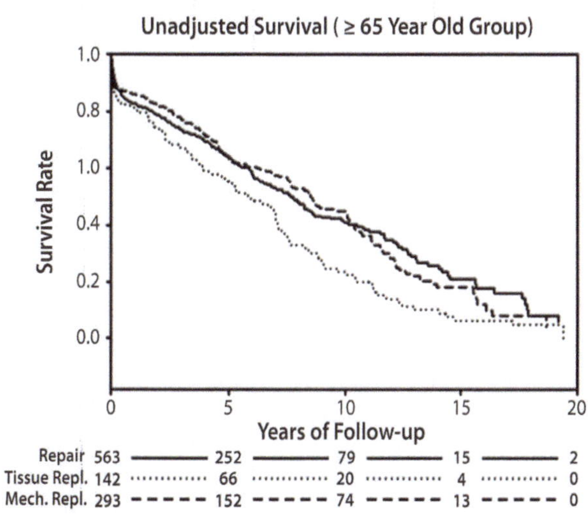

Fig. 16.4. In the elderly population >65 years of age, raw Kaplan–Meier survival was inferior with tissue valve replacement (p<0.001), whereas the higher risk repair group (containing most of the ischemic MR population) achieved equivalent survival to the lower-risk mechanical repair patients

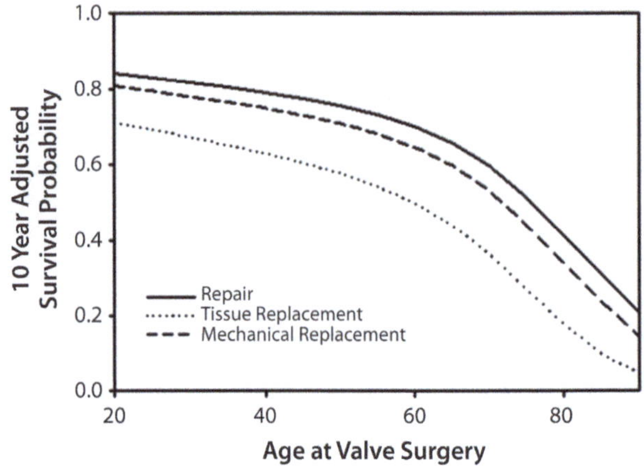

Fig. 16.5. After adjustment for differences in baseline characteristics, 10-year survival was best with repair, and worse with tissue valves, across the entire spectrum of patient age at implant

erative and intraoperative studies [7, 8]. These patients underwent coronary artery bypass alone. Group II consisted of coronary patients prospectively defined to have any degree of mitral regurgitation (MR), based on either preoperative or intraoperative studies (including preoperative dye ventriculography, transthoracic echocardiography, or transesophageal echocardiography), or by the surgeon in the operative note. Group II patients in turn were divided into patients who received CABG-only (IIa) (n=3,181), MV repair±CABG (IIb) (n=416), or MV replacement±CABG (IIc) (n=106). The hospital charts of all 522 patients having mitral valve procedures were audited to ensure proper categorization. Of the repairs, 30 patients received modified Kay annuloplasties, and the remaining 376 were managed with insertion of full annuloplasty rings. In the replacement group, 53% of patients received a bioprosthesis, while 47% received a mechanical valve.

With regard to baseline characteristics, patients with IMR (Group II) demonstrated worse preoperative risk factor profiles than Group I. Specific adverse factors in Group II included greater age, hyperlipidemia, diabetes, hypertension, and renal insufficiency, as well as advanced heart failure class, reduction in ejection fraction (EF), and history of myocardial infarction (MI). A higher percentage of females existed in Group II, suggesting that IMR may disproportionately affect women. Comparing Groups IIb and IIc, IIb patients displayed more class IV heart failure symptoms, worse EF, greater history of MI, as well as more diabetes, hypertension, and hyperlipidemia. The incidence of prior CABG was higher for Group II relative to Group I, but was similar between Groups IIb and IIc (16.8% versus 16.0% respectively). Mean follow-up was 8 years.

Raw Kaplan–Meier survival was best for patients undergoing CABG without evidence of preoperative IMR (Fig. 16.6, top panel). The presence of IMR (Group II) was associated with reduced unadjusted survival, regardless of treatment. Survival curves risk adjusted within the Cox model for differences in baseline characteristics are shown in Fig. 16.6 (bottom panel). Much of the reduced survival for Group II patients seemed to relate to worse preoperative risk factors, and adjusted Group IIa and IIb curves better approximated survival for Group I. After risk adjustment, IIb patients (valve repair) continued to demonstrate statistically and clinically better survival relative to IIc (valve replacement). In the area under the curve analysis, IIa patients (mild–moderate MR/no valve procedure) achieved 97.7% of Group I survival,

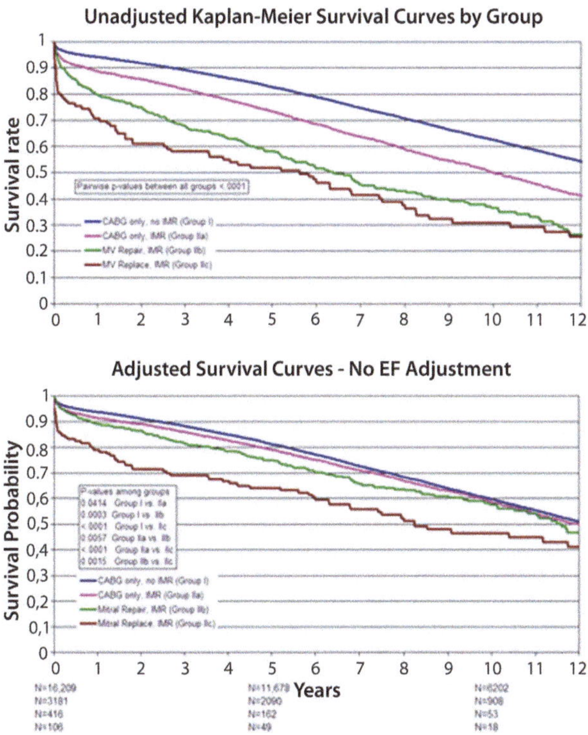

■ **Fig. 16.6.** Long-term survival for ischemic MR patients (Groups IIa, IIb, and IIc) relative to the standard coronary bypass population (*blue*, Group I). Ischemic MR patients are divided into Group IIa (i.e., patients with mild-to-moderated MR having coronary bypass only (*purple*)), Group IIb (i.e., patients having mitral valve repair (*green*)), and IIc (i.e., patients having mitral valve replacement (*brown*)). **a** The raw unadjusted Kaplan–Meier survival curves are shown, and **b** survival adjusted with the Cox model for differences in baseline characteristics are illustrated. Relative to standard coronary bypass patients, valve repair (*red*) achieved 93.7% of »potential long-term survival« observed after coronary bypass with no mitral valve disease, whereas mitral replacement (*brown*) was associated with a significantly worse risk-adjusted outcome, achieving only 79.1% of »potential survival«

and IIb patients 93.7% (mitral repair), while Group IIc patients achieved only 79.1% (mitral replacement). Thus, ischemic MR patients receiving mitral repair experienced an average of 14.1% better risk-adjusted survival over the follow-up time.

The most prominent difference between Group I and Group II was observed in the immediate postoperative period. The 30-day operative mortality for each of the cohorts was as follows: Group I 2.5%, Group IIa 4.6%, Group IIb 6.3%, and Group IIc 18.9%, respectively (all statistically different, $p<0.01$). To address late results, adjusted survival curves for patients surviving 90 days after the procedure in each of the groups were assessed. Even when perioperative mortality was eliminated, survival was different for all groups ($p<0.01$), favoring valve repair. Late cardiac-related mortality was similar in each of the groups; or stated differently, Group II patients did not experience greater late cardiac mortality, supporting the durability of the IMR treatment strategies, including MV repair [7, 8].

16.3.4 Degenerative mitral valve disease

The application of mitral valve repair versus replacement in degenerative disease increased steadily over the 20 years [9]. Analysis of baseline characteristics for 989 degenerative patients again subdivided into Group I (repair) and Group II (replacement) revealed worse risk factors for Group II vs Group I, included greater age (68 vs. 62 years), more CABG surgery (32% vs. 24%), and more nonelective surgery (34% vs. 25%), whereas Group I had worse congestive heart failure (68% vs. 43%) and lower ejection fractions (0.51 vs. 0.55) (all p<0.05). Categorization as severe regurgitation was worse for replacement patients (50% vs. 25%).

Unadjusted Kaplan–Meier survival was better for patients undergoing valve repair versus replacement (Fig. 16.7a). Survival curves risk adjusted with the Cox model for differences in baseline characteristics are shown in Fig. 16.7b. Part of the reduced survival for Group II was related to worse baseline risk factors in replacement patients, and Group II survival was more similar to Group I after risk adjustment. However, valve replacement patients continued to demonstrate statistically and clinically inferior adjusted survival relative to repair (p=0.04), with survival differences increasing over time. In the area under the curve analysis, replacement patients achieved an average of 92.7% of repair survival over 15 years; 99.3% for years 0–5, 95.1% for years 5–10, and 78.7% for years 10–15 (Fig. 16.7). In Group I, 24 of 705 (3.4%) patients subsequently underwent reoperation for valve procedure at Duke, whereas in Group II, 13 of 284 (4.6%) patients were reoperated. The proportion of late deaths that were categorized as cardiac-related was approximately 5% lower for Group I, consistent in magnitude with the survival differences observed.

Within the primary Cox model, the treatment interaction between repair versus replacement and age was negative (p=0.66), similar to the overall analysis. In Fig. 16.8, unadjusted survival curves for repair versus replacement, stratified for age greater than and less than 65 years, are shown to illustrate this point. In a logistic regression model examining factors determining referral propensity, year of surgery was by far the most important determinant of performing repair, with repair rates increasing in recent years (Fig. 16.1). Age was also significant, but less important, with elderly patients having a higher propensity for valve replace-

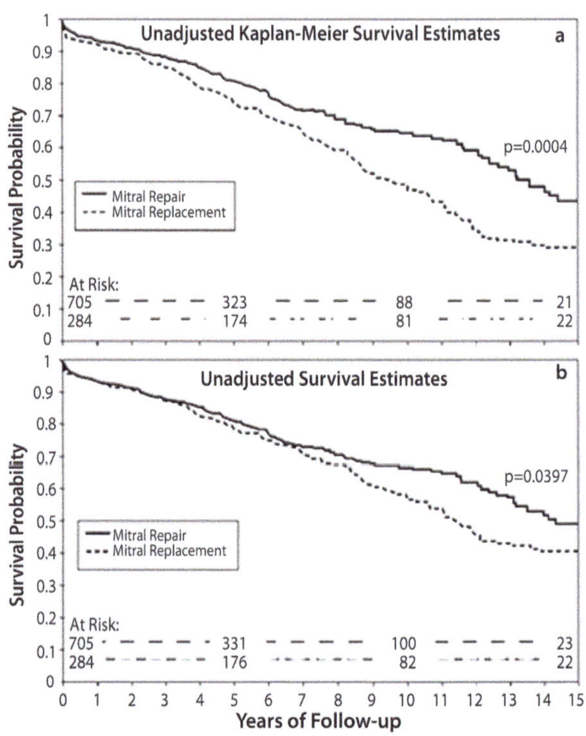

Fig. 16.7. In patients with degenerative mitral valve disease, unadjusted (**a**) and risk-adjusted (**b**) survival curves are presented for mitral valve repair (*solid line*) and valve replacement (*dotted line*). Outcomes were statistically and clinically better after mitral valve repair

ment. Risk adjustment then was accomplished using propensity stratification by dividing the population into quintiles based upon propensity for mitral repair and using the propensity classes (quintiles) as a stratification variable. Mitral replacement (versus repair) was still a significant predictor of mortality (p= 0.046; HR = 1.282; 95%CI [1.004, 1.636]), and specific survival differences for each quintile of propensity at each follow-up time are shown in ◘ Fig. 16.9 [9]. It is interesting that the Cox model and pure propensity analyses correlated so well.

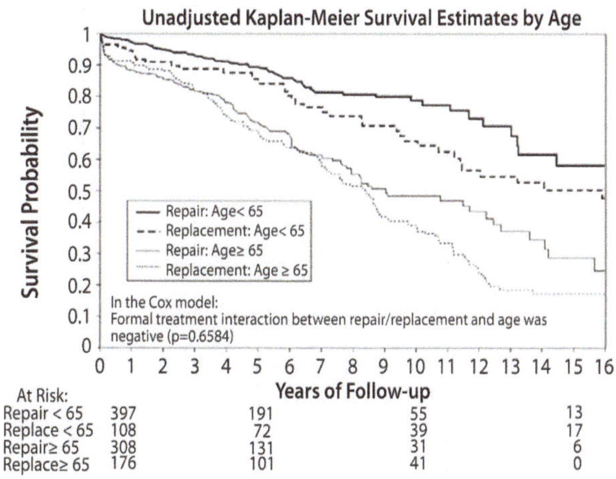

◘ **Fig. 16.8.** Unadjusted survival of degenerative valve disease patients greater than and less than age 65 years, stratified for mitral repair versus mitral replacement. In all categories, valve repair achieved superior results

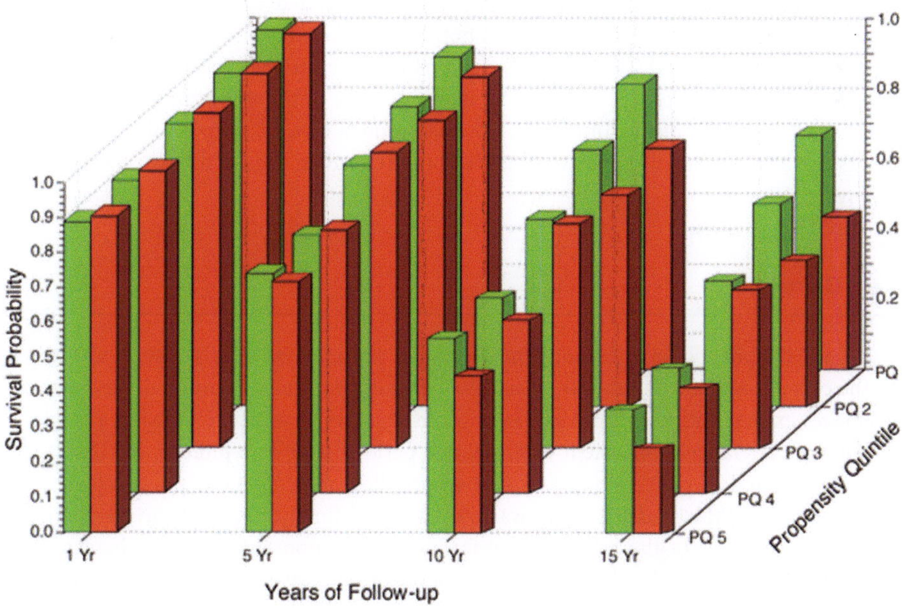

◘ **Fig. 16.9.** Raw survival outcomes of degenerative mitral disease patients categorized into five subgroups according to the propensity to perform repair (*green*) versus replacement (*red*) as determined by logistic regression. Long-term survival was better in all categories and also overall with mitral valve repair

16.3.5 Rheumatic disease

Baseline characteristics for the entire group of patients with rheumatic mitral valve disease (n=416) having mitral valve repair (n=47) and mitral valve replacement (n=369) were similar [10]. Patients undergoing mitral valve repair constituted 11% of the rheumatic population. The average age of patients undergoing mitral valve repair (57 years) was similar to that of patients undergoing mitral valve replacement (58 years). Interestingly, both groups were younger than the degenerative disease cohort (62 years). Mitral stenosis was the predominant lesion in both groups, comprising 68.1% of the repair group and 72.4% of the replacement group. The rates of diabetes, hypertension, dialysis, renal failure, peripheral vascular disease, infectious endocarditis, congestive heart failure, hyperlipidemia, chronic lung disease, cerebrovascular disease, prior PCI, prior CABG, ejection fraction, tricuspid valve disease, and nonelective operative status were not statistically different between the two groups. Repair patients had slightly more coronary disease (19.1% vs. 17.6%) and multivessel grafting. Patients in the replacement groups were more likely to have undergone a minimally invasive approach (31%) than patients in the repair groups (9%). Median follow-up was also longer in the repair group (13.2 years) than in the replacement group (5.4 years), indicating that repair was more common in earlier years.

Commissurotomy was the most frequently performed operation, constituting 28 (59.5%) of the 47 mitral valve repairs. This was followed by annuloplasty alone in 9 patients (19.1%), commissurotomy and annuloplasty in 4 patients (8.5%), and annuloplasty, chordal transfer, artificial chords in 3 patients (6.4%). Leaflet resection was rarely performed (2 patients), and annuloplasty and closure of mitral clefts was achieved in 1 patient. Mechanical mitral valve replacement was performed in 318 patients (86%) and bioprosthetic mitral valve replacement in 51 patients (14%). Mitral valve repair patients exhibited significantly better survival compared to mitral valve replacement in both unadjusted ($p<0.0001$) and risk-adjusted analyses ($p=0.008$, HR 1.94) (▪ Fig. 16.10). The preoperative variables with the greatest effects on survival were advanced age followed by dialysis. Nine of the 47 repair patients (19.1%) required reoperation at our institution at a median time of 6 years. Mitral valve replacement patients had a lower rate of reoperation (2.4%), but the median time of follow-up was shorter at 2.7 years [10].

16.4 Discussion

16

Once again, the purpose of embarking on the studies summarized in this chapter was to validate the current expansion of mitral repair into a greater percentage of mitral disease patients. Advantages existed with the approach used in this analysis. It was performed at a single institution with a relatively consistent technical and perioperative care philosophy. The sample size was good, and all patients had prospective recording of a consistent and complete set of baseline variables. Maximal follow-up was 20 years, and finally, the multivariable statistical approaches were state-of-the-art, adjusting for all known important baseline characteristics and propensity for procedural selection. This approach, however, is not without its limitations. An important issue is the validity of comparing procedures that may not have been equally applicable to all patients or all mitral disease pathologies. Because repair techniques have evolved so that reconstruction now can be performed in most patient categories, this point becomes less relevant at present, and late outcome comparisons become useful to guide

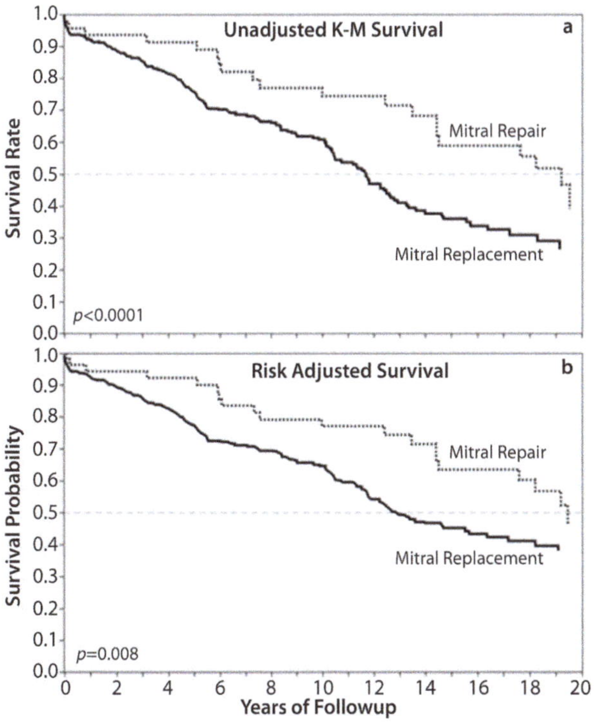

Fig. 16.10. Unadjusted (**a**) and risk-adjusted (**b**) survival for patients with rheumatic mitral disease undergoing mitral repair (*dotted line*) versus mitral valve replacement. Although valve anatomy was probably different between groups and reoperation rate was higher after repair, survival was best after mitral valve repair for rheumatic disease

future patient management. Another concern regards possible undefined treatment selection biases or confounding variables, such that some patients might have been selected for one treatment or another who were at higher risk than defined by baseline variables. After 25 years of work with this data set, however, the determinants of mortality in mitral surgery are pretty well understood, and although minor factors may have been omitted, the major determinants are likely accounted for. Eighteen different surgeons contributed patients over the 20 years, so that significant variability in procedural selection philosophies existed. Propensity regressions showed that surgeon of record accounted for most of the procedural selection decisions, rather than any sort of systematic bias based on patient characteristics. Thus, most surgeons »believed« in one approach or the other, and practiced accordingly and in a consistent way. It is also evident that individual surgeon philosophies changed over time, and as stability of repair with autologous tissues became more apparent, the proportion of repair procedures increased dramatically (Fig. 16.1). While a general selection bias existed toward employing bioprostheses in the elderly, *larger numbers* of sick elderly patients received mechanical valves and repair in the >65-year-old subgroup. In fact, the very sickest cohort, ischemic mitral regurgitation, was managed predominantly with repair. Thus, a spectrum of procedural selection philosophies existed among the 18 surgeons, supporting the appropriateness of the comparisons in this chapter. With a large sample size, long follow-up, a comprehensive and consistent variable set, and meticulous multivariable modeling, this type of observational analysis has been shown to be quite accurate even though possibilities for confounders always exist. Thus, like any observational analysis, the results of these studies should be qualified and interpreted within this context, but are probably the most precise performed to date.

Before and after risk adjustment for differences in preoperative baseline characteristics, mitral repair had the best predicted survival overall and in all categories of patients studied. Mechanical valve replacement was inferior to repair, but was always second in terms of survival prognosis. Surprisingly, tissue valves in the mitral position fared the worst and seemed inferior to both of the other options. This relationship was maintained in the older mitral disease population and far into the advanced age group. In the 90-day survival cohort, mitral repair still had better risk-adjusted outcomes, followed by mechanical then tissue valve replacement. Because nonfatal events were not available in these studies, the cause of this finding is unclear. However, it is likely related to worse valve-related complications after prosthetic replacement, including thromboembolism, anticoagulation complications, endocarditis, and valve degeneration (which occurs at a higher rate for tissue valves in the mitral position). Somewhat unexpected was the finding in the Cox model that tissue valve replacement had an associated hazard ratio of 1.8, second only to preoperative hemodialysis dependence. While the superiority of mitral repair relative to mechanical mitral replacement was definite but subtle, it seemed clear that tissue valve replacement was associated with inferior outcomes, independent of patient age. The findings of these studies suggest that valve repair should be the procedure of choice for most mitral valve disease and that tissue valves should be used only in specific situations.

The clinical outcomes observed in these studies are dependent on the quality of the mitral repairs. While valve replacement was fairly standardized during this period, repair techniques evolved significantly, enhancing both the applicability and stability of repair procedures. Repair results steadily improved, with »year of surgery« yielding a χ^2 value of 11.3 in the Cox model. Repair methods that have been shown to be less effective, such as pericardial bands, generally were avoided in the Duke practice, and utilization of inadequate repair techniques may account for some of the variability in the literature. In this series, full rings were used consistently, and management of chordal and leaflet abnormalities improved over time. Finally, it is probable that newer repair methods, such as artificial chordal replacement and autologous pericardial leaflet augmentation, will further enhance applicability and stability and that repair outcomes relative to valve replacement will continue to improve into the future.

The benefit of mitral repair on operative mortality seemed greater in acutely ill ischemic mitral regurgitation patients with adverse baseline characteristics. In contrast, differences in 30-day mortality after repair versus replacement in patients with degenerative disease were smaller, perhaps because of the more elective nature of the population. However, the long-term inferiority of valve replacement to repair was evident in both groups. Again, the reason for this difference will require further analysis of specific events, but it is now perhaps established that use of the body's own tissues to reconstruct heart valve function has significant long-term advantages. The tissue valve sample size in this study was marginal, and because of small numbers, comparison of early tissue valves with more recent designs was not possible. Therefore, further testing of the concluding hypotheses of this paper is suggested in other single institutional databases and potentially in the STS data set.

In summary, the results of multiple studies from the Duke University mitral surgery database support the concept that diseased mitral valves should be repaired regardless of etiology of valve disease or patient age. Based on these follow-up data, valves that are not amenable to repair should receive primarily mechanical mitral valve replacement. Utilization of tissue valves perhaps should be limited to irreparable patients who have contraindications to long-term systemic anticoagulation, although confirmation of these findings in other data sets seems indicated.

References

Papers referenced below are primarily the studies from which data in this chapter were generated. Within each paper, complete reference lists are given.

1. Rankin JS, Alfery DD, Orozcoa R, et al. (2008) Techniques of artificial chordal replacement for mitral valve repair: use in multiple pathologic disorders. Operat Tech Thorac Cardiovasc Surg 13:74–82
2. Rankin JS (2009) Artificial chordal replacement in complex mitral valve repair, at CTSNet: http://www.ctsnet.org/sections/clinicalresources/videos/vg2009_rankin_ACRinComplexMVR.html
3. Rankin JS, Burrichter CA, Walton-Shirley MK, et al. (2009) Trends in mitral valve surgery: a single practice experience. J Heart Valve Dis 18:359–366
4. Daneshmand MA, Milano CA, Rankin JS, et al. (2010) Influence of patient age on procedural selection in mitral valve surgery. Ann Thorac Surg 90:1479–1486
5. Blackstone EH (2002) Comparing apples and oranges. J Thorac Cardiovasc Surg 123:8–15
6. Cox D (1972) Regression model and life tables (with discussion). J R Stat Soc Ser B 34:187–220
7. Glower D, Tuttle R, Shaw L, et al. (2005) Patient survival characteristics after routine mitral valve repair for ischemic mitral regurgitation. J Thorac Cardiovasc Surg 129:860–868
8. Milano CA, Daneshmand MA, Rankin JS, et al. (2008) Survival prognosis and surgical management of ischemic mitral regurgitation. Ann Thorac Surg 86:735–744
9. Daneshmand MA, Milano CA, Rankin JS, et al. (2009) Mitral valve repair for degenerative disease: a 20-year experience. Ann Thorac Surg 88:1828–1837

V Inflammatory mitral valve disease

Repair of rheumatic mitral valve incompetence: surgical challenges and clinical results

C.A. Yankah, H. Siniawski, R. Hetzer

17.1 Introduction

Rheumatic heart valve disease (RHVD) is one of the sequelae of rheumatic fever (RF) triggered by autoimmune humoral and cellular responses [1, 2] and remains the predominant heart valve disease in developing countries [1–20]. It is seen in epidemic proportions in the preschool and school age groups but is also found in patients in their teens and early twenties. The youngest patient reported was 2 years old [10]. In addition, a number of patients present during adulthood at a mean age of 40 years in developing countries and in their early 50s and 60s in developed countries [4–20]. Rheumatic heart valve disease has become rare, virtually nonexistent in most affluent populations [3], but remains uncontrolled in developing countries with an incidence of 1.6/1000 in Liberia, 2.2/1000 in Cambodia, and 2.3/1000 in Mozambique, as determined by clinical diagnosis without echocardiograhic support [4, 5]. The global burden is estimated to be 15.6 million and about 282,000 new cases are registered each year with an annual mortality of 233,000 [6].

The disease occurs in the multicultural world as an acute or chronic rheumatic condition (burn-out RHVD) in varying degrees, including annulus dilatation, leaflet prolapse, tethering, restricted leaflet motion, shortened or elongated chordae, malformed papillary muscles, and left ventricular dysfunction. The mitral valve is involved in about 92% of the cases and mitral regurgitation is the most common lesion which requires surgical treatment [7–15, 19, 20, 28, 29].

Mitral valve repair as a surgical treatment for rheumatic mitral valve disease was first suggested by Sir Thomas Brunton in 1902 [21]. In 1923, Dr. Elliott Cutler of the Peter Bent Brigham Hospital, Boston, performed the world's first successful heart valve operation–a closed mitral valve *repair*. The patient was a 12-year-old girl with rheumatic mitral stenosis [22]. The introduction of the heart–lung machine by Gibbons in 1953 paved the way for open repair and *replacement* of the mitral valve with an artificial heart valve [23, 24].

With the support of a heart–lung machine, open mitral valve surgery to repair an incompetent mitral valve was performed by Lillehei and coworkers in 1957; however, the results were suboptimal [25, 26]. Thus, for decades, mitral valve replacement was the only surgical option for patients with a severely diseased mitral valve. Reproducible surgical repair of the diseased mitral valve apparatus was advocated by Carpentier to restore the interaction between the papillary muscle/the chordae and the leaflets and the mitral valve function [27]. The repair technique was conceived to obviate long-term anticoagulation, allow growth and uneventful pregnancy, and enable participation in active sports [9, 10, 27–31]. Echocardiography is recognized as a reliable diagnostic tool for predicting the possibility of repair of the mitral valve apparatus and for evaluating postrepair functional results [8–10, 19, 29, 30, 32]. In regions with endemic rheumatic fever and carditis, patients with a repaired mitral valve apparatus are under constant threat of recurrence of rheumatic fever and functional failure of the mitral valve. RHVD, therefore, presents a surgical and a medical challenge to surgeons not only in the developing world, but also in the developed world. This clinical report evaluates the different repair techniques for RHVD used in a single institution in Berlin and the impact of these different techniques on long-term results, followed by a review of the literature.

17.2 Patients and method

The clinical features of 50 out of 2,211 patients who underwent mitral valve repair for rheumatic valve disease between April 1986 and December 2009 at the Deustches Herzzentrum are shown in ◻ Table 17.1. Distribution of the patients by diagnosis and age groups is shown in ◻ Table 17.2. Indications for surgery were the following: (1) NYHA class III and IV (i.e., moderate to severe breathlessness on mild exertion or at rest), (2) atrial fibrillation uncontrolled by medication, (3) systemic embolization, or (4) echocardiographic evidence of reduced mitral valve opening area of below 1.5 cm^2/m^2 of body surface area. Frequency and pattern of valve involvement in rheumatic valve disease are shown in ◻ Table 17.3 [3].

◻ **Table 17.1.** Patients who underwent rheumatic mitral valve repair between April 1986 and December 2009 at the Deutsches Herzzentrum Berlin

Total mitral valve repair procedures	2,211
Rheumatic mitral valve repair	50 (2.3%)
Women	32
Men	18
Age (median)	45.6 years
Age range	5–82 years
<16 years	10 (20%)
≥16 years	40 (80%)
<20 years	13 (26%)
≥20 years	37 (74%)
Isolated mitral valve repair	20 (40%)
Concomitant procedures (CABG, re-CABG, AVR, re-AVR)	30 (60%)
Follow-up time	0.1–22 years
Patient–years	412
Median follow-up	6.0 years
Complete follow-up	100%

◻ **Table 17.2.** Rheumatic mitral valve disease. Distribution of patients by age and diagnosis. Deutsches Herzzentrum Berlin 1986–2009 (*n*=50). Reproduced from the Jornal of Heart Valve Disease (JHVD)

Lesions	*n*	<10 years	11–20 years	21–40 years	>40 years
Total	50	2	11	8	29
Pure MS	4	0	0	0	4
Pure MR	37	2	9	4	22
Mixed lesion (MS + MR)	9	0	2	4	3

MS mitral stenosis, *MR* mitral regurgitation

Table 17.3. Frequency and pattern of valve involvement at autopsy in rheumatic heart valve disease *n*=221 [20]

Valve involved	*n*	Percentage
Mitral alone	70	31.6
Mitral and aortic	57	25.7
Aortic alone	2	0.9
Mitral, aortic and tricuspid	60	27.1
Mitral and tricuspid	25	11.3
Mitral, aortic, tricuspid, and pulmonary	7[a]	3.2

[a]Acute rheumatic carditis

17.3 Establishing the diagnosis

The most common presenting signs and symptoms include fatigue, decreased exercise capacity, shortness of breath, and palpitations or supraventricular arrhythmias, such as atrial fibrillation. Auscultatory examination usually reveals a high-pitched systolic murmur radiating from the apex to the axilla. A holosystolic murmur suggests prolapse simultaneous with ejection typical of chordal rupture, whereas a murmur beginning in mid- or late systole favors billowing or chordal elongation. The electrocardiogram may be normal or show evidence of left atrial enlargement or atrial fibrillation. Radiographic findings may include left atrial and ventricular dilatation and prominent pulmonary vasculature in patients with long-standing severe mitral regurgitation.

Transesophageal echocardiography (TEE) is a useful adjunct to confirm the diagnosis and understand the mechanism of the rheumatic valve disease in the case of a nondefinitive transthoracic examination. Experience was also been gained with three-dimensional (3D) echocardiography in the assessment of annular geometry, leaflet coaptation, and leaflet dysfunction in the setting of mitral regurgitation, and it is predicted to have a more significant role in planning reparative procedures [8–10, 29, 30, 32].

The regurgitant volume and the effective orifice area of mitral regurgitation are measured and graded as mild, moderate, and severe. A biplane vena contracta width is measured to predict the regurgitant orifice area. Regurgitant jet geometry and area are assessed in multiple views, and mitral regurgitation severity is graded typically as a rank order variable, e.g., 1+=trace, 2+=mild, 3+=moderate, and 4+=severe mitral regurgitation (see Table 17.4) [(5, 8–10, 19].

17.4 Pathomorphology of rheumatic mitral valve disease

The pathogenesis of rheumatic heart disease and morphological changes of rheumatic mitral valve apparatus are shown in Figs. 17.1–17.3. The structural changes of a chorda tendineae (cross sectional and oblique views) of a rheumatic mitral valve are shown in Fig. 17.3. The

Table 17.4. Functional classification of mitral valve regurgitation. Data from [5, 8–10, 19]

Grading of MR	RV (ml)	EROA (cm²)
Mild (2+)	<30	<0.2
Moderate (3+)	30–59	0.2–0.39
Severe (4+)	≥60	≥0.4
Vena contracta width ≤0.3 cm ≥0.5 cm	 <60 ≥60	 <0.4 >0.4

RV regurgitant volume, *EROA* effective regurgitant orifice area

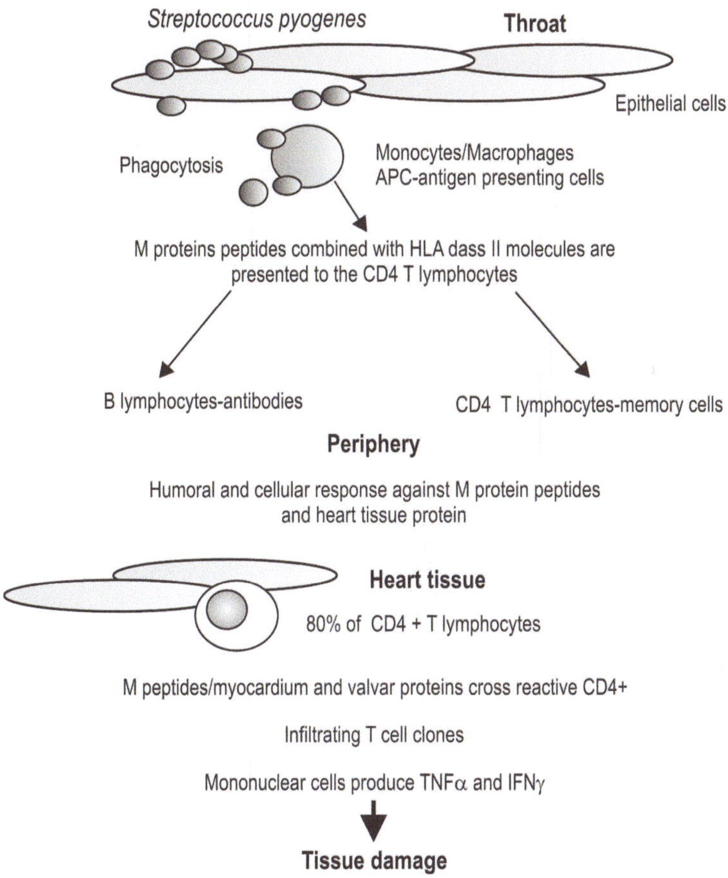

Fig. 17.1. Schematic representation of the pathogenesis of rheumatic heart disease. Streptococcal/self antigen cross reactive antibodies facilitate heart tissue T cells infiltrations. CD4 T cell clones recognize streptococcal antigens and heart tissue proteins (myosin, tropomyosin: peptides from the light meromyosin-LMM region, vimentin) by molecular mimicry. Inflammatory cytokines (TNF-alpha IFN-gamma) are produced by mononuclear cells. Few mononuclear cells produce IL-4 (regulatory cytokine), leading to the progression and maintenance of valvular lesions (carditis, valvulitis). ([1]; © Images Paediatr Cardiol)

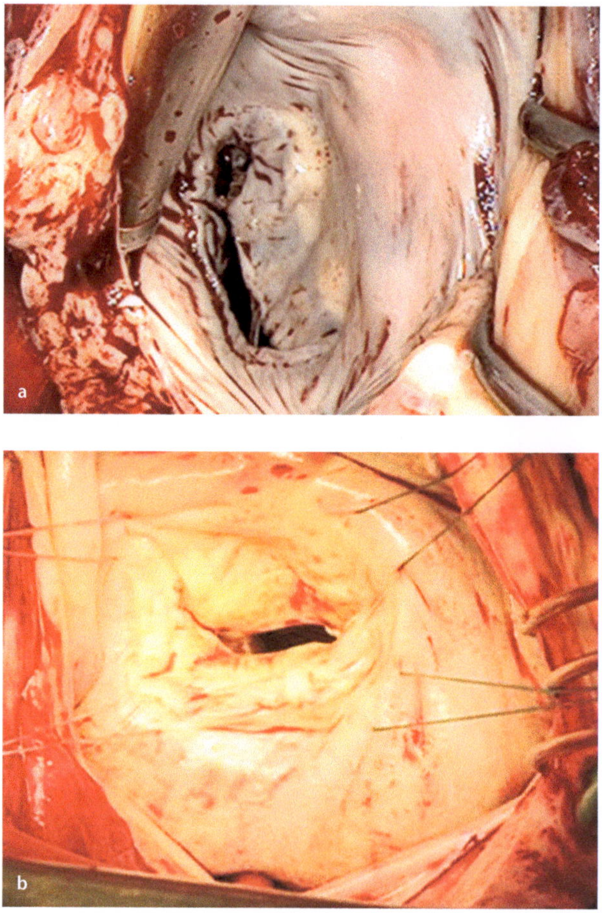

Fig. 17.2. Rheumatic mitral valve disease. **a** Pure rheumatic mitral valve incompetence in a child due to posterior annular dilatation and a mild deficient retracted anterior mitral leaflet. **b** Mixed lesion (mitral stenosis and incompetence): burn-out rheumatic mitral valve disease due to fibroelastic deficiency of the leaflet tissue (courtesy of Dr. El Oumeiri)

chords are thickened and scarred, which could obstruct complete opening and tether closure of the leaflets. Posterior leaflet retraction is a common feature of rheumatic disease.

17.4.1 Surgical techniques

The exposure of the heart is via a complete median sternotomy and cardiopulmonary bypass. The arterial inflow is facilitated by a single aortic cannula and venous drainage by bicaval cannulation. The mitral valve is exposed through a transseptal or interatrial groove. If there is echocardiographically evidence of atrial thrombus, the left atrial vent is inserted into the right superior pulmonary and left in place in the inferior pulmonary veins before the aorta is clamped. It is then placed in the left atrium to facilitate a clear visual operating field.

Options for the repair of rheumatic mitral valve disease include the following: (1) synthetic or autologous pericardial strip annuloplasty (PSA) for annular disease, (2) posterior plication annuloplasty suture, (3) leaflet remodeling by resection and sliding plasty of the

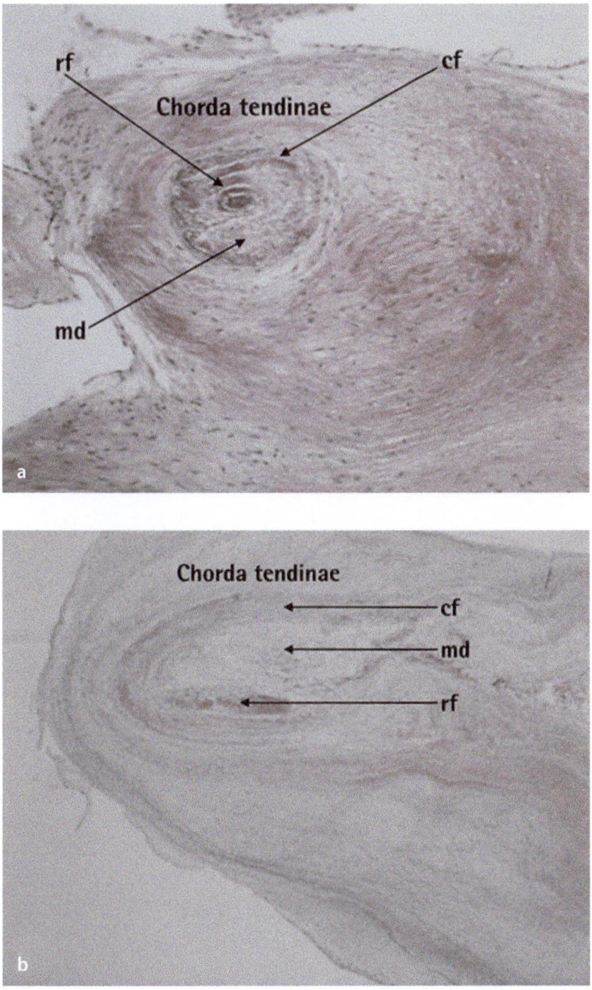

Fig. 17.3. Light microscopic view of the architecture of a chorda tendineae of a rheumatic mitral valve showing a structural deterioration: **a** Cross-sectional view. Elastica van Gieson: Collagen fibers (*cf*), residual fibrosa (*rf*), mucoid changes, **b** Oblique sectional view. Elastica van Gieson: Collagen fibers (*cf*), residual fibrosa (*rf*), mucinous degeneration (*md*). (courtesy of Dr. Dirsch, Cardiac Pathologist, Deutsches Herzzentrum Berlin)

posterior annulus or plication of the involved posterior leaflet, (4) leaflet augmentation with autologous pericardium (AP) for leaflet disease, (5) leaflet thinning (removal of fibrous tissue around the cusp), (6) partial replacement of the mitral valve apparatus with a segment of an autologous tricuspid valve apparatus, (7) incision of fused commissural chordae, (8) open mitral commissurotomy with or without papillary muscle split, (9) resection of secondary chordae, (10) shortening of elongated chordae, (11) transposition of elongated chordae, (12) expanded polytetrafluoroethylene (ePTFE, Gore-Tex®) artificial chordal replacement (ACR) for chordal disease (see Tables 17.5 and 17.6, Figs. 17.4–17.7).

The fibrous tissue of the confluence of the anterior mitral annulus and the aortic annulus forms a septum which is called the aortic mitral curtain or the intervalvular fibrous curtain. The area of the posterior segment of the mitral annulus is embedded in the ventricular myocardium and has limited fibrous tissue which dilates after rheumatic carditis. Posterior mitral annuloplasty requires a meticulous suturing technique to avoid suture obliteration of the neighboring circumflex artery (Fig. 17.4a)

Table 17.5. Surgical techniques for rheumatic mitral valve disease. Deutsches Herzzentrum Berlin 1986–2009 (*n*=50). Reproduced from the Jornal of Heart Valve Disease (JHVD)

		MR	MR + MS	MS
Repair techniques	*n*	*n*=38	*n*=9	*n*=5
Paneth annuloplasty	32	26	6	–
Autologous pericardial strip annuloplasty	17	12	5	–
PL plication	8	7	1	–
Kay-Wooler	6	3	3	–
Annuloplasty ring	1	1	–	–
Chordal transfer	1	1	–	–
Cleft closure	1	–	1	–
Commissuroplasty	1	–	1	–
PM splitting	2	–	–	2
Commissurotomy	12	–	7	5

PL posterior leaflet, *PM* papillary muscle

Table 17.6. Predictability of repair of rheumatic mitral valve incompetence, Carpentier classification and synopsis of repair of rheumatic mitral valve apparatus

Carpentier type	MV pathology	Repair technique
I. Normal leaflet motion	Annular dilatation	– Ring annuloplasty – Kay-Wooler – Paneth annuloplasty + autologous pericardial annuloplasty
II. Increased leaflet motion	Chordal elongation Leaflet prolapse	– Chordal shortening ?/replacement ± leaflet plication or quadrangular resection of prolapsed, redundant leaflet – Chordal transfer – Resection and commissuroplasty
	Chordal rupture PM rupture	– Chordal replacement/transfer – Refix the PM end-to-end or to neighboring PM or LV free wall
III. Restricted leaflet motion	Fibrosis of leaflet, fibroelastic deficiency (leaflet retraction)	– Bi-/unicommissurotomy – Augmentation of leaflet with pericardium ± chordal replacement – Partial leaflet replacement with tricuspid autograft/ mitral allograft

An average of two procedures including posterior leaflet plication, Paneth posterior suture annuloplasty and autologous pericardial strip as well as synthetic ring annuloplasty, chordal transfer, and papillary muscle splitting are used to repair a rheumatic mitral valve disease with leaflet prolapse, annulus dilatation, and elongated or restricted chordae and malformed papillary muscle (◘ Tables 17.5–17.8).

The various surgical techniques used for the valve repair and causes for reoperation are described in ◘ Tables 17.5–17.9. Preference card for mitral annulovalvuloplasty: 3-0 or 4-0 Prolene on an SH needle; 4-0 Prolene on an RB-1 needle; autologous pericardium, annuloplasty ring; 3-0 Ticron^{TM} suture for the ring; 4-0 or 5-0 expanded polytetrafluoroethylene (ePTFE, Gore-Tex®) CV-4 and -5 for chordae replacement.

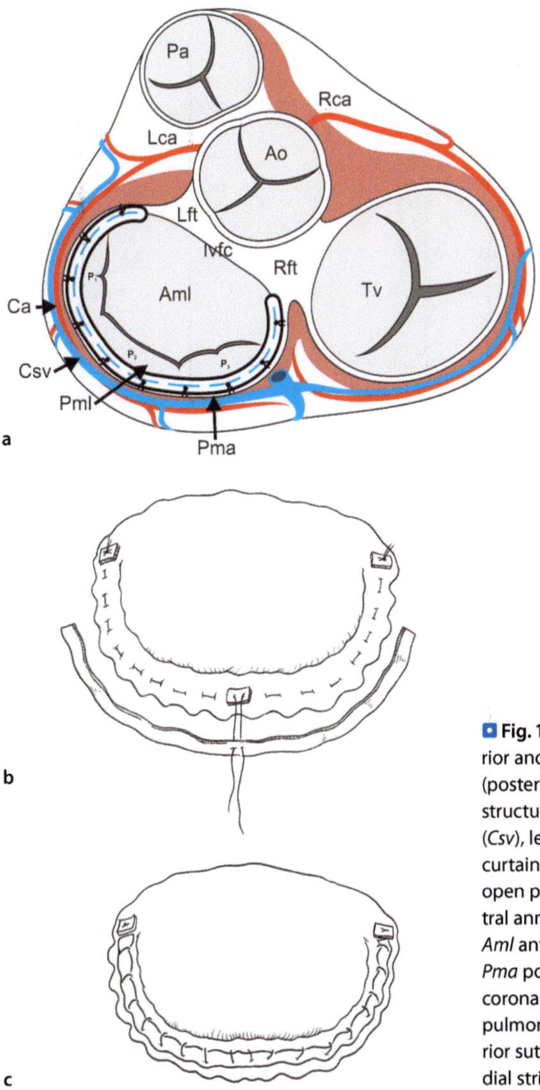

◘ **Fig. 17.4.** Mitral valve repair techniques: **a** the anterior and posterior mitral valve leaflets and the annulus (posterior mitral annulus, *Pma*) and the neighboring structures; circumflex artery (*Ca*), coronary sinus vein (*Csv*), left fibrous trigone (*Lft*), intervalvular fibrous curtain (*Ivfc*), right fibrous trigone (*Rft*). Insertion of open prosthetic annuloplasty ring at the posterior mitral annulus from the left to the right fibrous trigones. *Aml* anterior mitral leaflet, *Pml* posterior mitral leaflet, *Pma* posterior mitral annulus *P1,P 2 and P3*, *Lca* Left coronary artery, *Rca* right coronary artery, *Ao* aorta, *Pa* pulmonary artery, *Tv* tricuspid valve. **b** Paneth posterior suture annuloplasty (*PPSA*), **c** autologous pericardial strip annuloplasty (*PSA*)

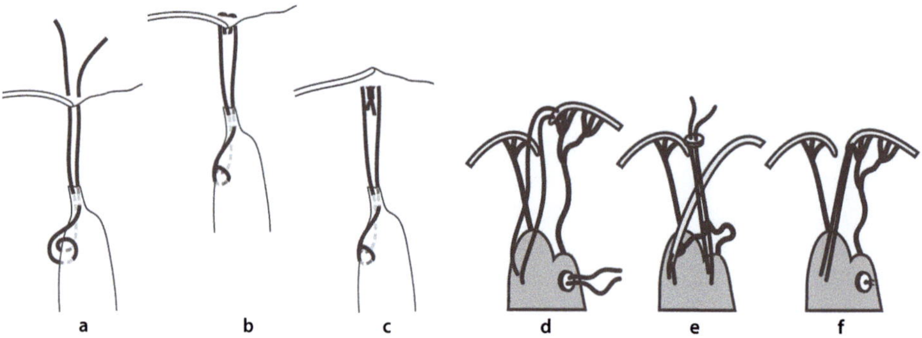

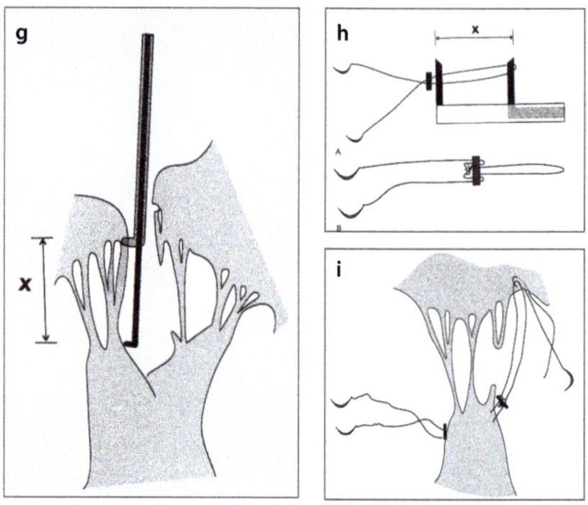

Fig. 17.5a–j. Techniques of chordal replacement with 4-0 or 5-0 expanded polytetrafluoroethylene (ePTFE), Gore-Tex®. (**a–i** [44], © Elsevier; **d–f** [48], © Elsevier; **g–j** ([73], © Elsevier, http//:ats.ctsnetjournals.org/cgi/content/full/70/6/2166)

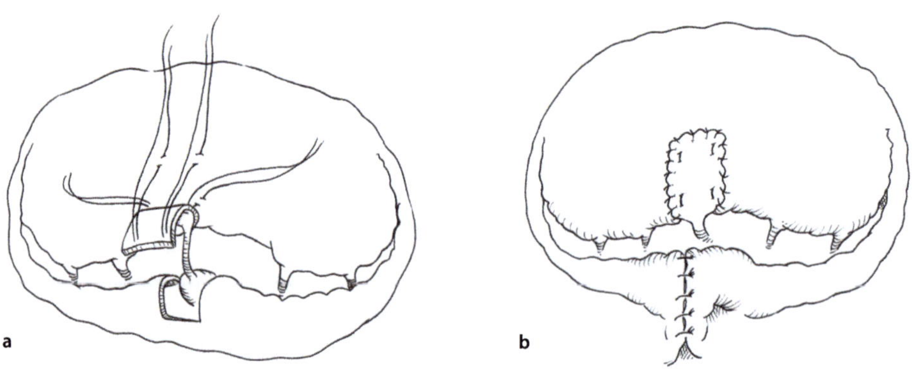

Fig. 17.6. a, b Chordal transfer to correct prolapsed anterior mitral leaflet (AML) or chordal rupture: a square piece of posterior mitral leaflet (quadrangular resection) with chordae of proper length is excised and marked with stay sutures at each angle. It is then transposed over onto the unsupported free edge or segment of the AML so that the atrial surfaces of the two leaflets oppose each other for fixation with a 5-0 polypropylene running suture. ([1]; © CTSNet Inc., Riley and Kon, http//:ctsnet.org/sections/clinicalresources/adultcardiac/expert_tech-2.html)

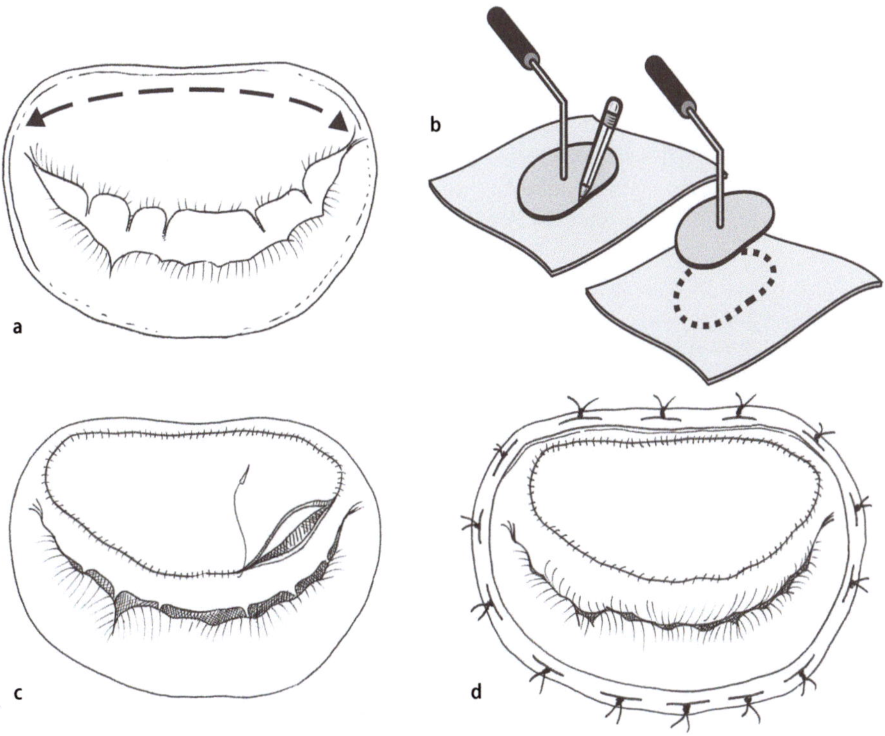

Fig. 17.7. Technique of augmentation of the anterior mitral leaflet ([72], © Elsevier). a The base of the anterior leaflet (AML) is detached and the length of the incision (L) is measured. Sutures for prosthetic ring annuloplasty have been already placed. b The flat side of a ring obturator is used to outline an ovoid shape on the sheet of the autologous pericardium. The obturator is then removed and the marked ovoid shape obtained on the sheet of the autologous pericardium is cut out as a patch for AML augmentation. c The pericardium is interposed between the anterior mitral annulus and the edge of the detached anterior mitral leaflet by a 5-0 Prolene running suture (Ethicon, Somerville, NJ, USA) starting at the posteromedial commissure. d After completion of the AML augmentation a prosthetic ring annuloplasty is performed by downsizing in order to achieve a perfect leaflet coaptation. Posterior leaflet augmentation with a glutaraldehyde-fixed autologous pericardial patch can be viewed at www.ctsnet.org (J. Scott Rankin, Rheumatic mitral valve repair, [70])

17.4.2 Data collection and postoperative follow-up

Patients were examined at our institution or were contacted by means of telephone interview and mailed questionnaire. Further patient data were obtained from hospital records, family doctors, and cardiologists. Patients with unknown addresses could be tracked through the district or state registry and the registry of births and deaths.

They underwent routine echocardiographic studies at 3 and 6 months after operation and thereafter annually. Transthoracic Doppler echocardiography was performed and some of the evaluations from different institutions were not comparable. The postoperative echocardiographic investigations were performed during the follow-up study period until 15 December 2008; however, they were inconsistent because various investigators were involved.

17.5 Statistical analysis

The guidelines for reporting morbidity and mortality after cardiac valvular operations approved by the Society of Thoracic Surgeons were used to analyze postoperative complications [33]. Continuous variables were expressed as mean±SEM and median. Actuarial curves were calculated by the Kaplan–Meier method. Linearized occurrence rate of events and confidence limits were calculated according to Poisson distribution. Actual competing risk analysis

Table 17.7. Rheumatic mitral regurgitation. Meta-analysis of repair techniques in 1,339 patients. Data from [8, 9, 19, 39]

Repair technique	Kumar *n*=898	Skoularigis *n*=254	ElOumeiri *n*=78	Bernal *n*=62	DHZB *n*=47
Leaflet					
– Excision/plication	4.5%	13.8%	21%	8.1%	17%
– Partial replacement	–	–	24.3%	–	–
Commissuroplasty	–	–	19.2%		2%
Annuloplasty					
– Plastic ring	88%	98.8%	80%	100%	2%
– Paneth	–	–	–	–	68%
– Autologous pericardium	–	–	–	–	36%
Chordae tendineae					
– Shortening	25%	68.1%	–	38%	–
– Transfer	1.4%	6.7%	3.2%	3.2%	0.9%
– Replacement	3.3%	–	30.7%	3.2%	–
PM splitting	–	–	–	27%	2%

PM papillary muscle, *DHZB* Deutsches Herzzentrum Berlin

Table 17.8. Rheumatic mitral regurgitation: 13 reoperations in 46 patients with pure MR and mixed lesions (MR + MS) according to the technique of repair of the mitral valve apparatus and age group. Deutsches Herzzentrum Berlin, 1986–2009. Reproduced from the Jornal of Heart Valve Disease (JHVD)

Technique of repair	Pure MR *n*=37	Mixed (MR + MS) *n*=9	Reoperation *n*=13
Pericardial strip annuloplasty	12	5/2[b]	2 (11.8%)[a]
Paneth posterior suture annuloplasty (+ 14 autologous pericardial strip annuloplasty)	26/7[b]	6/1[b]	8 (25.0%)[a]
PL plication + Paneth posterior suture annuloplasty (+ 3 autologous pericardial strip annuloplasty)	7/1[b]	1	1 (12.5%)[a]
Kay-Wooler commissurotomy	3	3/2[b]	2 (33.3%)

PL posterior leaflet plication (Gerbode technique), *MR* mitral regurgitation, *MS* mitral stenosis.
[a]Patients ≥20 years, [b]Primary operations/reoperation

(cumulative incidence) was performed. Differences in actuarial freedom between groups of patients are determined using the log-rank test. Differences in prognostic variables between two groups were evaluated by t-tests for continuous variables and the χ^2 or Fisher exact test for categorical variables. A p value <0.05 was considered as evidence of statistical significance. Predictors of events during follow-up were identified by means of Cox's proportional hazards regression.

17.6 Results

17.6.1 Hospital mortality and perioperative morbidity

Three patients (3/50, 6%) died during the hospital stay (30 days). There was no hospital mortality in patients under 16 years. The causes of early death on the 11th and 13th postoperative day were myocardial infarction and septic multiorgan failure in 2 patients with previous AVR+CABG and AVR, respectively, who required an intraaortic balloon pump before surgery due to a low output state. The third patient died of pneumonia due to aspiration. In reported series, isolated mitral valve repair has a hospital mortality of 1–2% in contrast to 2–8% for mitral valve repair with concomitant procedures in patients with a low ejection fraction [9–13].

17.6.2 Late mortality

There were 14 late deaths between 60 days and 14 years. Overall actuarial survival is shown in Fig. 17.8. Survival in the age group of patients over 16 years was 96.8±5.5%, 83.3±6.3%,

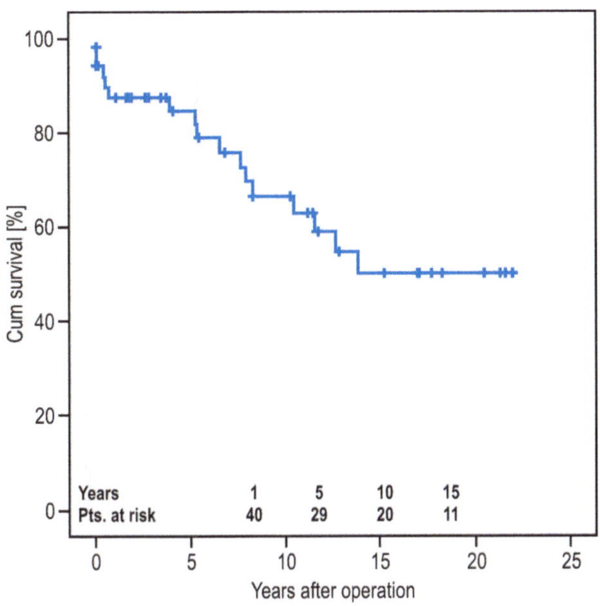

Fig. 17.8. Overall actuarial survival (Kaplan–Meier) after repair of rheumatic mitral valve. Reproduced from the Jornal of Heart Valve Disease (JHVD)

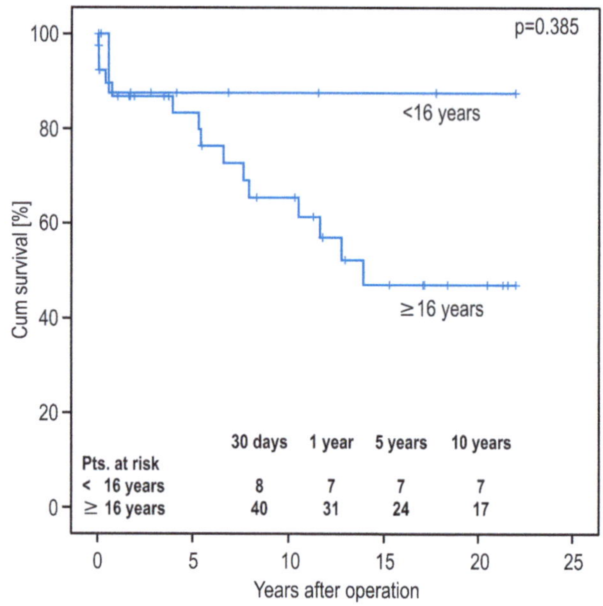

Fig. 17.9. Actuarial survival (Kaplan–Meier) after repair of rheumatic mitral valve by age group (<16 years and ≥16 years)

65.4±8.6% at 1, 5, and 10 years, respectively. It was 87.5±11.7% at 10 years in the age group under 16 years (p=0.385). Differences in survival in age groups <16 and ≥16 years are shown in Fig. 17.9. In the literature, actuarial survival at 10 years ranges from 81–97% [9, 10, 14, 15, 33, 54, 59]. It was 95.2±1.5% in young populations, whereas in adult populations, it was 65.8–75.3% at 20 years [8, 9, 14, 15].

17.6.3 Reoperation

Successful repair rate was 78%. Eighteen patients (18/50, 36%) underwent reoperation due to valve failure. While 3 (3/30, 6%) failures occurred within 1 year, 3 others occurred within 2–5 years and 12 (12/50, 24%) within 6–16 years after repair. Freedom from severe mitral regurgitation and reoperation at 1, 5, and 10 years was 92.7±4.1%, 77.3±7.2%, and 53.4±9.6%, respectively. Linearized rate for reoperation was 4.4%/patient-year (95% CI), and the range was 2.8–6.8%/patient-year. In other published series, it was 5.4%/patient-year [14]. Differences between the two age groups (<16 and ≥16 years) are demonstrated in the Kaplan–Meier curve (Fig. 17.10). Actuarial freedom from reoperation at 10 years in patients with the Paneth posterior suture and pericardial strip annuloplasty was 76.2±1.2%; in patients under 16 years it was 100% at 5 years (Fig. 17.11). Causes for reoperation by surgical technique in our series are shown in Tables 17.8 and 17.9. Three redo patients (3/18) underwent re-repair and 15 others (15/18) had replacement with biological and mechanical prostheses. Freedom from severe mitral regurgitation and reoperation at 10 years in other published series was 81–92.7% and 73% at 20 years (Table 17.10) [8–10, 15].

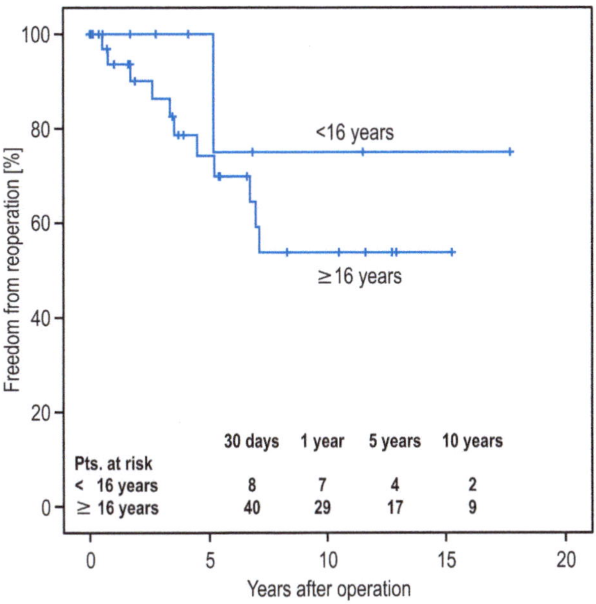

Fig. 17.10. Actuarial freedom from reoperation (Kaplan–Meier) after repair of rheumatic mitral valve by age group (<16 years and ≥16 years)

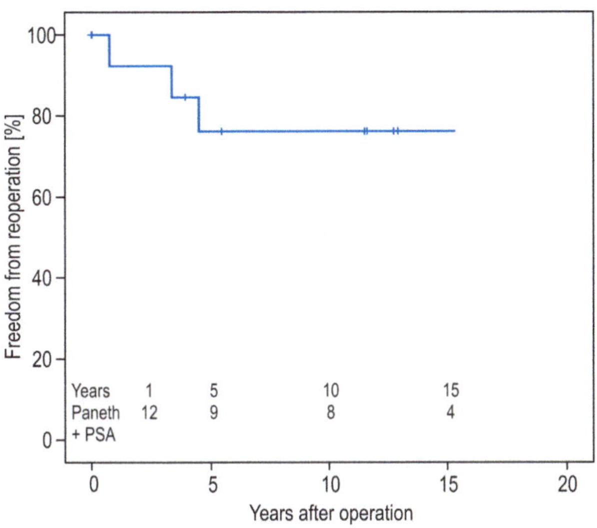

Fig. 17.11. Actuarial freedom from reoperation (Kaplan–Meier) after repair of rheumatic mitral valve by surgical technique using Paneth posterior suture annuloplasty (PPSA) and pericardial strip annuloplasty (PSA). Reproduced from the Jornal of Heart Valve Disease (JHVD)

17.7 Discussion

Rheumatic mitral valve disease is presented in young patients, who are generally in their teens and twenties, while in developed countries, it is a sequelae of previous episodes of rheumatic fever in patients who were living in endemic regions and require surgery for burn-out rheumatic heart valve disease, ventricular dysfunction, and pulmonary hypertension and in most cases these patients are in their early 50s and 60s. Mitral valve repair as

Table 17.10. Outcome of rheumatic mitral valve repair versus replacement. Actuarial freedom from reoperation after mitral valve repair and replacement and survival (Kaplan–Meier) after operation at 10 years (%). Data from [8–10, 14, 15, 34, 59]

Author	Freedom from reoperation and survival at 10 years (%)			
	Repair	Survival	Replacement	Survival
Bernal et al. 1996	97	85	na	na
Kumar et al. 2006	81	92	na	na
Talwar et al. 2005	86	95[b]	na	na
Kim et al. 2010	92	81.4	86.8	69.6
Kalangos et al. 2008	92	86.5[b]	na	na
Leyh et al. 2006	82	75	na	na
Yau et al. 2000	72	88.2	69–95[a]	70–73[a]

[a]Mechanical prosthesis, [b]Repair in children

advocated by Carpentier has become a well-established procedure in contemporary cardiac surgery and can be offered to all age groups, especially young patients. In addition to re-establishing the functional units of the mitral valve apparatus, mitral valve repair has a positive impact on left ventricular functional recovery and, consequently, survival benefits over valve replacement. The procedure especially benefits patients from a poor social background without health insurance because it would curtail the cost of long-term anticoagulation and frequent hospital visits for monitoring the international normalized ratio (INR) [9, 10, 14, 19].

In regions where the life expectancy is less than 60 years, repair of the native valve is preferred as an option to obviate serious valve-related complications of mechanical prosthesis, e.g., thromboembolic episodes and sudden death. Bioprostheses are an alternative device for replacement of a diseased mitral valve that is beyond repair. Bioprostheses are known to develop early structural valve deterioration and, therefore, have limited durability in younger age groups [16–18].

Not only the complexity of rheumatic mitral valve apparatus but also the unpredictability of successful repair and long-lasting results demand properly reproducible repair techniques in individual patients. Comprehensive mitral repair techniques that are reproducible and can be used to treat most pathologies of the mitral valve apparatus to restore the normal anatomy and function have evolved [7–15, 19, 27–31, 34–64].

17.7.1 Predictability of repair of rheumatic mitral valve disease

A good perioperative echocardiography was the most reliable method for predicting the possibility of successful mitral valve repair and durability and for identifying the potential risk factors for repair failure. The following criteria determine the possibilities of successful repair of the mitral valve apparatus [7–15, 27–31, 34–64].

- A pliable and a large anterior mitral leaflet, absence of gross abnormality of the chordae and extensive areas of calcification of the posterior leaflet were the most important echocardiographic criteria for satisfactory valvuloplasty with long-lasting results.
- Mixed lesions (mitral regurgitation and mitral stenosis) with rigid and retracted small posterior leaflet (P1, P2, and P3) might present unfavorable findings for adequate repair and this might fail afterwards. Therefore, deficient leaflet tissue poses a potential risk and is a predictive factor for early repair failure (hazard ratio 1.93, 95% confidence interval 1.29–2.6, p=0.004) [7–15, 38, 39, 63]. It is, therefore, mandatory to optimize the leaflet morphology to ensure optimal coaptation by pericardial augmentation to achieve long-term functional durability [38].
- An adequate reproducible repair technique (annulovalvuloplasty and chordal–papillary muscle reconstruction) is, therefore, mandatory in order to decrease immediate postoperative residual mitral valve regurgitation >1, because this is a major determinant of late failures that require redo mitral valve surgery.
- Presence of severe LV failure was a risk factor for MR (hazard ratio 5.2, 95% confidence interval 1.99–8.7, p=0.003) [9] and, therefore, favors mitral valvuloplasty because the LV function improves significantly as compared to prosthetic valve replacement and, thus, decreases the likelihood of thromboembolic events.
- Compliance of the patient to antirheumatic fever medication. Patients with rheumatic mitral repair, who are living in endemic areas, are constantly exposed to recurrent rheumatic activity postoperatively; thus, postrheumatic scarring and retraction of the structures of the mitral valve apparatus would result in regurgitation. Therefore, persistent or recurrent rheumatic carditis is a potential risk and a predictive factor for failure of rheumatic mitral valve repair. Consequently, long-term successful annuloplasty could be performed in a highly selected patient group, who could comply with postoperative antirheumatic medication therapy [9, 10].

A pure mitral stenosis with a pliable anterior and posterior leaflets and without extensive calcification and pathological changes of the submitral apparatus has a 60% probability of repair success as compared to 30% for a mixed lesion (hazard ratio 1.72; 95% confidence interval, p=0.006) [7, 10]. In young patients who have combined mitral stenosis with fused shortened chordae, the technique of fenestration described by Carpentier is used, whereby all fibrous tissue is removed and the papillary muscles are split down to the base to improve mobility of the anterior and posterior leaflets. However, the long-term results are suboptimal [7, 9, 28, 30].

The benefits of comprehensive mitral valvuloplasty have been demonstrated by its low incidence of valve-related morbid events; however, the results depend on the age at surgery and the mitral pathology. In reported series on young patients under 20 years, the reoperation rate for all type of repair techniques was between 5.9% and 23.6% [8, 9]. The actuarial freedom from reoperation at 15 years was 85.9±5.9% [9, 10]. Linearized rate of reoperation was 5.4% per patient–year [19]. In our series, the linearized rate of reoperation in the age group <20 years and ≥20 years was 4.5 (2.0–10.2)%/patient–year and 4.3 (2.5–7.2)%/patient–year, respectively. At the longest follow-up of over 20 years, freedom from reoperation for valve failure was 73.1% and freedom from thromboembolism was 74.3% [8]. The linearized rate of thromboembolism and endocarditis were 0.98% and 0.65% per patient–year, respectively [8].

Isolated mitral valve repair has a hospital mortality of 1–2% in contrast to 2–8% for mitral valve repair with concomitant procedures associated with a low ejection fraction [9, 10, 13,

59–62]. Survival was 95.2±1.5% in young populations, whereas in adult populations, it was 65.8–75.3% at 20 years [8, 9, 14, 15].

Immediate postoperative hemodynamic instability, cardiogenic shock, or difficulty in removing the patient from bypass after mitral valve repair could be related to myocardial ischemia by suture obliteration of the circumflex artery and left ventricular outflow obstruction by systolic anterior motion (SAM) [50, 53–55].

Incidence of mitral regurgitation due to annular dilation in patients with rheumatic disease is 10–80%, whereas chordal lesions (thickening, shortening, elongation, fusion, and rupture) occur in 94% and leaflet prolapse, retraction, and other leaflet dysfunction in 30% of patients [7–15, 38, 39, 63]. Consequently, an average of 2.7 procedures, including leaflet remodeling, chordal reconstruction, and annuloplasty (synthetic and biological), are required for the successful repair of a rheumatic mitral valve [7–9, 15, 27–31, 37–64, 68, 69]. The confluence of the anterior mitral annulus and the aortic annulus is called the aortic mitral curtain or the intervalvular fibrous curtain [66, 67]. The area of the posterior segment of the mitral annulus that has limited fibrous tissue dilates after rheumatic carditis unlike the anterior annulus, which is an integral part of the fibrous skeleton of the heart; hence, the Paneth posterior plication suture annuloplasty was introduced for stabilization [49, 50]. The Paneth posterior suture annuloplasty and pericardial strip annuloplasty for stabilization of the posterior mitral annulus are associated with a high incidence of failure in the long-term follow-up. This technique has been used in young patients in various modifications to allow annular growth, with mixed results [35, 49, 50].

Recently, a biodegradable annuloplasty ring has been introduced for pediatric mitral valve repair and is available in sizes 22–32 mm (mean: 26±6 mm) [10]. The midterm results appear more encouraging and the long-term results are still pending.

Synthetic ring annuloplasty is a gold standard in mitral valve repair in adults and has proven to be superior in the long term [7–15, 27–31, 37–64, 68, 69]. The ring sizers of synthetic annuloplasty and biodegradable rings have similar surface areas for adult sizes between 26 and 36 mm, but pediatric sizes below 26 mm do not exist for synthetic annuloplasty rings [47].

Chordal repair and transfer are preferred in selected groups of patients because of the excellent results, especially in young patients [8, 9, 15]. However, due to anticipated progression of the structural deterioration of the chordae tendineae in adults with a burn-out rheumatic mitral valve disease replacement with 5-0 expanded polytetrafluoroethylene (ePTFE), as advocated by Frater et al. and others, (a breaking strength of over 1 kg) is preferred by many contemporary surgeons [36, 39–46, 48, 51–64]. Reports with up to 20 years of clinical experience have demonstrated the efficacy and benefits of this chordal replacement technique in adults [43–46]. However, it is reported that 5-0 and 4-0 ePTFE chordal replacement will occasionally rupture; consequently, 2-0 ePTFE is preferred by some surgeons because it has proven to be still flexible and pliable after 10 years [51]. Professor James Gammie of the University of Maryland, Baltimore, USA, also reported a case of 5-0 ePTFE rupture after 2 years but he continues to use 4-0 and 5-0 ePTFE for chordal replacement. Proponents of 4-0 and 5-0 ePTFE criticize the use of 2-0 ePTFE as producing more friction going through the leaflet and the size of the knot tower as being bulky and unpleasant looking.

Recently, chordal replacement in children has been introduced and it has been demonstrated that it does not impede papillary muscle–mitral leaflet growth at the region of insertion as previously suggested. At a mean operation age of 4.7±5.3 years (range 1 month to 17.8 years) the actuarial freedom from reoperation at 5 and 8 years after chordal replacement was 94.8% and 89.5%, respectively [48]. However, long-term clinical data are needed before this technique is applied routinely in young populations with RHVD.

In the planning of mitral valve repair procedures where successful repair is predicted to be unlikely, there has been a resurgence of interest in augmentation of the shortened or retracted (fibroelastic deficient) anterior mitral leaflet caused by rheumatic disease with an autologous pericardium to restore its morphology, geometry, and function [38]. A further repair technique is a partial replacement of an unrepairable mitral valve segment with an allograft mitral valve from a donor heart unsuitable for transplantation or a segment of an autologous tricuspid valve [39].

The results of anterior mitral leaflet (AML) augmentation with autologous pericardium in Acar's series [38] have demonstrated the role of this technique in a subset of patients–in particular, in children with retracted deficient leaflet tissue. The rate of reoperation for leaflet augmentation versus no augmentation was 2.5% versus 12.9%, respectively, at 2.8 years of follow-up ($p<0.05$) [38].

In addition to inadequate stabilization of the dilated posterior annulus, the major causes for repair failure of the mitral valve are improper repair of deficient leaflet tissue and failure to re-establishing effective long-lasting functioning chords. Therefore, a more liberal application of pericardial patches and chordal replacement or transfer (in children) procedures might reduce reoperations, expand application, and extend the survival benefits of repair to a larger percentage of patients [38, 70, 71]. The technique could contribute to improved survival after rheumatic repair, which is enhanced by fewer valve-related complications at the expense of a higher rate of late reoperations [59–64, 68].

For mitral allograft and tricuspid autograft implantation, freedom from recurrent mitral regurgitation at 5 years was 98% and from reoperation at 10 years it was 94% [39]. The benefits of these techniques include avoidance of anticoagulants and a reduced risk of valve-related complications, but the results are suboptimal.

17.7.2 Time-related repair failure

Failures resulting in a mild mitral regurgitation (MR), as evidenced by intraoperative transesophageal echocardiography, which occur within 2–3 years after repair are related to improper indication, inadequate repair, and technical factors [55–64, 68, 69]. Consequently, to avoid early reoperation, an inadequate leaflet coaptation of less than 8 mm in length with a mild MR in the operating room should not be accepted. Reoperations that occur beyond 7 years were found to be due to recurrent rheumatic activity, which leads to a progressive structural deterioration of the mitral apparatus. Regular postoperative echocardiographic and clinical studies and penicillin prophylaxis (1.2 million units i.m. every 4 weeks, in high-risk groups every 3 weeks) in endemic regions are highly recommended [9, 10, 19].

17.8 Conclusion

Mitral valve repair in rheumatic disease is feasible, but the long-term functional results are suboptimal. It has become the preferred surgical method over replacement because of its good functional results, rapid recovery of the left ventricle, socioeconomic benefits, and positive impact on quality of life. Pure mitral incompetence may be reparable and long-lasting, while valves with mixed lesions may be reparable but fail afterwards. A successful repair is based on profound knowledge of the complex pathology of the mitral valve apparatus and application of an appropriate repair technique; thus, better understanding of the natural history of the disease contributes to functional stability of the valve in endemic regions. Predictability of repair and long-term functional results are determined by perioperative echocardiographic evaluation and early surgical repair before the onset of significant left ventricular dysfunction. An adequate reproducible repair technique (annulovalvuloplasty and chordal–papillary muscle reconstruction) is mandatory in order to decrease immediate postoperative residual mitral valve regurgitation to less than grade 1 as this is a main determinant of late failures requiring redo mitral valve surgery. Therefore, a more liberal application of pericardial patches, chordal replacement, and transfer procedures might reduce early reoperations, expand application, and extend the survival benefits of repair to a larger percentage of patients. Postoperative regular penicillin prophylaxis is required to prevent rheumatic activity in endemic regions in order to achieve a long-lasting competent mitral valve.

Acknowledgments

The authors are grateful to Anne M. Gale, ELS, for editorial assistance, Julia Stein, MSc, for statistical analysis, Christine Detschades, SRN, for computing the data for evaluation and statistical analysis, and Astrid Benhennour for bibliographic support. Similarly we are indebted to Carla Weber and Helge Haselbach for the graphic design work.

References

1. Binotto MA, Guilherme L, Tanaka AC (2002) Rheumatic fever. Images Paediatric Cardiol 11:12–15
2. Guilherme L, Ramasawmy R, Kalil J (2007) Rheumatic fever and rheumatic heart disease: Genetics and pathogenesis. Scand J Immunol 66:199–207
3. Ayoub EM (1992) Resurgence of rheumatic fever in the United States. The changing picture of a preventable illness. Postgrad Med 92:133–136,139–142
4. Yankah AC, Marshall R, Van Reken D, Boakye E, Sasraku SD (1981) Cardiovascular diseases in Liberia. Cardiologie Tropicale, Tropical cardiology 7:15–20
5. Marijon E, Ou P, Celermajer DS, Ferreira B, Mocumbi AO, Jani D, Paquet C, Jacob S, Sidi D, Jouven X (2007) Prevalence of rheumatic heart disease detected by echocardiographic screening. N Engl J Med 357:470–476
6. Carapetis JR, Steer AC, Mulholland EK, Weber M (2005) The global burden of group A streptococcal diseases. Lancet Infect Dis 5:685–694
7. Antunes MJ, Magalhaes MP, Colsen PR, Kinsley RH (1987) Valvuloplasty for rheumatic mitral valve disease. A surgical challenge. J Thorac Cardiovasc Surg 94:44–56
8. Bernal JM, Rabasa JM, Olalla JJ, Carrión MF, Alonso A, Revuelta JM (1996) Repair of chordae tendineae for rheumatic mitral valve disease. A twenty-year experience. J Thorac Cardiovasc Surg 111:211–217
9. Kumar AS, Talwar S, Saxena A, Singh R, Velayoudam D (2006) Results of mitral valve repair in rheumatic mitral regurgitation. Interact Cardiovasc Thorac Surg 5:356–361
10. Talwar S, Rajesh MR, Subramanian A, Saxena A, Kumar AS (2005) Mitral valve repair in children with rheumatic heart disease. J Thorac Cardiovasc Surg 129:875–879
11. Phan KP, Nguyen vP, Pham NV, Dao HT, Dang tT, Le HD, Chu TH, Tri Ho HQ, Carpentier A (1999) Mitral valve repair in children using Carpentier's techniques. Semin Thorac Cardiovasc Surg Pediatr Card Surg Annu 2:111–120
12. Ho HQ, Nguyen VP, Phan KP, Pham NV (2004) Mitral valve repair with aortic valve replacement in rheumatic heart disease. Asian Cardiovasc Thorac Ann 12:341–345
13. Fedakar A, Sasmazel A, Bugra O, Sarikaya S, Büyükbayrak F, Erdem H, Baysal A, Zeybek R (2010) Results of mitral valve repair in rheumatic mitral lesions. Heart Surg Forum 13:E86–90

14. Kim JB, Kim HJ, Moon DH, Jung SH, Choo SJ, Chung CH, Song H, Lee JW (2010) Long-term outcomes after surgery for rheumatic mitral valve disease: valve repair versus mechanical valve replacement. Eur J Cardiothorac Surg 37:1039–1046
15. Kalangos A, Christenson JT, Beghetti M, Cikirikcioglu M, Kamentsidis D, Aggoun Y (2008) Mitral valve repair for rheumatic valve disease in children: midterm results and impact of the use of a biodegradable mitral ring. Ann Thorac Surg 86:161–169
16. Alsoufi B, Manlhiot C, McCrindle BW, Al-Halees Z, Sallehuddin A, Al-Oufi S, Saad E, Fadel B, Canver CC (2010) Results after mitral valve replacement with mechanical prostheses in young children. J Thorac Cardiovasc Surg 139:1189–1196
17. Alsoufi B, Manlhiot C, McCrindle BW, Canver CC, Sallehuddin A, Al-Oufi S, Joufan M, Al-Halees Z (2009) Aortic and mitral valve replacement in children: is there any role for biologic and bioprosthetic substitutes? Eur J Cardiothorac Surg 36:84–90
18. von Oppell UO, Zilla P (2001) Prosthetic heart valves: why biological? J Long Term Eff Med Implants 11:105–113
19. Skoularigis J, Sinovich V, Joubert G, Sareli P (1994) Evaluation of the long-term results of mitral valve repair in 254 young patients with rheumatic mitral regurgitation. Circulation 90:II167–174
20. Chopra P, Bhatia ML (1992) Chronic rheumatic heart disease in India: a reappraisal of pathologic changes. J Heart Valve Dis 1:92–101
21. Brunton L (1902) Preliminary note on the possibility of treating mitral stenosis by surgical methods. Lancet 1:352
22. Ross FP (1979) Master surgeon, teacher, soldier, and friend: Elliott Carr Cutler, MD (1888–1947). Am J Surg 137:428–432
23. Gibbons JH Jr (1954) The application of a mechanical heart and lung apparatus to cardiac surgery. Minn Med 37:171–174
24. Hill JD. John H. Gibbon, Jr. (1982) Part I. The development of the first successful heart-lung machine. Ann Thorac Surg 34:337–341
25. Lillehei CW, Gott VL, De Wall RA, Varco RL (1957) Surgical correction of pure mitral insufficiency by annuloplasty under direct vision. Lancet 77:446–449
26. Gott VL (2005) Lillehei, Lewis, and Wangensteen: the right mix for giant achievements in cardiac surgery. Ann Thorac Surg 79:S2210–2213
27. Carpentier A (1983) Cardiac valve surgery – the »French correction«. J Thorac Cardiovasc Surg 86:323–337
28. Carpentier A, Deloche A, Dauptain J (1971) A new reconstructive operation for correction of mitral and tricuspid insufficiency. J Thorac Cardiovasc Surg 61:1–13
29. Duran CG, Pomar JL, Revuelta JM (1980) Conservative operation for mitral insufficiency: critical analysis supported by postoperative hemodynamic studies of 72 patients. J Thorac Cardiovasc Surg 79:326–337
30. Duran CM, Gometza B, De Vol EB (1991) Valve repair in rheumatic mitral disease. Circulation 84(Suppl):III125–132
31. Duran CM, Gometza B, Balasundaram S, al Halees Z (1991) A feasibility study of valve repair in rheumatic mitral regurgitation. Eur Heart J 12 (Suppl B):34–38
32. Siniawski H, Grauhan O, Hofmann M, Pasic M, Weng Y, Yankah C, Lehmkuhl H, Hetzer R (2004) Factors influencing the results of double-valve surgery in patients with fulminant endocarditis: the importance of valve selection. Heart Surg Forum 7:E405–410
33. Akins CW, Miller DC, Turina MI, Kouchoukos NT, Blackstone EH, Grunkemeier GL, Takkenberg JJ, David TE, Butchart EG, Adams DH, Shahian DM, Hagl S, Mayer JE, Lytle BW; Councils of the American Association for Thoracic Surgery; Society of Thoracic Surgeons; European Assoication for Cardio-Thoracic Surgery; Ad Hoc Liaison Committee for Standardizing Definitions of Prosthetic Heart Valve Morbidity (2008) Guidelines for reporting mortality and morbidity after cardiac valve interventions. J Thorac Cardiovasc Surg 135:732–738
34. Leyh RG, Jakob H (2006) Current aspects of mitral valve repair in the surgical treatment of mitral valve insufficiency. Herz 31:47–52
35. Hillman ND, Tani LY, Veasy LG, Lambert LL, Di Russo GB, Doty DB, McGough EC, Hawkins JA (2004) Current status of surgery for rheumatic carditis in children. Ann Thorac Surg 78:1403–1408
36. Erez E, Kanter KR, Isom E, Williams WH, Tam VK (2003) Mitral valve replacement in children. J Heart Valve Dis 12:25–29
37. Padala M, Powell SN, Croft LR, Thourani VH, Yoganathan AP, Adams DH (2009)Mitral valve hemodynamics after repair of acute posterior leaflet prolapse: quadrangular resection versus triangular resection versus neochordoplasty. J Thorac Cardiovasc Surg 138:309–315

38. Acar C, de Ibarra JS, Lansac E (2004) Anterior leaflet augmentation with autologous pericardium for mitral repair in rheumatic valve insufficiency. J Heart Valve Dis 13:741–746
39. El Oumeiri B, Boodhwani M, Glineur D, De Kerchove L, Poncelet A, Astarci P, Pasquet A, Vanoverschelde JL, Verhelst R, Rubay J, Noirhomme P, El Khoury G (2009) Extending the scope of mitral valve repair in rheumatic disease. Ann Thorac Surg 87:1735–1740
40. Frater RW, Berghuis J, Brown AI, Jr, Ellis FH Jr (1965) The experimental and clinical use of autogenous pericardium for the replacement and extension of mitral and tricuspid vave cusps and chordae. J Cardiovasc Surg 6:214–228
41. Frater RW, Gabbay S, Shore D (1983) Reproducible replacement of elongated or ruptured mitral valve chordate. Ann Thorac Surg 35:14–28
42. Vetter HO, Burack JH, Factor SM, Maculso F, Frater RWM (1986) Replacement of chordate tendinae of the mitral valve using the new expanded PTFE suture in sheep. In: Bodnar E, Yacoub M (eds) Biologic and bioprosthetic valves. York Medical Books, New York, pp 772–785
43. Frater RW, Vetter HO, Zussa C, Dahm M (1990) Chordal replacement in mitral valve repair. Circulation 82(Suppl):IV125–130
44. David TE, Bos J, Rakowski H (1991) Mitral valve repair by replacement of chordae tendineae with polytetrafluoroethylene sutures. J Thorac Cardiovasc Surg 101:495–501
45. Salvador L, Mirone S, Bianchini R, Regesta T, Patelli F, Minniti G, Masat M, Cavarretta E, Valfrè C (2008) A 20-year experience with mitral valve repair with artificial chordae in 608 patients. J Thorac Cardiovasc Surg 135:1280–1287
46. Zussa C, Polesel E, Da Col U, Galloni M, Valfré C (1994) Seven-year experience with chordal replacement with expanded polytetrafluoroethylene in floppy mitral valve. J Thorac Cardiovasc Surg 108:37–41
47. Kalangos A, Sierra J, Vala D, et al. (2006) Annuloplasty for valve repair with a new biodegradable ring: an experimental study. J Heart Valve Dis 15:783–790
48. Minami K, Kado H, Sai S, Tatewaki H, Shiokawa Y, Nakashima A, Fukae K, Hirose H (2005) Midterm results of mitral valve repair with artificial chordae in children. J Thorac Cardiovasc Surg 129:336–342
49. Hetzer R, Delmo Walter EB, Hübler M, Alexi-Meskishvili V, Weng Y, Nagdyman N, Berger F (2008) Modified surgical techniques and long-term outcome of mitral valve reconstruction in 111 children. Ann Thorac Surg 86:604–613
50. Scrofani R, Moriggia S, Salati M, Fundaro P, Danna P, Santoli C (1996) Mitral valve remodeling: long-term results with posterior pericardial annuloplasty. Ann Thorac Surg 61:895–899
51. Rankin JS, Sharma MK, Teague SM, McLaughlin VW, Johnston TS, McRae AT (2008) A new approach to mitral valve repair for rheumatic disease: preliminary study. J Heart Valve Dis 17:614–619
52. Adams DH, Anyanwu AC, Rahmanian PB, Filsoufi F (2006) Current concepts in mitral valve repair for degenerative disease. Heart Fail Rev 11:241–257
53. Virmani R, Chun PK, Parker J, McAllister HA (1982) Suture obliteration of the circumflex coronary artery in three patients undergoing mitral valve operation: role of left dominant or nondominant coronary artery. J Thorac Cardiovasc Surg 84:773–778
54. Tavilla G, Pcini D (1998) Damage to the circumflex coronary artery during mitral valve repair with sliding leaflet technique. Ann Thorac Surg 66:2090–2093
55. Shah PM, Ranney AA (2001) Echocardiographic correlates of left ventricular outflow obstruction and systolic anterior motion following mitral valve repair. J Heart Valve Dis 10:302–306
56. Rankin JS (2010) Mitral valve repair for Barlow's syndrome using adjustable artificial chordal replacement. http://www.ctsnet.org/sections/clinicalresources/videos/vg2010_RankinS_ACR_Barlows.html (Accessed: Nobember 29, 2010)
57. Butany J, Collins MJ, David TE (2004) Ruptured synthetic expanded polytetrafluoroethylene chordae tendineae. Cardiovasc Pathol 13:182–184
58. Farivar RS, Shernan SK, Cohn LH (2009) Late rupture of polytetrafluoroethylene neochordae after mitral valve repair. J Thorac Cardiovasc Surg 137:504–506
59. Yau TM, El-Ghoneimi YAF, Armstrong S, Ivanov J, David TE (2000) Mitral valve repair and replacement for rheumatic disease. J Thorac Cardiovasc Surg 119:53–61
60. Shahin GM, van der Heijden GJ, Kelder JC, Boulaksil M, Knaepen PJ, Six AJ (2006) Long-term follow-up of mitral valve repair: a single-center experience. Med Sci Monit 12:308–314
61. Talwalkar NG, Earle NR, Earle EA, Lawrie GM (2004) Mitral valve repair in patients with low left ventricular ejection fractions: early and late results. Chest 126:709–715
62. Shahian DM, O'Brien SM, Filardo G, Ferraris VA, Haan CK, Rich JB, Normand SL, DeLong ER, Shewan CM, Dokholyan RS, Peterson ED, Edwards FH, Anderson RP (2009) The Society of Thoracic Surgeons 2008 cardiac surgery risk models: part 3–valve plus coronary artery bypass grafting surgery. Society of Thoracic Surgeons Quality Measurement Task Force. Ann Thorac Surg 88(Suppl):S43–62

63. Adams DH, Anyanwu A (2006) Pitfalls and limitations in measuring and interpreting the outcomes of mitral valve repair. J Thorac Cardiovasc Surg 131:565–573
64. Shuhaiber J, Anderson RJ (2007) Meta-analysis of clinical outcomes following surgical mitral valve repair or replacement. Eur J Cardiothorac Surg 31:267–275
65. Farivar RS, Shernan SK, Cohn LH (2009) Late rupture of polytetrafluoroethylene neochordae after mitral valve repair. J Thorac Cardiovasc Surg 137:504–506
66. Yacoub MH, Kilner PJ, Birks EJ, Misfeld MI (1999) The aortic outflow and root: a tale of dynamism and crosstalk. Ann Thorac Surg 68:S37–43
67. Yacoub MH, Cohn LH (2004) Novel approaches to cardiac valve repair: from structure to function: Part II. Circulation 109:1064–1072
68. DiBardino DJ, ElBardissi AW, McClure RS, Razo-Vasquez OA, Kelly NE, Cohn LH (2010) Four decades of experience with mitral valve repair: analysis of differential indications, technical evolution, and long-term outcome. J Thorac Cardiovasc Surg 139:76–83
69. Rankin JS, Burrichter CA, Walton-Shirley MK, Whiteside JH, Teague SM, McLaughlin VW, Sharma MK, Johnston TS, McRae AT, Myers PR (2009) Trends in mitral valve surgery: a single practice experience. J Heart Valve Dis 18:359–366
70. Rankin JS, Sharma MK, Teague SM, McLaughlin VW, Johnston TS, McRae AT (2008) A new approach to mitral valve repair for rheumatic disease: preliminary study. J Heart Valve Dis 17:614–619
71. Romano MA, Patel HJ, Pagani FD, Prager RL, Deeb GM,Bolling SF (2005) Anterior leaflet repair with patch augmentation for mitral regurgitation. Ann Thorac Surg 79:1500–1504
72. Aubert S, Flecher E, Rubin S, Acar C, Gandjbakhch I (2007) Anterior mitral leaflet augmentation with autologous pericardium. Ann Thorac surg 83:1560–1561.
73. von Oppell UO, Mohr FW (2000) Chordal replacement for both minimally invasive and conventional mitral valve surgery using premeasured Gore-Tex loops. Ann Thorac Surg 70:2167–2168

Mitral valve repair in rheumatic disease

J.S. Rankin, M.A. Daneshmand, J.G. Gaca

18.1 Introduction

Rheumatic mitral valve disease was the earliest indication for cardiac surgery [1], and techniques have evolved progressively since the first mitral »valvotomy« by Elliot Cutler in 1923 [2]. Worldwide, rheumatic heart disease remains a major cause of cardiac morbidity and mortality with the incidence exceeding 50 per 100,000 children [3]. After decades of declining incidence in North America and Europe, current data suggest that rheumatic disease is increasing [4] even in developed countries. In most cardiac surgical centers, rheumatic valve dysfunction remains a significant clinical entity comprising approximately 20% of current mitral practice [5].

In recent years, prosthetic valve replacement has been the dominant procedure for treatment of rheumatic mitral valve disease. With recent improvements in reconstructive techniques, however, the overall rate of mitral valve repair in North America is increasing steadily, and repair is expanding into more complex pathologies [6, 7]. Multiple clinical studies have demonstrated the general advantages of mitral valve repair over valve replacement, including lower operative mortality, improved left ventricular function, lower risk of stroke and infection, improved freedom from reoperation, freedom from anticoagulation, and superior long-term survival [8–11]. Given the documented clinical benefits of autologous valve reconstruction, it may be time to extend mitral repair into more patients with rheumatic disease.

18.2 Outcomes

Limited data are available to compare late outcomes after rheumatic mitral repair versus valve replacement. In the study by Yau and associates [12], 25% of 573 patients with rheumatic mitral disease had repair, and after risk adjustment with a Cox model, operative mortality was better with repair (0.7% after repair vs 5.1% for replacement) as was late survival (Fig. 18.1). Valve-related complications were lower after repair, although late reoperation was higher. At a mean follow-up of 68 months, 16% of repair patients required reoperation, although no reoperative mortalities occurred. Similar data were reported by Gaca et al. [13]. Of 416 patients having mitral surgery for rheumatic disease over a 20-year period, 11% underwent repair. While baseline characteristics of repair and replacement patients were similar, valve pathology almost certainly was worse in the replacement cohort. Risk-adjusted survival was significantly better after repair (Fig. 18.2), although reoperation was higher, being required in 19% at a median of 6 years. Although both studies employed repair methods that were rudimentary by today's standards, these data do suggest a consistent survival benefit of mitral repair for rheumatic disease, albeit with a higher reoperation rate. These data support the current effort to repair more rheumatic valves, and hopefully, newer repair methods will reduce reoperation rates as well. The following sections will describe repair methods for rheumatic mitral valves that have been highly successful in recent practice [14].

18.3 Repair techniques

In early experience, mitral surgery was limited to »closed commissurotomy« for mitral stenosis, and this procedure was effective in properly selected patients [15]. Later, »open commissurotomy« became the standard for patients with mitral stenosis [16], and ring annuloplasty together with submitral chordal procedures were introduced for patients with insufficiency

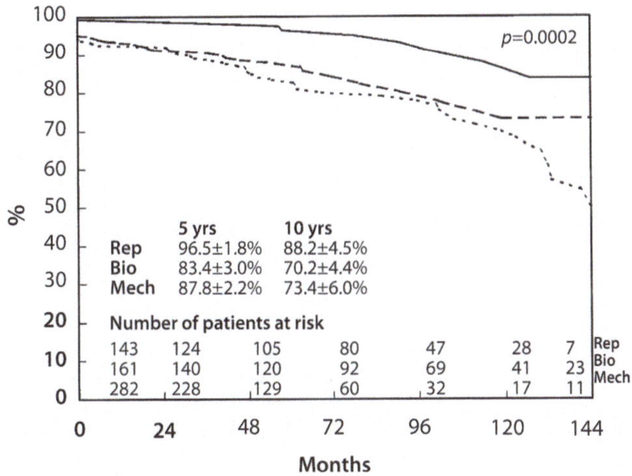

Fig. 18.1. Survival (y-axis) in rheumatic mitral surgery patients after repair (*Rep*), tissue valve replacement (*Bio*), and mechanical valves (*Mech*). Repair produced significantly better outcomes ([12]; © The American Association for Thoracic Surgery)

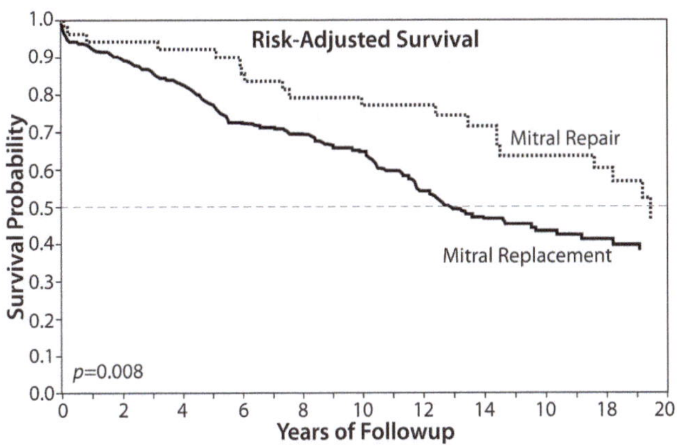

Fig. 18.2. Risk-adjusted survival after mitral surgery for rheumatic disease consisting of repair versus replacement. Repair produced significantly better outcomes. ([13]; © Elsevier Publishing)

[17]. However, repair with these techniques failed in up to 20% of patients–because of continued retraction of the posterior leaflet causing worsening leak–or because of persistent submitral disease producing continued valve obstruction. As a result, many surgeons abandoned rheumatic valve repair because the pathology was prone to »progress« [18–21]; but in fact, the underlying pathology was often not adequately corrected at the original operation. It was later shown that gluteraldehyde-fixed autologous pericardial patches were effective in repairing valves with scarred retracted leaflet tissue, and good long-term results were published from a number of sources [22–27]. It also became clear that late results of rheumatic repair were better if submitral obstruction was adequately relieved, and several methods were utilized for accomplishing this objective [28, 29]. Finally, with perfection of artificial chordal replacement using Gore-Tex® sutures [30–42], it became possible to resect even the most diseased of submitral structures to the anterior leaflet, and after reattachment of the anterior leaflet to the papillary muscles with artificial chords, excellent anterior leaflet mobility could be re-established [43]. Using combinations of these techniques, the vast majority of rheumatic valves now can

be repaired, and the benefits of valve repair can be extended to most rheumatic patients [44]. Preoperative concomitant atrial fibrillation is usually treated with the Cox–Maze IV atrial ablation procedure [45]. The goal is to complete surgical therapy with a long-term functional repair of the patient's own mitral valve and normal sinus rhythm, so that the patient can be maintained only on aspirin, with the attendant lower complication rates of autologous repair. The following sections will describe multiple minor variations in reconstructive approaches that are used for the different varieties of rheumatic mitral disease.

18.4 Pure mitral regurgitation

A common pathology in rheumatic disease is pure mitral regurgitation, especially with the acute disease variety seen in developing countries. The defect is caused by scarring and retraction of the posterior leaflet, or scarring and tethering of the chordae, or both. Early in the mitral repair experience, these lesions were treated with ring annuloplasty alone, and because of inadequate posterior leaflet surface area, recurrence rates were high. The Europeans then reported using gluteraldehyde-fixed autologous pericardial patches to augment the scarred posterior leaflet with excellent long-term results [23–25]. This approach is now the standard for treating pure rheumatic mitral regurgitation. An example is a 67-year-old male with pure rheumatic mitral regurgitation, NYHA Class IV heart failure, atrial fibrillation, normal coronaries, and normal LV function (◘ Fig. 18.3). The echocardiogram shows the *characteristic scarred retracted posterior leaflet* and a central regurgitant jet. A segment of the patient's own pericardium was excised and immersed in 0.6% glutaraldehyde for 10 minutes. It should be emphasized that glutaraldehyde can harbor bacteria, so it is important for the pharmacy to filter it during preparation. In ◘ Fig. 18.4, the posterior leaflet has been incised from the annulus throughout its length, leaving 1 cm intact at each commissure. The patch of autologous pericardium is sewn to the annular side of the leaflet incision, using 4-0 Prolene and starting in the center of the incision and working toward both ends. The patch is then trimmed anteriorly to fit the incision, judging the size so that the leaflet-side suture line will form the line of coaptation after completion. The suture line is completed anteriorly, starting in the center and working laterally, and then both sutures are tied at the ends of the leaflet incision. Thus, the original posterior leaflet moves down into the ventricle and forms the entire posterior surface of coaptation. After simple insertion of a posterior leaflet pericardial patch and an annuloplasty ring, the valve has a large surface area of coaptation and margin of safety, and no residual leak (◘ Fig. 18.3). Most of the competent leaflet tissue shown in ◘ Fig. 18.4 is actually pericardial patch. In pure rheumatic mitral regurgitation, this method is all that is required and achieves excellent long-term results [24]. Sinus rhythm has been maintained in this patient after the Cox–Maze IV ablation.

18.5 Pure mitral stenosis

A common form of rheumatic disease in North America is pure mitral stenosis. In ◘ Fig. 18.5 is shown a valve of a 55-year-old woman with a long history of mitral stenosis, NYHA class III heart failure, normal coronaries, and normal LV function. The valve is quite stenotic with completely fused left and right commissures, but no leak. Both commissures are developed using sharp and blunt dissection, and chordal attachments to the posterior leaflet are main-

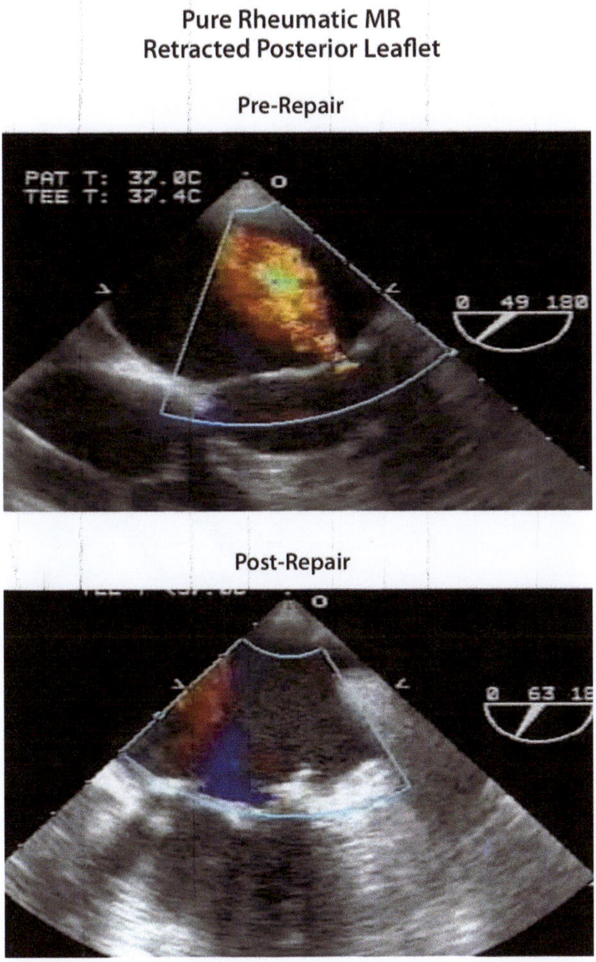

Fig. 18.3. Operative transesophageal echocardiogram in a patient with regurgitation due to posterior leaflet retraction undergoing posterior leaflet pericardial patch augmentation. The valve is completely competent at the conclusion of the procedure

tained. Commonly, the anterior leaflet is fused directly to the papillary muscles, and these attachments are transected, leaving the anterior leaflet free of the submitral obstruction. Any calcium in the commissures or anterior leaflet is resected. Usually, calcification involves the endocardial layer, and a normal appearing anterior leaflet emerges with careful dissection (Fig. 18.5). As in the previous example, the posterior leaflet is incised from the annulus throughout its length, leaving 1 cm intact at each commissure. Then an autologous pericardial patch is inserted, and after ring placement, two sets of artificial chords are run from both papillary muscles to the right and left corners of the anterior leaflet (Fig. 18.5). In Fig. 18.6a, preoperative leaflet fusion and stenosis are evident. After repair (Fig. 18.6b), the valve closes normally without leak. With mobilization and artificial chordal replacement of the anterior leaflet (Figs. 18.6c, d), the valve exhibits excellent leaflet motion, no leak, insignificant gradient, and laminar flow. The combination of posterior leaflet pericardial patching and anterior leaflet mobilization/chordal replacement routinely produces an adequate physiological result, even in the most diseased rheumatic valves.

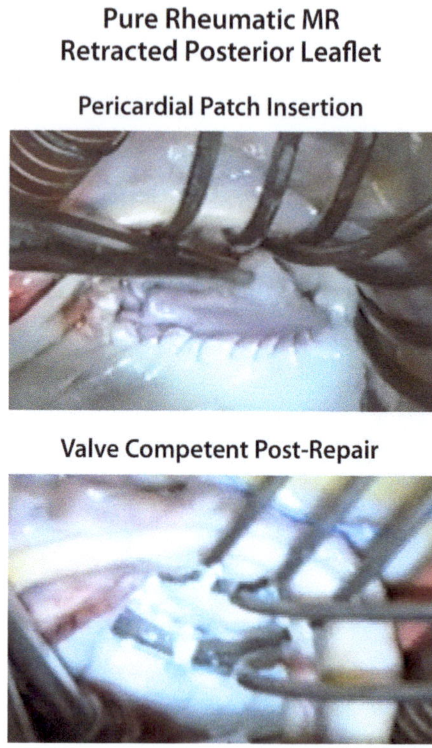

Fig. 18.4. Appearance of a regurgitant valve due to rheumatic posterior leaflet retraction during pericardial patch augmentation, and after repair, showing complete valve competence. Most of the leaflet visible after repair is the pericardial patch

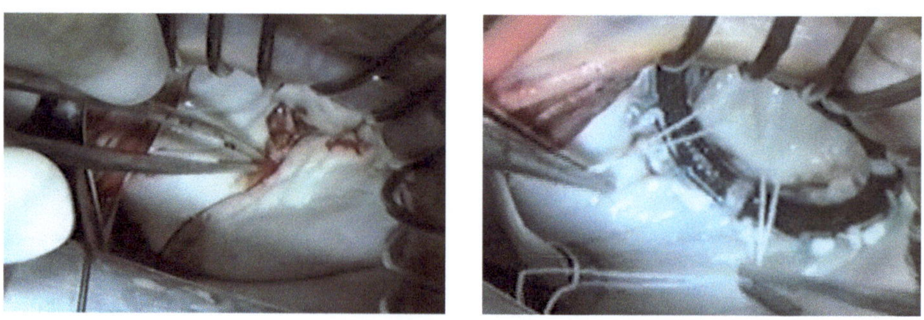

Fig. 18.5. Appearance of a rheumatic mitral valve with stenosis before and after repair. Notice the emergence of a fairly normal appearing anterior leaflet after complete mobilization and artificial chordal replacement

18.6 Complex mixed lesions–advanced calcification and predominant stenosis

The next patient is a 62-year-old woman with long-standing mixed mitral stenosis and regurgitation, chronic atrial fibrillation, clear coronaries, and moderate left ventricular dysfunction. She had limited leaflet mobility and significant stenosis, but also concurrent mitral regurgitation (Fig. 18.7). At the beginning of the case, she underwent a Cox–Maze IV procedure, and then the valve was approached. The calcium in the commissures was debrided, and

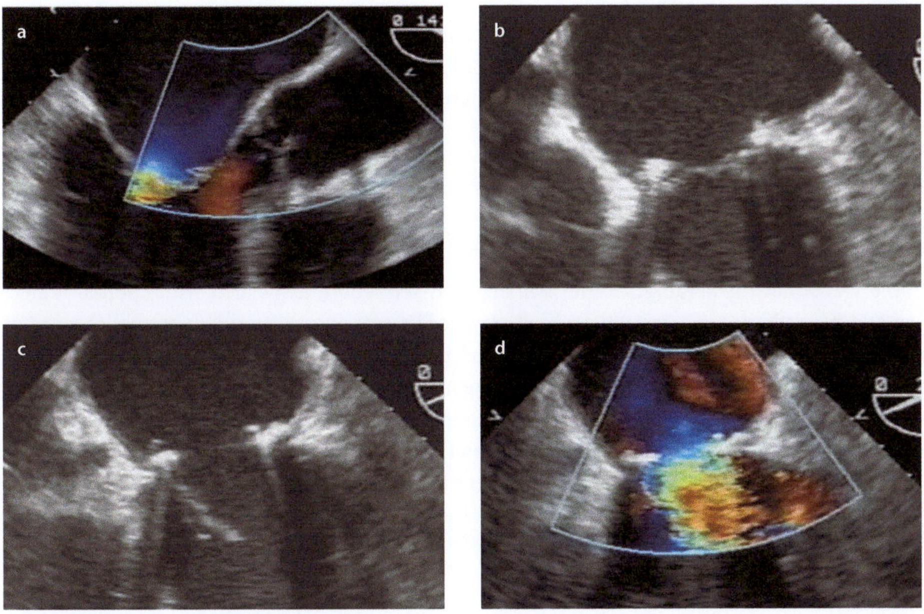

Fig. 18.6. Operative transesophageal echocardiogram during rheumatic repair for mitral stenosis: preoperative valve (**a**) and frames obtained after repair (**b–d**)

the commissures were developed using sharp and blunt dissection. The chordal attachments to the posterior leaflet were maintained, but the primary and secondary chords to the anterior leaflet were disconnected. Pledgeted anchor sutures and 2-0 Gore-Tex® artificial chords were passed through both papillary muscles and left untied. The chords were stuffed into the ventricle for later retrieval. In Fig. 18.8a, the posterior leaflet was disconnected from the annulus throughout most of its length. In Fig. 18.8b, the pericardial patch was inserted into the posterior leaflet with a running 4-0 Prolene suture. A pledgeted valve suture was placed in the left fibrous trigone, and then also in the right, and a Carpentier ring was true-sized. The posterior ring sutures were completed using an interrupted pledgeted technique, and the ring was moved into position. Full rigid Carpentier rings are used in all cases, since it is sometimes difficult to bring annular shape into proper geometry. The anterior leaflet was further debrided as necessary to ensure free hinge movement and good mobility. After ring annuloplasty placement (Fig. 18.8c), the artificial chords were retrieved and run from both papillary muscles to the front corners of the anterior leaflet. Finally, the neochordal lengths were adjusted and tied, and the valve was completely competent with saline pressurization (Fig. 18.8d). The posterior leaflet patch and tied anterior leaflet artificial chords are evident. On the postoperative echocardiogram (Fig. 18.7), the anterior leaflet opens well, the gradient is negligible, and there is no residual leak. A 1-year transesophageal echocardiogram also is shown, and the hemodynamic result has remained stable. The atrial ablation was also successful, and the patient achieved an excellent valve repair and sinus rhythm long term. Echocardiograms have been obtained in all patients on a yearly basis and have been stable in over 20 patients at this point, beyond 5 years. These findings suggest that a more rigorous valve reconstruction will not only allow most rheumatic valves to be repaired, but also will reduce late failure/reoperation rates. It is highly probable that late outcomes will improve over those observed with prosthetic valve replacement. The transesophageal echocardiogram from a similar patient is shown in ◘ Fig. 18.9, and videos from this patient's operation can be viewed at: http://www.ctsnet.org/sections/clinicalresources/videos/vg2010_RankinS_MVR_Rheumatic.html

18.7 Advanced mixed lesions–predominant leaflet tethering and regurgitation

Some valves have generalized leaflet scarring and retraction, associated with chordal tethering and regurgitation (◘ Fig. 18.10a). Multiple chordal scarring can produce virtual absence of chords, with leaflets inserting directly into the papillary muscles. The basic operation is the same as described above, with pericardial augmentation of the posterior leaflet and mobilization of the anterior leaflet together with artificial chordal replacement. In ◘ Fig. 18.10b, the finished repair shows the posterior leaflet patch, the anterior leaflet chords, and complete valve competence. It is rarely necessary to resect or augment the anterior leaflet, although this can be done

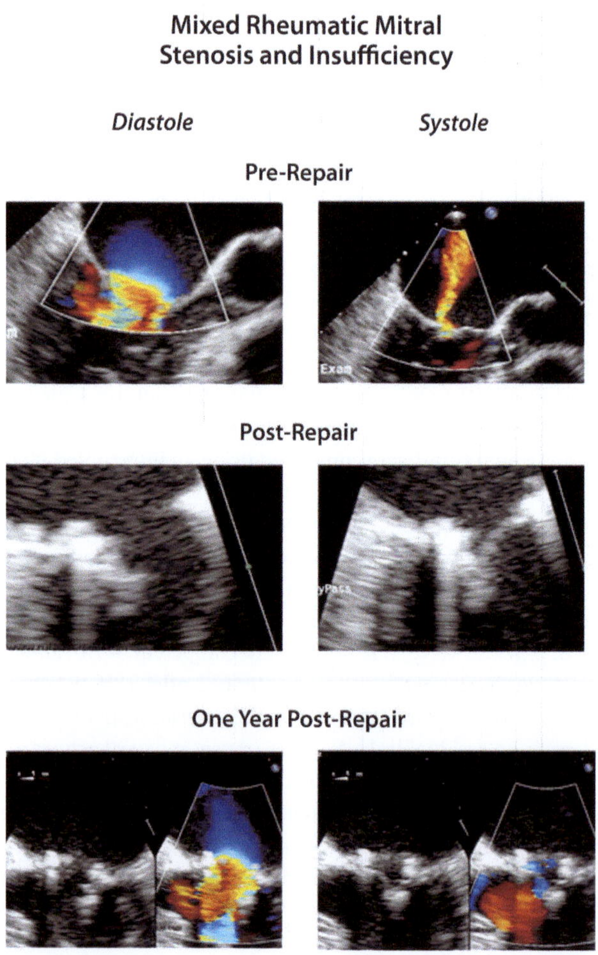

◘ **Fig. 18.7.** Operative transesophageal echocardiogram before, after, and 1-year after rheumatic mitral repair

18

if necessary [44]. In some cases, chordal scarring can involve only one or two chords and make the chordal tethering abnormality more subtle. In such cases, single chords can be resected and replaced with Gore-Tex® neochordae. However, virtually all rheumatic abnormalities now can be corrected with techniques utilizing autologous tissues, as described in this report.

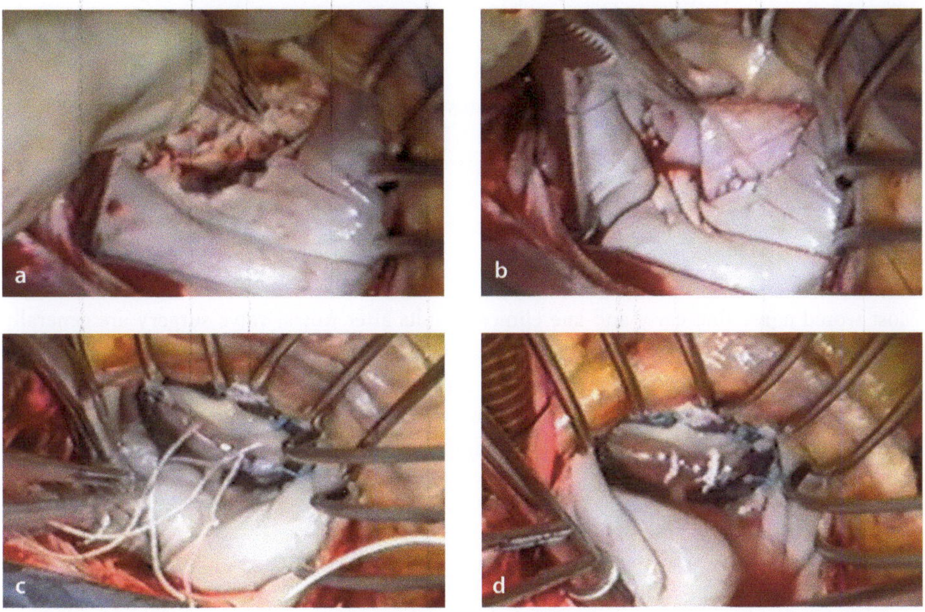

Fig. 18.8. Operative appearance of valve during successive stages of rheumatic repair. See text for details

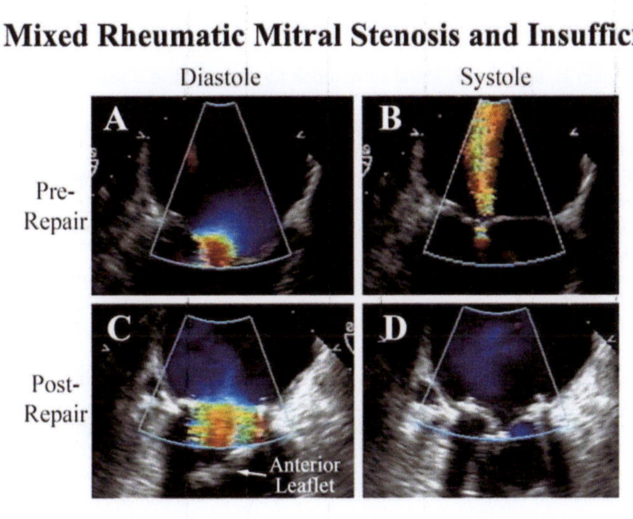

Fig. 18.9. Operative transesophageal echocardiogram before and after rheumatic mitral repair. See text for details

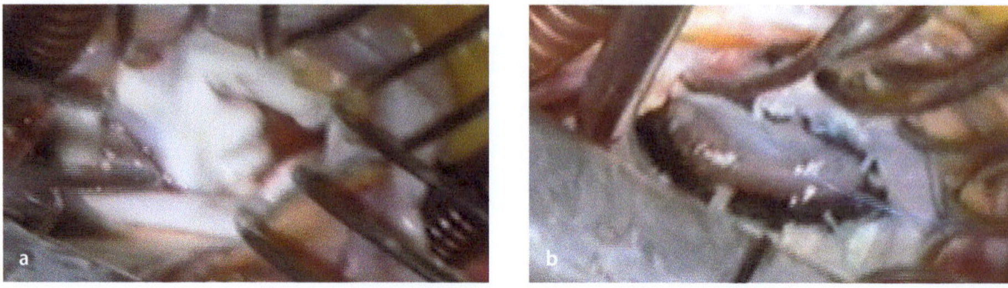

Fig. 18.10. Operative appearance of a scarred and retracted rheumatic valve before (**a**) and after repair (**b**). See text for details

18.8 Conclusion

Most would agree that early and late clinical results after mitral valve surgery are generally better with repair, compared to replacement, in most forms of mitral disease. Given recent advances in leaflet and chordal replacement, it may now be time to reassess the role of valve repair in rheumatic disease. The combination of posterior leaflet pericardial patching and anterior chordal replacement appears promising, but longer follow-up will be required to fully validate this approach.

References

1. Rankin JS (1986) Mitral and tricuspid valve disease: historical aspects. In: Sabiston DC, Jr. (ed) Textbook of surgery. WB Saunders Company, Philadelphia, pp 2345ff
2. Cutler EC, Levine SA, Beck CS (1924) The surgical treatment of mitral stenosis: experimental and clinical studies. Arch Surg 689–698
3. Carapetis JR, McDonald M, Wilson NJ (2005) Acute rheumatic fever. Lancet 366:155–168
4. Lee GM, Wessels MR (2006) Changing epidemiology of acute rheumatic fever in the United States. Clin Infect Dis 42:448–450
5. Daneshmand MA, Milano CA, Rankin JS, et al. (2009) Mitral valve repair for degenerative disease: a 20-year experience. Ann Thorac Surg 88:1828–1837
6. Gammie JS, Sheng S, Griffith BP, et al. (2009) Trends in mitral valve surgery in the United States: results from The Society of Thoracic Surgeons Adult Cardiac Database. Ann Thorac Surg 87:1431–1439
7. Rankin JS, Alfery DD, Orozco RE, et al. (2008) Techniques of artificial chordal replacement for mitral valve repair: use in multiple pathologies. Op Tech Thorac Cardiovasc Surg 13:74–82
8. Rankin JS, Hammill BG, Ferguson JTB, et al. (2006) Determinants of operative mortality in valvular heart surgery. J Thorac Cardiovasc Surg 131:547–557
9. Daneshmand MA, Milano CA, Rankin JS (2010) Influence of patient age on procedural selection in mitral valve surgery. Ann Thorac Surg 90:1479–1486
10. Braunberger E, Deloche A, Berrebi A, et al. (2001) Very long-term results (more than 20 years) of valve repair with Carpentier's techniques in nonrheumatic mitral valve insufficiency. Circulation 104:I8–I11
11. Milano CA, Daneshmand MA, Rankin JS, et al. (2008) Survival prognosis and surgical management of ischemic mitral regurgitation. Ann Thorac Surg 86:735–744
12. Yau TM, El-Ghoneimi YAF, Armstrong S, et al. (2000) Mitral valve repair and replacement for rheumatic disease. J Thorac Cardiovasc Surg 119:53–61
13. Gaca JG, Daneshmand MA, Rankin JS, et al. (2010) Re-examination of mitral valve repair in rheumatic heart disease. Ann Thorac Surg (in press)
14. Rankin JS, Burrichter CA, Walton-Shirley MK, et al. (2009) Trends in mitral valve surgery: a single practice experience. J Heart Valve Dis 18:359–366
15. Bailey CP, Glover RP, O'Neill TJE (1950) The surgery of mitral stenosis. J Thorac Surg 19:16–25

16. Housman LB, Bonchek L, Lambert L, et al. (1977) Prognosis of patients after open mitral commissurotomy: Actuarial analysis of results in 100 patients. J Thorac Cardiovasc Surg 73:742–749
17. Carpentier A (1983) Cardiac valve surgery – the »French correction«. J Thorac Cardiovasc Surg 86:323–337
18. Duran CM, Gometza B, Saad E (1994) Valve repair in rheumatic mitral disease: an unsolved problem. J Card Surg 9:282–285
19. Kuwaki K, Kawaharada N, Morishita K, et al. (2007) Mitral valve repair versus replacement in mitral and aortic valve surgery for rheumatic disease. Ann Thorac Surg 83:558–563
20. Kumar AS, Talwar S, Saxena A, et al. (2006) Results of mitral valve repair in rheumatic mitral regurgitation. Interact Cardiovasc Thorac Surg 5:356–361
21. Shin HJ, Lee YJ, Choo SJ, et al. (2005) Analysis of recurrent mitral regurgitation after mitral valve repair. Asian Cardiovasc Thorac Ann 13:261–266
22. Frater RWM (1964) Anatomical rules for the plastic repair of a diseased valve. Thorax 19:458–464
23. Chauvaud S, Jebara V, Chachques JC, et al. (1991)Valve extension with gluteraldehyde-preserved autologous pericardium. J Thorac Cardiovasc Surg 102:171–177
24. Chauvaud S, Fuzellier JF, Berrebi A, et al. (2001) Long-term (29 years) results of reconstructive surgery in rheumatic mitral valve insufficiency. Circulation 104(Suppl I):I12–I15
25. Ng CK, Nesser J, Punzengruber C, et al. (2001) Valvuloplasty with glutaraldehyde-treated autologous pericardium in patients with complex mitral valve pathology. Ann Thorac Surg 71:78–85
26. Romano MA, Patel HJ, Pagani FD, et al. (2005) Anterior leaflet repair with patch augmentation for mitral regurgitation. Ann Thorac Surg 79:1500–1504
27. Acar C, de Ibarra JS, Lansac E (2004) Anterior leaflet augmentation with autologous pericardium for mitral repair in rheumatic valve insufficiency. J Heart Valve Dis 13:741–746
28. Bernal JM, Rabasa JM, Olalla JJ, et al. (1996) Repair of chordae tendineae for rheumatic mitral valve disease: a twenty-year experience. J Thorac Cardiovasc Surg 111:211–217
29. Pomerantzeff PM, Brandão CM, Faber CM (2000) Mitral valve repair in rheumatic patients. Heart Surg Forum 3:273–276
30. Vetter HO, Burack JH, Factor SM, et al. (1986) Replacement of chordae tendineae of the mitral valve using the new expanded PTFE suture in sheep. In: Bodnar E, Yacoub M (eds) Biologic bioprosthetic valves. Yorke Medical Books, New York, pp 772–784
31. Frater RWM, Vetter HO, Zussa C, et al. (1990) Chordal replacement in mitral valve repair. Circulation 82 (Suppl IV):125–130
32. David TE, Bos J, Rakowski H (1991) Mitral valve repair by replacement of chordae tendineae with polytetrafluoroethylene sutures. J Thorac Cardiovasc Surg 101:495–501
33. David TE, Omran A, Armstrong S, et al. (1998) Long-term results of mitral valve repair for myxomatous disease with and without chordal replacement with expanded polytetrafluoroethylene sutures. J Thorac Cardiovasc Surg 115:1279–1285
34. Duebener LF, Wendler O, Nikoloudakis N, et al. (2000) Mitral-valve repair without annuloplasty rings: results after repair of anterior leaflet versus posterior-leaflet defects using polytetrafluoroethylene sutures for chordal replacement. Eur J Cardiothorac Surg 17:206–212
35. von Oppell UO, Mohr FW (2000) Chordal replacement for both minimally invasive and conventional mitral valve surgery using premeasured Gore-Tex loops. Ann Thorac Surg 70:2166–2168
36. Nigro JJ, Schwartz DS, Bart RD, et al. (2004) Neochordal repair of the posterior mitral leaflet. J Thorac Cardiovasc Surg 127:440–447
37. Rankin JS, Orozco RE, Addai TR, Rodgers TL, Tuttle RH, Shaw LK, Glower DD (2004) Several new considerations in mitral valve repair. J Heart Valve Dis 13:399–409
38. Rankin JS, Orozco RE, Rodgers TL, et al. (2006) »Adjustable« artificial chordal replacement for repair of mitral valve prolapse. Ann Thorac Surg 81:1526–1528
39. Lawrie GM, Earle EA, Earle NR (2006) Feasibility and intermediate term outcome of repair of prolapsing anterior mitral leaflets with artificial chordal replacement in 152 patients. Ann Thorac Surg 81:849–856
40. Rankin JS, Alfery DD, Orozco R, et al. (2008) Techniques of artificial chordal replacement for mitral valve repair: use in multiple pathologic disorders. Op Tech Thorac Cardiovasc Surg 13:74–82
41. Chiappini B, Sanchez A, Noirhomme P, et al. (2006) Replacement of chordae tendineae with polytetrafluoroethylene (PTFE) sutures in mitral valve repair: early and long-term results. J Heart Valve Dis 15:657–663
42. Salvador L, Mirone S, Bianchini R, et al. (2008) Twenty-year experience of mitral valve repair with artificial chordae in 608 patients. J Thorac Cardiovasc Surg 135:1280–1287
43. Rankin JS, Sharma MK, Teague SM, et al. (2008) A new method of mitral valve repair for rheumatic disease: preliminary study. J Heart Valve Dis 17:614–619
44. El Oumeiri B, Boodhwani M, Glineur D, et al. (2009) Extending the scope of mitral valve repair in rheumatic disease. Ann Thorac Surg 87:1735–1740
45. Lall SC, Melby SJ, et al. (2007) The effect of ablation technology on surgical outcomes after the Cox–Maze procedure: a propensity analysis. J Thorac Cardiovasc Surg 133:389–396

Autologous pericardial patch leaflet augmentation in the setting of mitral valve repair

J. Chikwe, A.B. Goldstone, A. Akujuo, J. Castillo, D.H. Adams

19.1 Introduction

Mitral valve repair is the standard of care for correction of significant mitral regurgitation for a wide range of etiologies as it confers a significant survival advantage in selected patients, has demonstrated equivalent or superior durability compared to bioprosthetic replacement particularly in young patients, reduces the thromboembolic complications of mechanical replacement, and avoids the need for anticoagulation [1]. Leaflet augmentation with glutaraldehyde-fixed autologous pericardium is a useful adjunct when there is insufficient leaflet tissue to produce a reliable repair using standard techniques, as it is a cheap and readily available substrate with excellent resistance to infection and calcific degeneration. Autologous pericardial patch augmentation has been described in the setting of rheumatic mitral insufficiency [2], ischemic mitral regurgitation [3], endocarditis [4], congenital mitral valve disease [5], and re-repair [6]. Here, we provide a brief overview of the historical background, a technical description of our approach to mitral valve repair requiring pericardial patch leaflet augmentation, followed by a summary of the operative technique and results reported according to etiology.

19.2 History

Among the earliest attempts to use pericardium as a substrate for mitral valve repair were those by John Gibbon of Jefferson College in Philadelphia in the pre- cardiopulmonary bypass era of cardiac surgery. He managed to reduce mitral regurgitation using a pedicled piece of autologous pericardium, which he passed around the mitral annulus using a finger in the left atrial appendage, suturing the free ends with sufficient tension to reduce regurgitation. His use of pedicled pericardium, as opposed to a free graft, was aimed at reducing late shrinkage, and he claimed success with this technique in 6 patients.

Early approaches to mitral valve surgery permitted by the advent of cardiopulmonary bypass included use of a wide variety of substitutes, including autologous pericardium, dura mater and fascia-lata in both repair and valve replacement (Fig. 19.1) [7]. Early shrinkage and rapid thickening and calcification of all these tissues were observed. Preshinking these tissues in formaldehyde appeared to offer some increased longevity, but long-term outcomes remained unsatisfactory, and it was not until the 1960s when Dr Alain Carpentier discovered the unique ability of glutaraldehyde to cross-link collagen fibers, eliminating the early shrinkage and greatly reducing the rapid thickening [8], that pericardium began to be seen as a viable long-term substitute for leaflet tissue. Initially applied to xenograft valve replacement, glutaraldehyde fixation of autologous pericardium has become a useful adjunct in complex mitral valve repair where leaflet tissue is deficient.

19.3 Glutaraldehyde fixation

Following sternotomy, a piece of pericardium approximately 5 cm by 5 cm is freed from any pleural and mediastinal adhesions. The pericardial patch is unfolded onto cardboard from a suture packet, secured in place with surgical clips, and immersed in 0.625% buffered glutaraldehyde solution (Poly Scientific, Bay Shore, NY) for 15 minutes. The patch is then rinsed in saline for a minimum of 15 minutes. Fixing tissue beyond 20 minutes provides minimal extra cross-linkage. Tissue elasticity and handling is preserved. Fixation not only stabilizes the

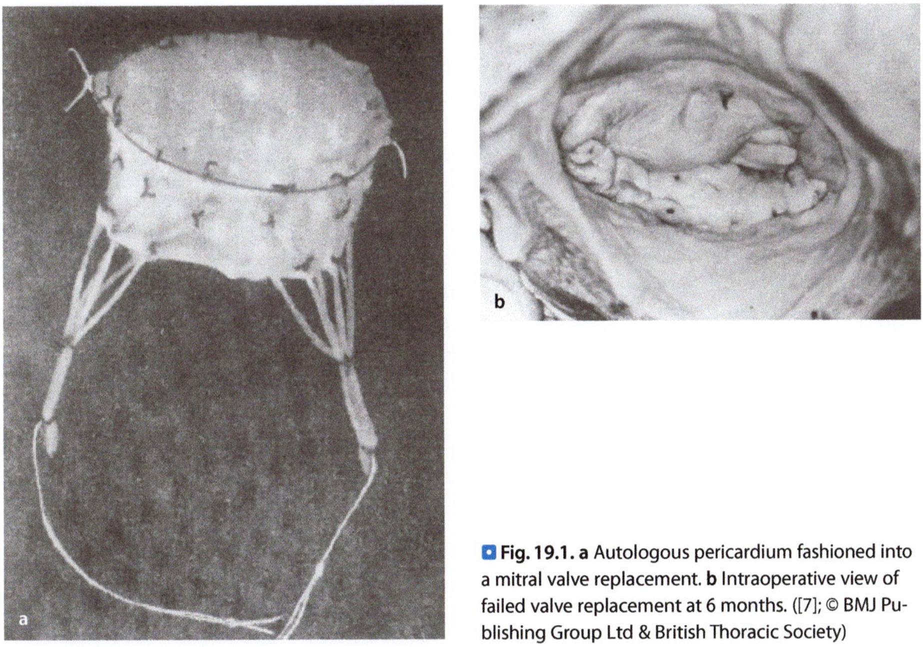

Fig. 19.1. **a** Autologous pericardium fashioned into a mitral valve replacement. **b** Intraoperative view of failed valve replacement at 6 months. ([7]; © BMJ Publishing Group Ltd & British Thoracic Society)

collagen cross-linkages preventing early shrinkage, but also reduces tissue antigenicity (relevant in heterologous pericardium), and reduces enzymatic degradation and cell viability [9]. The latter becomes relevant many years after implantation as, in the absence of normal cell mechanisms for transporting calcium, the pericardium eventually calcifies. The same process in bioprosthetic tissue valves eventually results in structural degeneration.

19.4 Principal of repair

The mitral valve is exposed through a sternotomy or thoracotomy, using bicaval cannulation, via Sondergaard's groove and systematically analyzed to identify valvular lesions. Usually abnormal leaflet tissue is completely resected, leaving margins supported by normal length chordae wherever possible. If the defect is in the anterior leaflet, sizing and sewing the patch is facilitated by a traction stitch securing the margin of A2 to the pericardial well above the right pulmonary veins. The pericardial patch is sized 4–5 mm larger than the defect, so that it can sewn in without tension. A running 4-0 Prolene suture is generally used, taking care not to purse-string it. Where the patch forms the leaflet margin without the support of native chordae, chordal transfers or neochorade are employed. At completion of reconstruction, a saline test is employed to reveal any residual mitral regurgitation. After the valve is deemed competent, the surface of coaptation is evaluated with an intraoperative »ink test« [10]. The coaptation line is delineated with a Gentian violet marking pen (Codman, Raynham, MA), and subsequent aspiration of intraventricular saline permits inspection of each leaflet. A coaptation depth of greater than 4 mm below the marked line (but less 10 mm with respect to the anterior leaflet) is judged satisfactory. Frequently, most of the area of the patch is below the coaptation line. Occasionally, it is not possible to harvest autologous pericardium that is suitable for use in this context: alternative substrates that have been employed using the same principals include bovine pericardium, and Core matrix.

19.5 Long-term results of repair

Chauvaud et al. [11] provide long-term results for 64 patients who underwent leaflet augmentation using autologous glutaraldehyde-fixed pericardium between 1980 and 1989. Their patients ranged from 3–60 years (mean 19±15 years), and etiology included rheumatic fever (69%), bacterial endocarditis (17%), congenital (8%), endomyocardial fibrosis (4.5%), and trauma (1.5%). Posterior leaflet augmentation was performed more frequently than anterior leaflet augmentation for all etiologies, except for endocarditis where anterior and posterior leaflets were equally likely to be affected. Adjunctive techniques included chordal techniques (shortening, transposition, and fenestration), and commissurotomy, with almost 80% of patients receiving a remodeling annuloplasty ring. The mean follow-up was 3±2.5 years. There were no operative deaths, 1 late death, and 6 reoperations—at which the pericardium was found to be free of calcification in all cases. There was 80% freedom from mild or greater mitral insufficiency.

19.6 Endocarditis

19.6.1 Technique

All infected and necrotic material is carefully debrided, including leaflet tissue, annulus and subvalvular apparatus, taking care to spare leaflet margin and associated chords wherever possible. A thoracoscopic camera is used to look for vegetations on the ventricular side of the valve. The feasibility of repair depends on how much leaflet tissue remains: if extensive augmentation is required of both leaflets, then a durable repair is unlikely. A pericardial patch is sewn to defects in the native leaflet using a 5-0 polypropylene suture. Additional techniques depend on the extent of debridement: most commonly the free leaflet margin requires additional support and where chordal transfer is not possible, we place 5-0 polytetrafluoroethylene chordae neochordae. In the case of small perforations of either leaflet, adjunctive repair techniques are not usually required. We routinely employ a true-sized annuloplasty ring in most patients, although in very young patients, we either do not use an annuloplasty ring, if the repair is competent, or perform a horizontal compression annuloplasty buttressed by a strip of glutaraldehyde-fixed autologous pericardium.

19.6.2 Results

Zegdi et al. [12] report the results of mitral valve repair for endocarditis in 37 patients, including 16 (43%) patients who required pericardial patch augmentation (◘ Fig. 19.2). In 4 patients (11%), it was possible to close a leaflet perforation primarily. In long-term follow-up, 1 patient required reoperation for patch dehiscence, and the 10-year rates of survival and freedom from reoperation were 80% (95% CI 66–94) and 95% (95% CI 81–100), respectively. Associated repair techniques included mitral annuloplasty in 31 patients (84%), chordal shortening or transposition procedures included aortic valve repair or replacement in 11 (30%), and tricuspid repair in 2 (6%) patients.

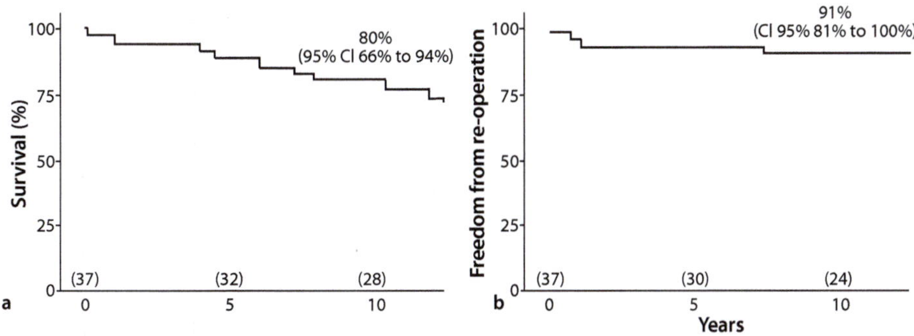

Fig. 19.2. The results from a series of 236 patients undergoing mitral repair for endocarditis, of whom just under half underwent glutaraldehyde-fixed autologous = pericardial parch augmentation: **a** survival (numbers in parentheses indicate numbers of patients alive), **b** freedom from reoperation (numbers in parentheses indicate number of patients at risk). ([12]; © American Heart Association)

19.7 Rheumatic valve disease

19.7.1 Technique

Rheumatic mitral valve disease results in a range of lesions that cause mitral regurgitation and/or stenosis through a variety of mechanisms, including Carpentier type I regurgitation due to annular dilatation, type II regurgitation resulting from leaflet prolapse, type IIIa regurgitation due to restricted leaflet motion as a result of thickening and calcification, and type IIa/IIIp (combined anterior leaflet prolapse with retraction of the posterior leaflet). Augmentation, most commonly of the posterior leaflet (although anterior leaflet augmentation has also been described [2, 13]), is performed to increase leaflet surface area in type IIIa lesions, or where resection of calcified areas has left a defect in leaflet tissue that cannot be closed primarily. In this case, the decision to repair the valve is based on the pliability of the anterior leaflet: Zegdi et al. [14] describe pushing the anterior leaflet with a pair of forceps to evaluate this—if the leaflet rebounds into position then fibrosis likely precludes repair. The posterior leaflet is detached from the posterior annulus (Fig. 19.3) and the secondary chordae are removed. A crescent shaped piece of autologous pericardium, sized 4–5 mm larger than the defect, is sewn into place using 5-0 continuous polypropylene suture. Adjunctive procedures usually required include commissurotomy for chordal fusion, and chordal fenestration to increase the mobility of fused chordae, or resection of fused chordae and replacement with PTFE neochordae.

19.7.2 Results

One of the largest reported series of rheumatic mitral valve repair which included 951 patients with mitral insufficiency, of which 65 underwent pericardial patch augmentation, reported excellent freedom from reoperation and long-term survival using these techniques (Fig. 19.4) [15]. Although the functional type was pure type III (restricted leaflet motion), where pericardial patch augmentation would be expected to be most commonly used, the freedom from reoperation was only 46% at 20 years, compared to 65% for rheumatic mitral regurgitation due to leaflet prolapse. Results of anterior leaflet augmentation with autologous pericardium for rheumatic mitral insufficiency were described in 62 patients operated on between 1995 and 1999. Significant associated stenosis was present in 19% of patients and all patients underwent ring annuloplasty. Mean follow-up was 3 years; reoperation was necessary in 1 case for early failure for patch dehiscence.

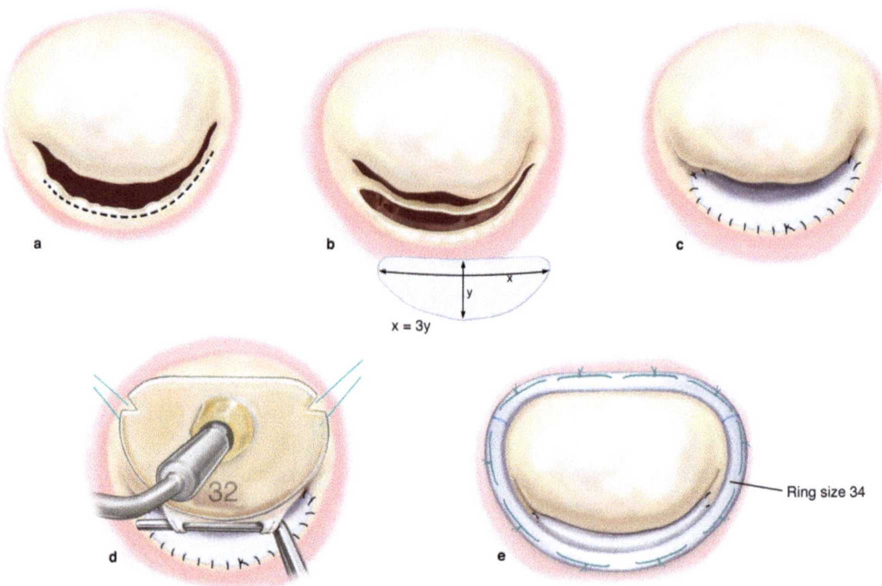

Fig. 19.3. Posterior leaflet augmentation. Mitral regurgitation is due to a type III a lesion with retracted posterior leaflet (**a**). This is excised, preserving the leaflet margin (**b**). The defect is repaired with a pericardial patch (**c**) and the ring sized according to the intercommissural distance and surface area of the anterior leaflet (**d**). The finished repair is shown (**d**) with a symmetrical closure line towards the posterior annulus and much of the patch providing coaptation area (**e**). ([18]; © Elsevier)

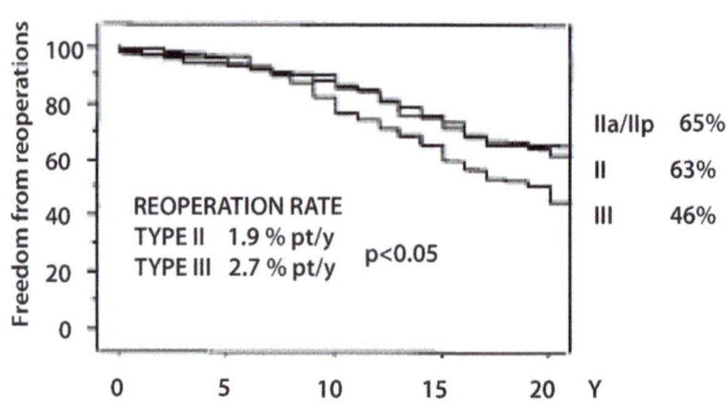

Fig. 19.4. Comparison between reoperation rates for rheumatic mitral valve repair, showing that type III lesions (in which leaflet augmentation techniques are most likely to be required) have lower freedom from reoperation than type II lesions, where leaflet prolapse is the mechanism of mitral regurgitation. ([15]; © American Heart Association)

19

19.8 Re-repair

19.8.1 Technique

The previous annuloplasty ring, associated pledgets, and remaining suture material are removed via sharp dissection with a scalpel (#15 blade) (◘ Fig. 19.5a and b). Particular care is taken not to damage the hinge leaflet tissue. If present, calcified areas, vegetations, and dehisced leaflet suture lines are completely debrided. Annular sutures are placed to improve exposure, thereby allowing attention to be turned to the subvalvular apparatus. Any abnormally shortened or fused chordae are resected, and wherever possible, leaflet margins with chordae of normal length are preserved. Leaflet margins are secured with 5-0 Prolene (Ethicon Inc., Piscataway, NJ) stay sutures to enable accurate assessment of the size of the leaflet defect. The decision is made to use a pericardial patch when a sliding plasty and compression annuloplasty will not suffice to approximate the leaflet edges without tension. The pericardial patch is sized 4–5 mm in diameter larger than the residual defect and attached to the native leaflets using a running 4-0 Prolene suture (◘ Fig. 19.5c). Chordal reconstruction using a combination of chordal transfer and 5-0 polytetrafluoroethylene (Gore-Tex®, Flagstaff, AZ) to create neochordae may

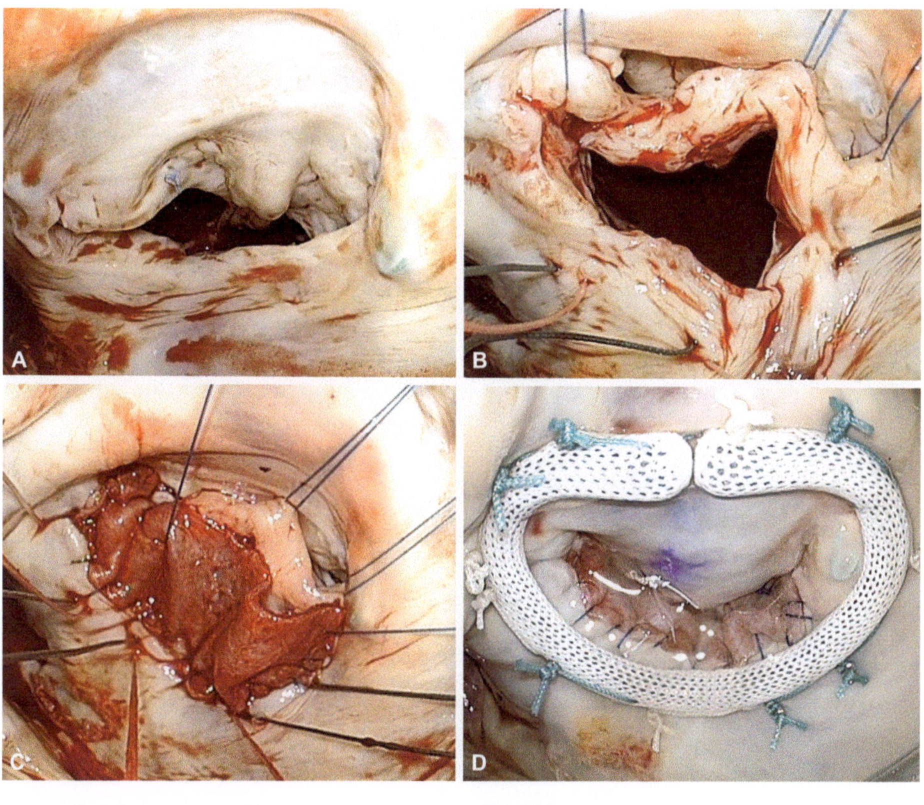

◘ **Fig. 19.5.** Pericardial patch augmentation used to treat failed primary repair (**a**), abnormal posterior leaflet tissue including the dehisced suture line resected preserving the laflet margin (**b**), pericardial patch sewn in situ (**c**), and a satisfactory saline test showing the finished repair with a Carpentier Classic annuloplasty ring, and a PTFE neo-chordae to support the P1 margin.

be performed where leaflet margins are unsupported by native chordae, or where native leaflet margins are absent. The valve is sized by comparing the height of the anterior leaflet and the intertrigonal distance to the valve sizer, and a true-sized complete remodeling annuloplasty ring implanted (◘ Fig. 19.5d), which is often several sizes smaller than the original implant, over-sizing of which is frequently a contributing factor in the failure of the primary repair. Additional mitral valve repair techniques, including commissural sutures, triangular resection, and cleft closure are often required to obtain a competent repair.

19.8.2 Results

Mitral valve re-repair provides an effective and durable treatment option when faced with recurrent mitral regurgitation. The preservation of left ventricular function and reduction of valve-related complications are associated with significantly improved survival in comparison with reoperative mitral valve replacement [6, 14]. Failure of mitral repair is attributable to procedure-related factors (e.g., suture and prosthetic ring dehiscence, excessive tension on leaflet suture lines, failure to take full-thickness bites, rupture of previously shortened chordae, or incomplete primary correction) or valve-related factors (e.g., progression of disease or endocarditis) [16]. Most mitral valve failures are valve-related in rheumatic disease and procedure-related in degenerative disease [16]. In both cases, resection of the diseased or damaged valvular components may be required for successful re-repair, leaving inadequate native tissue to complete a tension free, competent repair. Glutaraldehyde-treated pericardium represents a readily available, durable, and inexpensive substrate that is relatively resistant to infection which can be fashioned to reconstruct the valve leaflets as needed.

The durability of mitral re-repair compares favorably with bioprosthetic mitral valve replacement. In a study of 64 patients who underwent redo mitral repair, freedom from reoperation was 83% at the 5-year follow-up [6]. In the study, Zegdi et al. [14] noted that recurrent mitral regurgitation resulted from posterior leaflet retraction in 2 of 3 patients following re-repair, and proposed liberal pericardial augmentation of retracted posterior leaflets at the time of initial mitral re-repair. In our own patient series, a quarter of cases were third time mitral re-repairs for recurrent mitral regurgitation due to leaflet shortening.

19.9 Ischemic mitral regurgitation

19.9.1 Technique

Severe leaflet restriction is encountered in ischemic mitral regurgitation and probably results from a combination of ventricular dilatation leading to papillary muscle displacement posteriorly, myocardial dysfunction, and annular dilatation in the setting of severe ischemic cardiomyopathy. The most effective method of repair involves rigid down-sized remodeling annuloplasty rings, some of which are designed to facilitate asymmetrical down-sizing of the P3 area of the mitral annulus, together with dividing secondary chordae restricting leaflet motion. The small size of annuloplasty ring sometimes required to achieve a satisfactory area of coaptation has been associated with functional mitral stenosis postoperatively. Kincaid et al. [3] describe their experience in 25 adult patients operated on for ischemic mitral regurgitation between 2002 and 2003, using posterior leaflet augmentation with bovine pericardium, with the aim of avoiding the need to downsize the annuloplasty ring to achieve a competent repair. A 1 cm by 3 cm patch is sewn lengthways into a linear incision made in the anterior leaflet, parallel to the anterior annulus, approximately 5 mm from the hinge area. A flexible annuloplasty band is then secured after true-sizing the intertrigonal distance. This approach has not seen wide-spread uptake, possibly because of good results that can more reliably be obtained with the simpler approach of down-sized rigid ring and chordal cutting.

19.9.2 Results

Operative mortality reported by Kincaid et al. [3] for pericardial patch augmentation in ischemic mitral regurgitation in their small series was 12%, and on intraoperative transesophageal echocardiography all patients had mild or less residual mitral regurgitation. At mean follow-up of 13 months, 2 patients had at least moderate mitral regurgitation, including 1 patient with partial dehiscence of the pericardial patch. Mitral stenosis and abnormal systolic anterior motion were not observed in any patients, and no patients underwent reoperation.

19.10 Congenital mitral valve disease

Two groups have described satisfactory midterm outcomes with pericardial patch leaflet augmentation in congenital valve lesions, including cleft mitral leaflet, »hammock« mitral valve, annular dilatation, and chordal shortening [5, 17]. Long-term follow-up was not specifically provided for mitral repairs involving pericardial patches, but overall durability of repair appeared superior to that of replacement in this age group.

19.11 Summary

Autologous glutaraldehyde-fixed pericardial patch augmentation pericardium is an effective and reliable adjunct to standard mitral valve repair techniques, for mitral regurgitation due to a variety of etiologies which result in inadequate leaflet tissue to otherwise permit a competent and durable repair.

References

1. Bonow RO, Carabello BA, Kanu C, et al. (2006) ACC/AHA 2006 guidelines for the management of patients with valvular heart disease: a report of the American College of Cardiology/American Heart Association Task Force on Practice Guidelines (writing committee to revise the 1998 Guidelines for the Management of Patients With Valvular Heart Disease): developed in collaboration with the Society of Cardiovascular Anesthesiologists: endorsed by the Society for Cardiovascular Angiography and Interventions and the Society of Thoracic Surgeons. Circulation 114:e84–231
2. Romano MA, Patel HJ, Pagani FD, Prager RL, Deeb GM, Bolling SF (2005) Anterior leaflet repair with patch augmentation for mitral regurgitation. Ann Thorac Surg 79:1500–1504; discussion 1504
3. Kincaid EH, Riley RD, Hines MH, Hammon JW, Kon ND (2004) Anterior leaflet augmentation for ischemic mitral regurgitation. Ann Thorac Surg 78:564–568; discussion 568

4. Ushijima T, Kikuchi Y, Takata M, Yamamoto Y, Kawachi K, Watanabe G (2009) Commissural autologous pericardial patch repair: a novel technique for active mitral valve endocarditis involving the mitral annulus. Ann Thorac Surg 88:e29–30
5. Chauvaud S, Fuzellier JF, Houel R, Berrebi A, Mihaileanu S, Carpentier A (1998) Reconstructive surgery in congenital mitral valve insufficiency (Carpentier's techniques): long-term results. J Thorac Cardiovasc Surg 115:84–92; discussion 93
6. Suri RM, Schaff HV, Dearani JA, et al. (2006) Recurrent mitral regurgitation after repair: should the mitral valve be re-repaired? J Thorac Cardiovasc Surg 132:1390–1397
7. van der Spuy JC (1972) Mitral valve pericardioplasty—a long-term follow-up study. Thorax 27:207–211
8. Carpentier A (2007) Lasker Clinical Research Award. The surprising rise of nonthrombogenic valvular surgery. Nat Med 13:1165–1168
9. Vincentelli A, Zegdi R, Prat A, et al. (1998) Mechanical modifications to human pericardium after a brief immersion in 0.625% glutaraldehyde. J Heart Valve Dis 7:24–29
10. Anyanwu AC, Adams DH (2007) The intraoperative »ink test«: a novel assessment tool in mitral valve repair. J Thorac Cardiovasc Surg 133:1635–1636
11. Chauvaud S, Jebara V, Chachques JC, et al. (1991) Valve extension with glutaraldehyde-preserved autologous pericardium. Results in mitral valve repair. J Thorac Cardiovasc Surg 102:171–177; discussion 177–178
12. Zegdi R, Debieche M, Latremouille C, et al. (2005) Long-term results of mitral valve repair in active endocarditis. Circulation 111:2532–2536
13. Aubert S, Flecher E, Rubin S, Acar C, Gandjbakhch I (2007) Anterior mitral leaflet augmentation with autologous pericardium. Ann Thorac Surg 83:1560–1561
14. Zegdi R, Khabbaz Z, Chauvaud S, Latremouille C, Fabiani JN, Deloche A (2007) Posterior leaflet extension with an autologous pericardial patch in rheumatic mitral insufficiency. Ann Thorac Surg 84:1043–1044
15. Chauvaud S, Fuzellier JF, Berrebi A, Deloche A, Fabiani JN, Carpentier A (2001) Long-term (29 years) results of reconstructive surgery in rheumatic mitral valve insufficiency. Circulation 104:I12–15
16. Gillinov AM, Cosgrove DM, Lytle BW, et al. (1997) Reoperation for failure of mitral valve repair. J Thorac Cardiovasc Surg 113:467–473; discussion 473–475
17. Oppido G, Davies B, McMullan DM, et al. (2008) Surgical treatment of congenital mitral valve disease: midterm results of a repair-oriented policy. J Thorac Cardiovasc Surg 135:1313–1320; discussion 1320–1321
18. Carpentier A, Adams DH, Filsoufi F (2010) Carpentier's Valve Reconstruction. Elsevier

Mitral valve repair for active infective endocarditis

A 20-year, single center experience

M. Musci, M. Hübler, A. Amiri, M. Pasic, Y. Weng, R. Hetzer

20.1 Introduction

In the treatment of degenerative severe mitral regurgitation, there is a general consensus and well-accepted class 1 grade A level evidence for preferring mitral valve (MV) repair over MV replacement [1]. If MV repair is feasible, it has been shown to reduce operative mortality and improve long-term survival and functional status in the comparison with MV replacement [2].

In the mid 1960s, valve replacement was proposed for patients with MV endocarditis by Robicsek and coauthors [3]. In 1990, Dreyfus et al. [4] were the first to demonstrate the feasibility of MV repair in active infective endocarditis (AIE), introducing the concept of early surgery to prevent further destruction of the valve. Since this report, others have confirmed the feasibility of MV repair and better survival than with MV replacement in patients undergoing surgery for either active or healed endocarditis [5, 6]. However, these observations, which are based on data derived from studies with small sample sizes and limited follow-ups, are mostly not comparable with each other because of their heterogeneity [7–9]. For these reasons, this study was undertaken to review the 20-year experience of surgical treatment for isolated active infective MV endocarditis undergoing MV repair at the Deutsches Herzzentrum Berlin. Goals of this retrospective study were to (1) analyze early and long-term survival, (2) identify reinfection rate and freedom from reoperation, (3) find clinical differences between MV repair and replacement patients, and finally (4) determine independent risk factors for early mortality (≤30 days) by the application of univariate and multivariate analyses.

20.2 Patients and methods

20.2.1 Patient population

Between May 1986 and December 2007, a total of 1,163 patients with active infective endocarditis (AIE) were operated on at the Deutsches Herzzentrum Berlin (see ◘ Table 20.1 for an overview of the patient population). Of these, 497 patients showed endocarditis involvement of the mitral valve (MV). To exclude the effect of other associated valve operations on outcome, only patients with isolated MV repair (*n*=61) were enrolled in the study. The comparison group for the analysis of the clinical differences consisted of consecutive patients undergoing single MV replacement (*n*=219) during the same period.

◘ **Table 20.1.** Patient population. Demographic and clinical differences between patients with MV repair and MV replacement

Period 05/86–12/2007 Patients with AIE	MV repair (*n*=61)	MV replacement (*n*=219)	p value
Men	40 (66%)	134 (61%)	
Women	21 (34%)	85 (39%)	
Total	61	219	0.485
Age in years			
Median	49	58	
Mean	47.7±2.4	56.2±1.03	<0.001
Range	11–80	7–84	

Table 20.1. *Continued*

Endocarditis			
Native AIE	61	166 (76%)	–
Prosthetic AIE	–	53 (24%)	
Preoperative status			
Cardiogenic shock	–	15 (7%)	0.045
High-dose catecholamines	4 (6%)	41 (19%)	0.024
Pulmonary edema	4 (6%)	45 (20%)	0.010
Intubation	6 (10%)	56 (25%)	0.008
Septic shock	2 (3%)	21 (9%)	0.107
Renal insufficiency	19 (31%)	71 (32%)	0.906
Fever	12 (20%)	80 (36%)	0.053
Cerebral embolization	24 (39%)	54 (25%)	0.028
Spleen embolization	4 (6%)	33 (15%)	0.077
Abscess formation	6 (10%)	43 (20%)	0.069
Intravenous drug abuse	4 (6%)	9 (4%)	0.744
Days from infection until operation			
Median (range)	38 (4–324)	32 (1–315)	0.043
Operation performed as			
Elective	14 (23%)	35 (16%)	
Urgent	38 (62%)	113 (52%)	
Emergency	9 (15%)	71 (32%)	0.023
Type of prosthesis			
Bioprosthesis	–	127 (58%)	–
Mechanical prosthesis	–	92 (42%)	–
Concomitant bypass operation	4 (6%)	24 (11%)	0.145
Microbiological epidemiology			
Staphylococci	18 (30%)	79 (36%)	0.307
S. aureus	*15 (25%)*	*53 (24%)*	0.993
S. coag. neg.	–	*13 (6%)*	0.050
S. epidermidis	–	*8 (4%)*	0.127
MRSA	*2 (3%)*	*3 (1%)*	–
Others	*1 (2%)*	*2 (1%)*	–
Streptococci	27 (44%)	46 (21%)	<0.001
S. viridans	*8 (13%)*	*14 (6%)*	0.091
S. ß-hemolys.	*5 (8%)*	*4 (2%)*	0.014
S. general	*14 (23%)*	*26 (12%)*	0.032
S. epidermidis	–	*2 (1%)*	–
Enterococcus	3 (5%)	22 (10%)	0.205
Culture negative	10 (16%)	31 (14%)	0.692
Others	1 (2%)	13 (6%)	–
Unknown	2 (3%)	28 (13%)	0.032
Follow-up			
Completed (%)	97	96	
Median (years)	4	2	
Range (years)	0–21	0–19	
Patient–years	348	810	

AIE Active infective endocarditis, *MV* Mitral valve, *MRSA* multiresistant Staphylococcus aureus

Follow-up was completed by telephone contact with the patient, by analyzing standardized mail questionnaires sent to the patients, by consulting the population registry, and by contacting peripheral hospitals. In the repair group, 2 patients were lost to follow-up, while 97% of all survivors were followed up for a median of 4 years (range 0–21 years) and 348 patient–years. In the replacement group, 8 patients were lost to follow-up. Thus, 96% of all survivors were followed up for a median of 2 years (range 0–19 years) and 810 patient–years.

20.2.2 Indications for surgery and operations performed

An overview of the main operative indications during the acute phase of AIE is given in Table 20.2. In general, patients had several indications for surgery during antibiotic treatment for AIE. The majority had to be operated on due to suspected MV vegetations, progressive heart failure, severe mitral insufficiency due to leaflet destruction, recurrent septic embolism, or therapy-resistant infections.

20.2.3 Surgical strategy for active infective MV endocarditis

All operations were performed through a median sternotomy on full cardiopulmonary bypass between the two caval veins and the ascending aorta. Until 1999, antegrade cold crystalloid cardioplegia with topical ice slush and with mild systemic hypothermia (32 °C) was used; later this was replaced by normothermic blood cardioplegia.

Our surgical strategy for active infective endocarditis is based on three principles:

- Intensive and wide debridement of all macroscopically involved tissue without concern for the possibility of repair. If the infected process is localized on the valve, vegetectomy followed by intensive irrigation of the infected area with polyvidone iodine solution is performed. Excision of a vegetation alone is limited to patients with a well-circumscribed vegetation and a well-defined shaft in an otherwise normal valve. If the vegetation has a wide base and no well-defined shaft, the base is also excised.
- Whenever possible, valve defects which emerge from vegetectomy are repaired with homologous or autologous pericardium using monofilament sutures reinforced with horse pericardium and preserved in polyvidone-iodine solution. To ensure leaflet coaptation, annuloplasty with pericardium is performed. In order to avoid artificial material in an infected field, no prosthetic ring annuloplasty device is used.
- If valve replacement is unavoidable because of extensive endocarditic destruction of the leaflets or due to the poor quality of the remaining tissue, MV replacement is performed. Until 1999, either biological or mechanical prostheses were implanted in the patients depending on the surgeon's decision. Over the past 8 years, the Shelhigh® MV bioprosthesis, which is a biological substitute without any artificial material on the surface that might become infected, has been used in all cases [10].

A summary of surgical techniques used for MV repair in our study population is given in Table 20.3. Depending on the various pathologies found in the patients, several techniques of leaflet and ring plasty were applied to achieve MV continence. At our institution, the classical techniques (Gerbode, Kay-Wooler, Paneth) were used (Table 20.3). A limitation of our technique is posed by extensive endocarditic destruction of the leaflets, especially of the

Table 20.2 Summary of main indications for surgery

Indication	MV repair	MV replacement
Suspected MV vegetations	54 (88%)	134 (61%)
Progressive heart failure	32 (52%)	153 (70%)
Severe mitral insufficiency due to leaflet destruction	25 (40%)	98 (45%)
Recurrent septic embolism	30 (49%)	81 (37%)
Therapy-resistant septic infection	8 (13%)	50 (23%)
Abscess formation	6 (10%)	43 (20%)
Prosthetic endocarditis	0	53 (24%)
Prosthetic reinfection	0	13 (6%)
– Early ≤60 days	0	4
– Late >60 days–1 year	0	5
– 1–2 years	0	4

MV mitral valve

Table 20.3. Summary of surgical techniques used for MV repair in active infective MV endocarditis

Surgical techniques	Patients
Leaflet plasty	**61 (100%)**
Gerbode	25 (40%)
Commissuroplasty	10 (16%)
Resection of leaflet parts	42 (69%)
Simple suture	10 (16%)
Pericardial patch reconstruction	4 (6%)
Ring plasty	**37 (61%)**
Paneth + posterior annulus pericardial strip plasty	29 (487%)
Kay-Wooler	5 (8%)
Others	3 (5%)

anterior leaflet. There was no insertion of new chordae in these patients. Posterior annulus pericardial strip plasty with autologous pericardium, which was used in 61% of our study patients, has become the standard technique for all patients undergoing MV repair to ensure leaflet coaptation.

An intraoperative view of a posterior leaflet vegetation with infected posterior annulus is shown in Fig. 20.1a, while a schematic drawing and an operative view of the Gerbode plasty and the posterior annulus pericardial strip plasty after vegetectomy and debridement of the infected tissue of the posterior annulus are shown in Fig. 20.1b and 20.1c.

An intraoperative view of an anterior leaflet defect is shown in Fig. 20.2a. After reconstruction of the defect with homologous pericardium (Fig. 20.2b), a posterior annulus pericardial strip plasty is performed to ensure MV reconstruction (Fig. 20.2c).

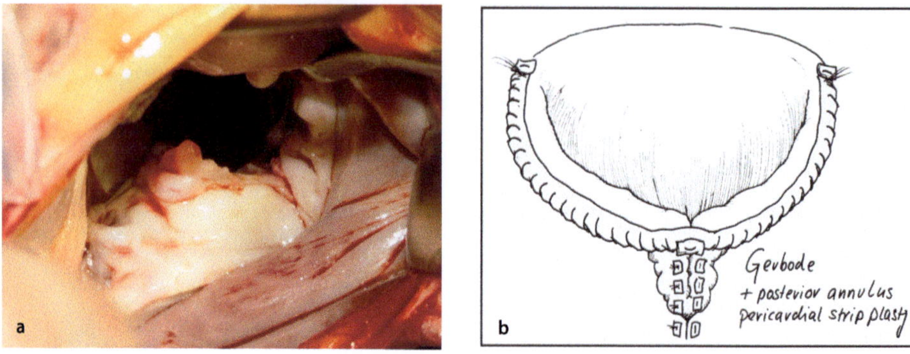

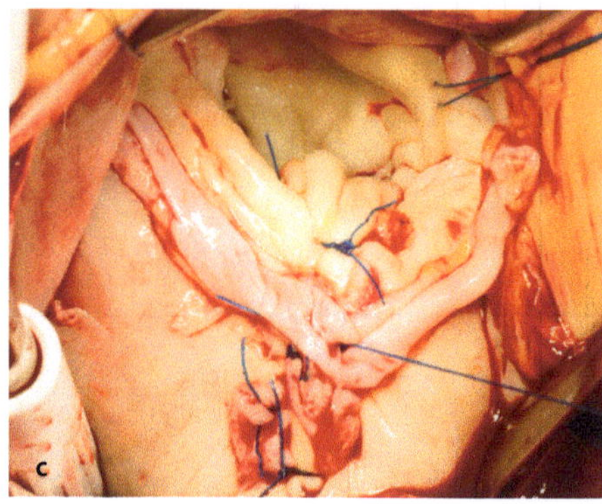

Fig. 20.1. Intraoperative view of a posterior leaflet vegetation with infected posterior annulus(**a**). Drawn (**b**) and operative view (**c**) of the Gerbode plasty and the posterior annulus pericardial strip plasty after vegetectomy and debridement of the infected tissue of the posterior annulus

20.2.4 Definition of active infective endocarditis

AIE was defined on the basis of vegetations or an abscess in the echocardiogram and accompanied by positive blood cultures or intraoperatively harvested valve cultures, on the basis of clinical evidence of persistent sepsis or recurrent septic embolism, or on the basis of the intraoperative diagnosis.

It has to be taken into consideration that our hospital is a referral surgical center receiving patients who have already been medically treated elsewhere and sometimes coming for an operation as salvage therapy. All patients enrolled in the study had evidence of and were operated on during an active infective endocarditis process. Postinfectious MV endocarditis patients were excluded from the study.

20.2.5 Statistical analysis

SPSS for Windows version 12.01 was used. Qualitative data are presented as number (*n*) and percent. For quantitative data means±standard error were calculated. Analyses of survival and freedom from endpoints were performed according to Kaplan–Meier estimation. Survival in different patient groups was compared using the Gehan test.

A logistic regression model was applied to investigate possible risk factors for early mortality (<30 days). First, all possible risk factors were evaluated with a univariate approach,

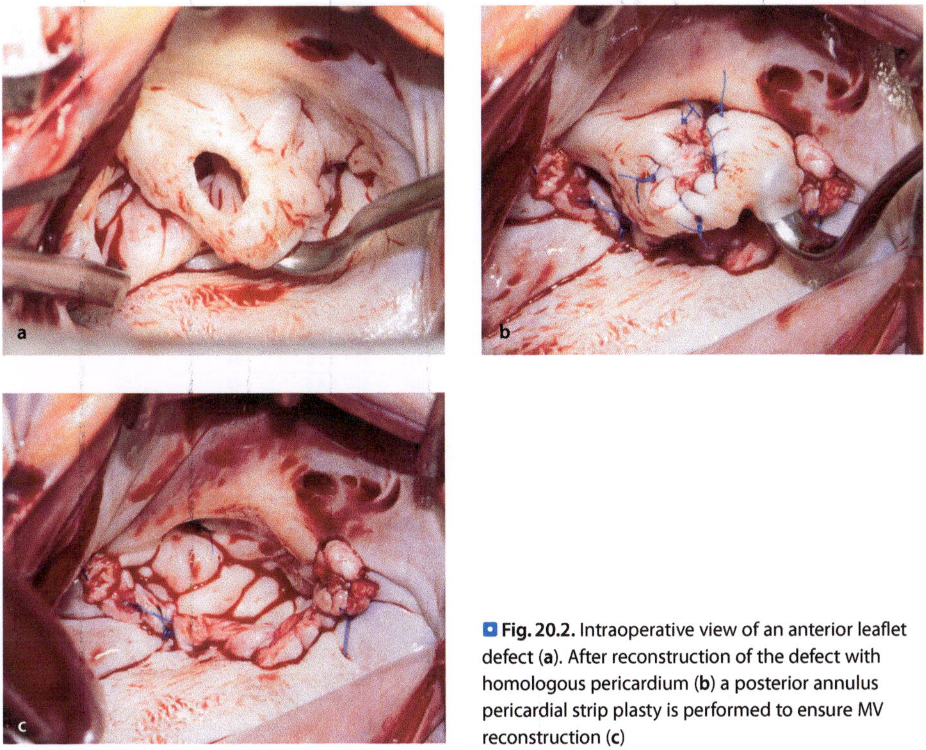

■ **Fig. 20.2.** Intraoperative view of an anterior leaflet defect (**a**). After reconstruction of the defect with homologous pericardium (**b**) a posterior annulus pericardial strip plasty is performed to ensure MV reconstruction (**c**)

followed by multivariate logistic regression with backward elimination procedure. Survivors and nonsurvivors were compared by Pearson's χ^2 test or Student's t test accordingly. A p value <0.05 was considered statistically significant.

20.3 Results

20.3.1 Early and long-term survival after MV repair

The 30-day, 1, 5, 10, and 15-year survival for the whole MV repair study population were 90.1±3.9%, 83.2±4.8%, 77.0±5.7%, 60.5±8.0%, and 60.5±8.0%, respectively (■ Fig. 20.3).

There was 1 intraoperative death due to myocardial failure (1.6%) and 6 (9.8%) early deaths (≤30 days), 2 from myocardial failure and 4 from septic multiorgan failure (MOF). After the period of between 1 month and 1 year, the survival curves run nearly parallel.

20.3.2 Freedom from reoperation after MV repair

Only 3 patients developed reinfection leading to reoperation following MV repair, thus resulting in excellent 30-day, 1, 5, 10, and 15 year freedom from reoperation rates due to reinfection of 100%, 96.3±2.6%, 96.3±2.6%, 89.4%±7.0%, and 89.4±7.0%, respectively (■ Fig. 20.4).

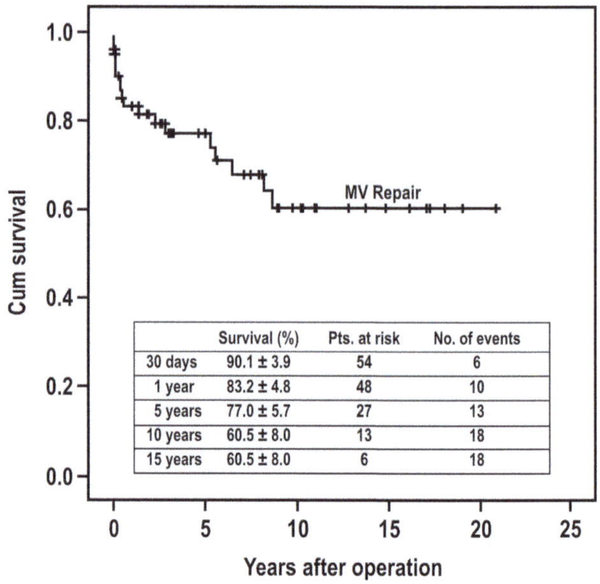

	Survival (%)	Pts. at risk	No. of events
30 days	90.1 ± 3.9	54	6
1 year	83.2 ± 4.8	48	10
5 years	77.0 ± 5.7	27	13
10 years	60.5 ± 8.0	13	18
15 years	60.5 ± 8.0	6	18

Fig. 20.3. Early and long-term survival after MV repair for active infective endocarditis

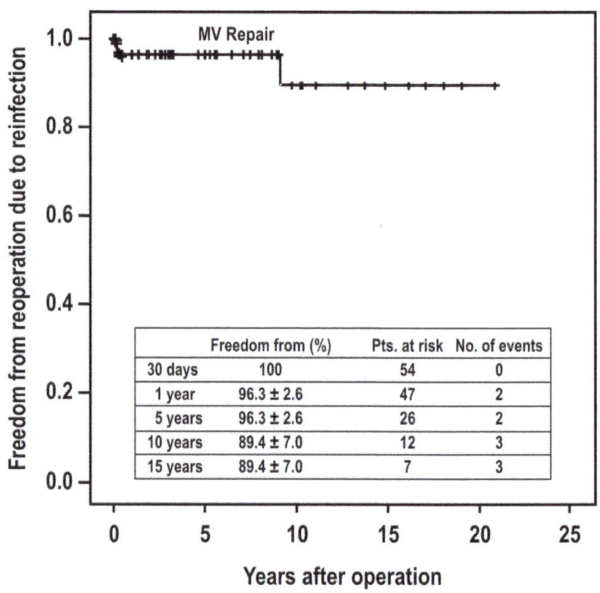

	Freedom from (%)	Pts. at risk	No. of events
30 days	100	54	0
1 year	96.3 ± 2.6	47	2
5 years	96.3 ± 2.6	26	2
10 years	89.4 ± 7.0	12	3
15 years	89.4 ± 7.0	7	3

Fig. 20.4. Freedom from reoperation due to reinfection after MV repair for active infective endocarditis

Analysis showed early reinfection (≤60 days) in 2 patients (3.2%) and late reinfection in the long-term follow-up (up to 10 years) in 1 patient (1.6%).

Analysis of reoperation due to valve-related events showed that another 8 patients required MV replacement due to insufficiency leading to a 30-day, 1, 5, 10, and 15-year freedom from reoperation due to all events after MV repair due to AIE of 96.5%±2.5%, 86.9%±4.6%, 84.8%±5.0%, 73.4%±8.8%, and 66.1%±10.5%, respectively (Fig. 20.5).

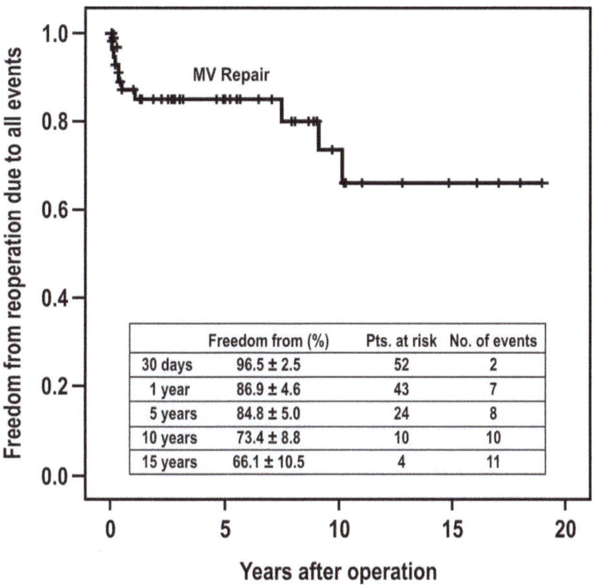

Fig. 20.5. Freedom from reoperation due to all events after MV repair for active infective endocarditis

20.3.3 Demographic and clinical differences between patients undergoing MV replacement and MV repair

Table 20.1 summarizes the demographic and clinical differences between patients undergoing MV replacement and MV repair. In summary, patients requiring MV replacement were significantly older (mean age 56 vs. 47 years, $p \leq 0.001$) and were, on average, more critically ill showing advanced endocarditis with annular destruction.

Analysis of the preoperative status showed replacement patients to more often have advanced cardiac decompensation ($p=0.045$), high-dose catecholamines ($p=0.024$), pulmonary edema ($p=0.010$), artificial ventilation ($p=0.008$), and emergency operation ($p=0.023$). They were operated on significantly earlier ($p=0.043$), whereas fever ($p=0.053$), spleen embolization ($p=0.077$), and abscess formation ($p=0.069$) showed only nonsignificant tendencies. In contrast, MV repair patients showed preoperative cerebral embolization and infection with Streptococci significantly more often ($p=0.028$).

20.3.4 Risk factors for early mortality

Univariate logistic regression analysis found 12 statistically significant risk factors for early mortality (≤30 days; Table 20.4). Not only the preoperative development of septic shock (OR 8.8), necessity of ventilation (OR 6.1), and high doses of catecholamines (OR 5.9), but also MV abscess formation (OR 5.4) and emergency operation (OR 4.0) showed the highest odds ratios. In the final step, multivariate analysis identified preoperative ventilation (OR 6.3), MV abscess formation (OR 5.3), prosthetic endocarditis (OR 3.1), and age ≥60 years (OR 2.8) as independent risk factors for early mortality.

Table 20.4. Risk factors for early mortality (≤30 days) in the univariate and multivariate logistic regression analysis after MV repair and MV replacement in active infective endocarditis

Risk factors	Odds Ratio	95% CI	p value
Univariate			
Preop. septic shock	8.8	3.5–21.8	≤0.001
Preop. ventilation	6.1	3.1–11.8	≤0.001
Preop. catecholamines	5.9	2.9–12.0	≤0.001
MV abscess formation	5.4	2.7–10.1	≤0.001
Emergency operation	4.0	1.2–13.6	≤0.001
Preop. cardiac shock	3.5	1.1–10.6	0.026
Preop. fever	3.1	1.7–5.8	≤0.001
Preop. renal insufficiency	2.7	1.4–5.0	0.002
Age >60 years	2.5	1.3–4.6	0.005
Prosthetic endocarditis	2.3	1.1–4.9	0.027
Preop. diabetes mellitus	2.2	1.1–4.4	0.020
Staphylococcal infection	2.0	1.1–3.8	0.024
Multivariate			
Preop. ventilation	6.3	3.0–13.1	≤0.001
MV abscess formation	5.3	2.4–11.5	≤0.001
Prosthetic endocarditis	3.1	1.3–7.3	0.009
Age >60 years	2.8	1.4–5.8	0.005

CI confidence interval, *Preop* preoperative, *Intraop* intraoperative, *MV* mitral valve

20.4 Discussion

Our study presents 20-year single center results in a group of high-risk patients with active infective MV endocarditis and analyzes the outcome of the patients who underwent MV repair. It has been shown that MV repair for AIE can be performed not only with low operative mortality and satisfactory early and long-term survival, but also with excellent freedom from recurrent infection and repeat operation. Our results are in accord with the well-accepted class 1 grade A level of evidence of better outcome after MV repair [1, 2] despite the fact that our patients were compromised preoperatively by AIE. Analysis of the survival curve demonstrates that there is a particularly clear difference in the first 30 days and in the period between 1 month and 1 year postoperatively, whereby after this period the curves nearly run parallel. In our study, causes of the 6 early deaths (9.8%) after MV repair were septic multiorgan failure in 4 patients (4/6, 66%) and myocardial failure in 2 patients (2/6, 34%) reflecting the poorer preoperative clinical condition of these patients. However, these results suggest that early outcome could have been improved if patients had been operated upon before heart failure or septic shock had developed [11, 12]. For the risk stratification and survival in our study, it has to be taken into consideration that our hospital is a referral surgical center receiving patients who have already been medically treated elsewhere and sometimes coming for an operation as ultima ratio therapy. This fact also explains the long median time between diagnosis and surgery observed in our study.

It can be argued that our good results after MV repair are related to the fact that there is a selection of the patients and that the patients undergoing MV replacement in general had more advanced endocarditis and were more critically ill. In our study, patients undergoing MV replacement were not only significantly older but preoperatively they had a significantly higher prevalence of advanced cardiac decompensation, high-dose catecholamines, pulmonary edema, and artificial ventilation. MV replacement patients were not only operated on earlier than repair patients but they had to undergo an emergency operation significantly more often. Each of these factors increases the clinical variability and complexity of active infective MV endocarditis and may represent an additional possible explanation.

Such data were confirmed by the results of our uni- and multivariate analyses of risk factors for early mortality (≤30 days) which showed correlations between the preoperatively compromised status of the patients arriving at our hospital and their outcome. But it is noteworthy that the inhospital period may not be an appropriate time frame to evaluate the mortality rate and clinical outcome of surgery in infective endocarditis and that the benefit may be seen in the long-term follow-up [13].

Our study is also in accord with recently published data by Feringa et al. [7] who presented a metaanalysis of 24 studies involving 470 patients undergoing MV repair and 724 patients undergoing MV replacement for endocarditis in the last decade. This review found that patients undergoing MV replacement had significantly poorer outcome not only with regard to early mortality (14% vs. 2%) and late mortality (40% vs. 8%) but also with regard to early (11% vs. 5%) and late cerebrovascular events (24% vs. 2%), need for reoperation (12% vs. 2%), and late recurrence of endocarditis (7% vs. 2%).

Potential concerns with MV repair are the possibility of recurrent infection due to incomplete resection of the infected field, the feasibility of the repair due to the extent of the infection, and the safety and long-term durability of the repair. In our study, we report not only a low early reinfection rate after MV repair but also excellent long-term freedom from operation due to reinfection. Our 10- and 15-year freedom from reoperation are supported by the results of various groups in the literature in which equivalent or even better long-term results have been reported. In addition, it has to be considered that the preoperative status of the patients also influences the surgeon's decision to repair or replace an infected MV [7, 14, 15]. Also it has to be mentioned that the degree of leaflet destruction is an important correlate of the likelihood of repair, with greater leaflet tissue destruction associated with a lower likelihood of repair.

Although it is a generally accepted principle to avoid placing prosthetic material in an infected field and in our group a pericardial band was used to stabilize the annulus in repair, the low reinfection rate leads to the advice in the literature that prosthetic ring annuloplasty may be used when the annulus is dilated to stabilize complex repair [9, 11].

20.5 Study limitations

The present study is retrospective. Clinical endpoints such as exercise capacity and echocardiographic hemodynamic control could not be assessed. There is a natural bias in the clinical selection of patients undergoing MV repair. Despite these limitations, the present study represents a unique attempt to collect and analyze a single-center experience and to investigate the outcome after MV repair in patients with AIE over a period of 20 years.

20.6 Conclusion

MV repair for AIE shows low operative mortality and provides excellent freedom from reoperation rates due to recurrent infection and satisfactory rates related to repeat operation due to all events.

If all infected material can be resected and the remaining tissue allows reshaping of a competent valve, we also recommend repairing the MV in the setting of AIE in line with the general recommendations for MV surgery. Thereby, after reconstruction we recommend performing a posterior annulus pericardial strip plasty with autologous or homologous pericardium to ensure leaflet coaptation. This has become the standard technique for all patients undergoing MV repair at our institution. In order to avoid artificial material in an infected field, we do not use any prosthetic ring annuloplasty devices.

Compared to the MV repair group, patients requiring MV replacement had more advanced endocarditis and were more critically ill. Patients with replacement were not only significantly older but preoperatively they had a significantly higher prevalence of advanced cardiac decompensation, high-dose catecholamines, pulmonary edema, and artificial ventilation. Our results suggest that early outcome could have been improved if patients had been operated upon before heart failure or septic shock developed.

Acknowledgments

We thank Ms. S. Kosky for her great help with data acquisition, Ms. J. Stein for statistical work, Ms. A. Benhennour for bibliographic assistance, Ms. K. Weber for photographic work, Dr. T. Komoda for the intraoperative photographs, and Ms. A. Gale for editorial assistance.

References

[1] Bonow RO, Carabello BA, Kanu C, et al. (2006) ACC/AHA 2006 guidelines for the management of patients with valvular heart disease: a report of the American College of Cardiology/American Heart Association Task Force on Practice Guidelines. Circulation 114:e84–231

[2] Moss RR, Humphries KH, Gao M, et al. (2003) Outcome of mitral valve repair or replacement: a comparison by propensity score analysis. Circulation 108:II90–97

[3] Robicsek F, Payne RB, Daugherty HK, Sanger PW (1967) Bacterial endocarditis of the mitral valve treated by excision and replacement. Ann Surg 166:854–857

[4] Dreyfus G, Serraf A, Jebara VA, et al. (1990) Valve repair in acute endocarditis. Ann Thorac Surg 49:706–713

[5] Fuzellier JF, Acar C, Jebara VA, et al. (1993) Plasties mitrales au cours de la phase aigue de l'endocardite. Arch Mal Coeur Vaiss 86:197–201

[6] Hendren WG, Morris AS, Rosenkranz ER, et al. (1992) Mitral valve repair for bacterial endocarditis. J Thorac Cardiovasc Surg 103:124–129

[7] Feringa HH, Shaw LJ, Poldermans D, et al. (2007) Mitral valve repair and replacement in endocarditis: a systematic review of literature. Ann Thorac Surg 83:564–570

[8] Iung B, Rousseau-Paziaud J, Cormier B, et al. (2004) Contemporary results of mitral valve repair for infective endocarditis. J Am Coll Cardiol 43:386–392

[9] Zegdi R, Debieche M, Latremouille C, et al. (2005) Long-term results of mitral valve repair in active endocarditis. Circulation 111:2532–2536

[10] Musci M, Siniawski H, Pasic M, et al. (2008) Surgical therapy in patients with active infective endocarditis: seven-year single centre experience in a subgroup of 255 patients treated with the Shelhigh® stentless bioprosthesis. Eur J Cardiothorac Surg 34:410–417

[11] de Kerchove L, Vanoverschelde JL, Poncelet A, et al. (2007) Reconstructive surgery in active mitral valve endocarditis: feasibility, safety and durability. Eur J Cardiothorac Surg 31:592–599

[12] Hill EE, Herregods MC, Vanderschueren S, Claus P, Peetermans WE, Herijgers P (2008) Outcome of patients requiring valve surgery during active infective endocarditis. Ann Thorac Surg 85:1564–1569

[13] Musci M, Siniawski H, Pasic M, et al. (2007) Surgical treatment of right-sided active infective endocarditis with or without involvement of the left heart: 20-year single center experience. Eur J Cardiothorac Surg 32:118–125

[14] Aranki SF, Adams DH, Rizzo RJ, et al. (1995) Determinants of early mortality and late survival in mitral valve endocarditis. Circulation 92:II143–149

[15] Moon MR, Miller DC, Moore KA, et al. (2001) Treatment of endocarditis with valve replacement: the question of tissue versus mechanical prosthesis. Ann Thorac Surg 71:1164–1171

VI Atlas of mitral and tricuspid annuloplasty rings

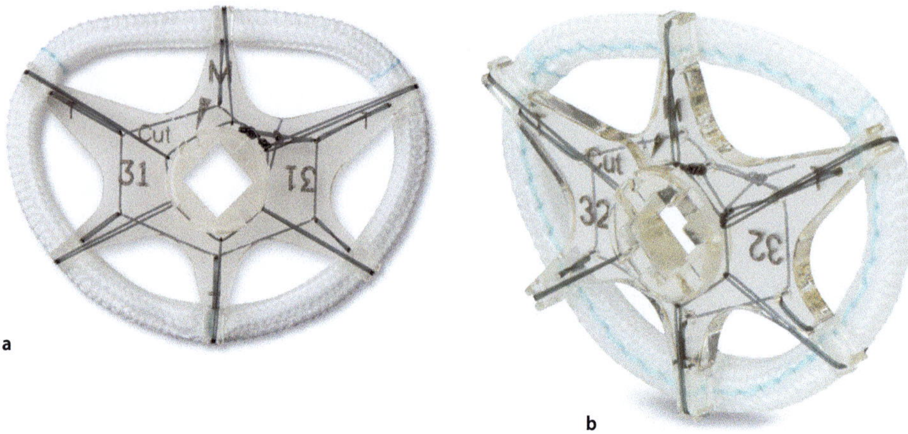

a

b

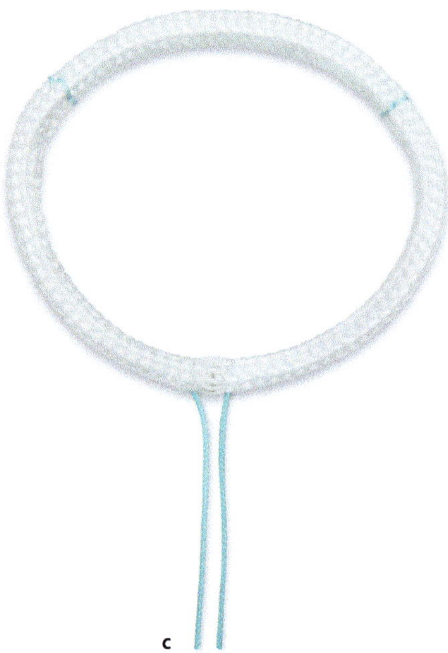

c

Fig. 21.1. ATS-Medtronic mitral annuloplasty rings
a Flexible mitral annuloplasty ring – 2006
b Semi-rigid mitral annuloplasty ring – 2008
c Adjustable mitral annuloplasty ring – under clinical investigation

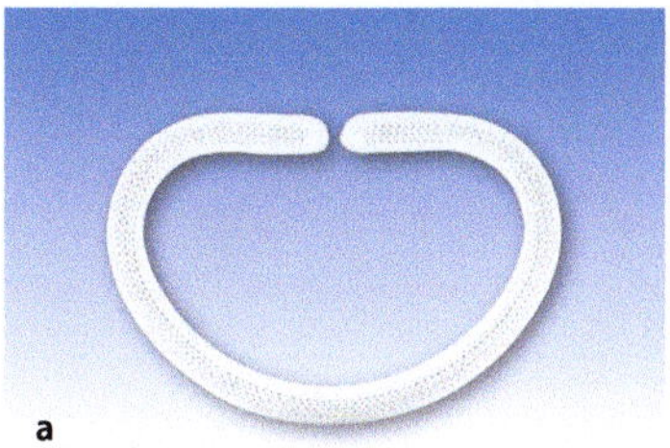

a

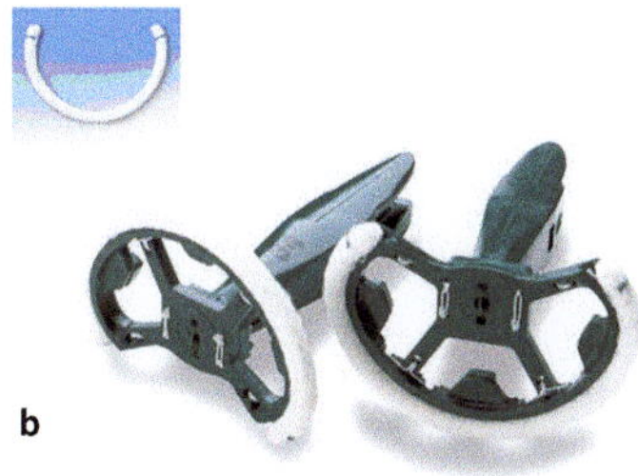

b

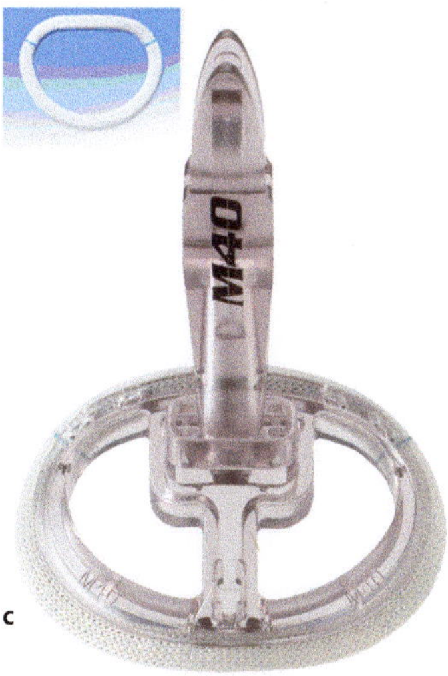

c

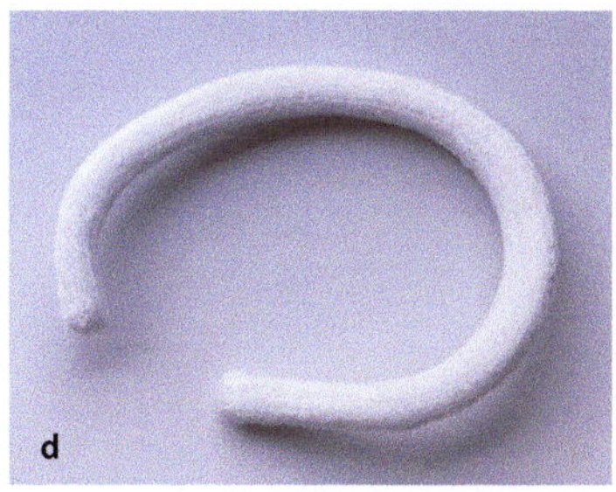

d

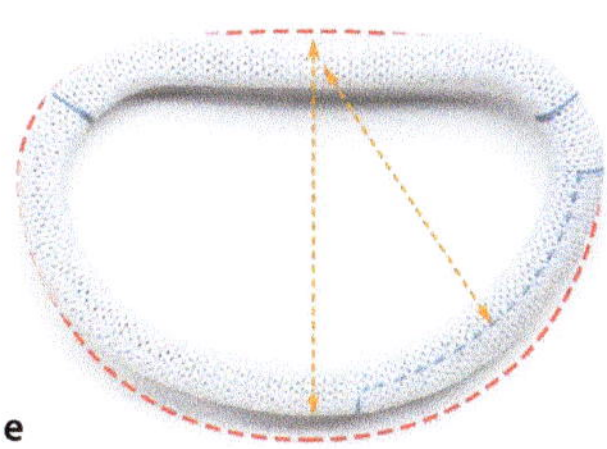

e

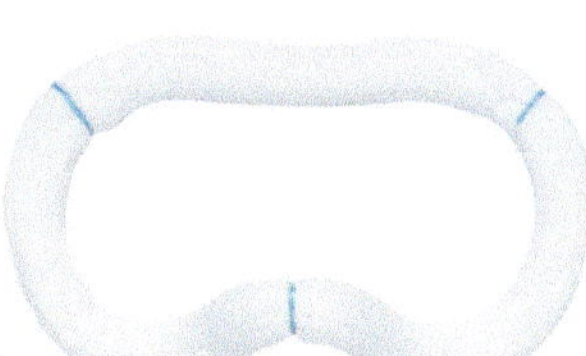

f

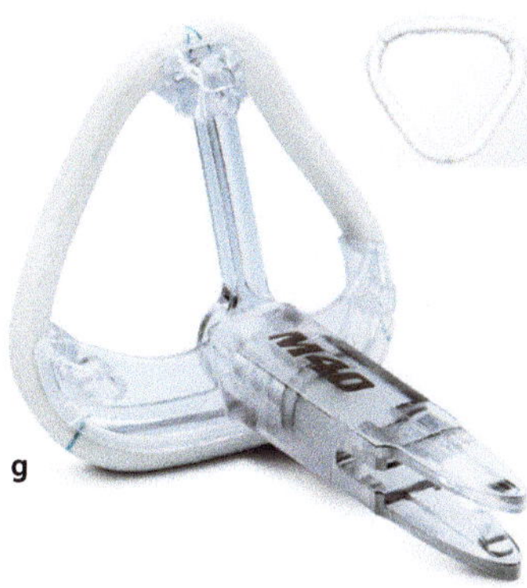

g

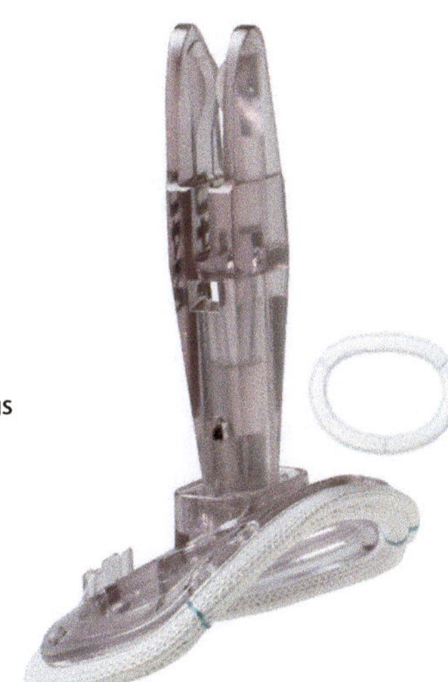

h

Fig. 21.2. Edwards Lifesciences mitral and tricuspid annuloplasty rings
a Carpentier–Edwards classic mitral annuloplasty ring – 1968
b Cosgrove–Edwards Band – 1993
c Carpentier Edwards Physio annuloplasty ring – 1993
d Edwards MC3 Tricuspid annuloplasty system – 2001
e Carpentier–McCarthy–Adams IMR Etlogix ring – 2004
f GeoForm ring – 2005
g Edwards 133 Myxo Etlogix – 2007
h Carpentier Edwards Physio II annuloplasty ring – 2009

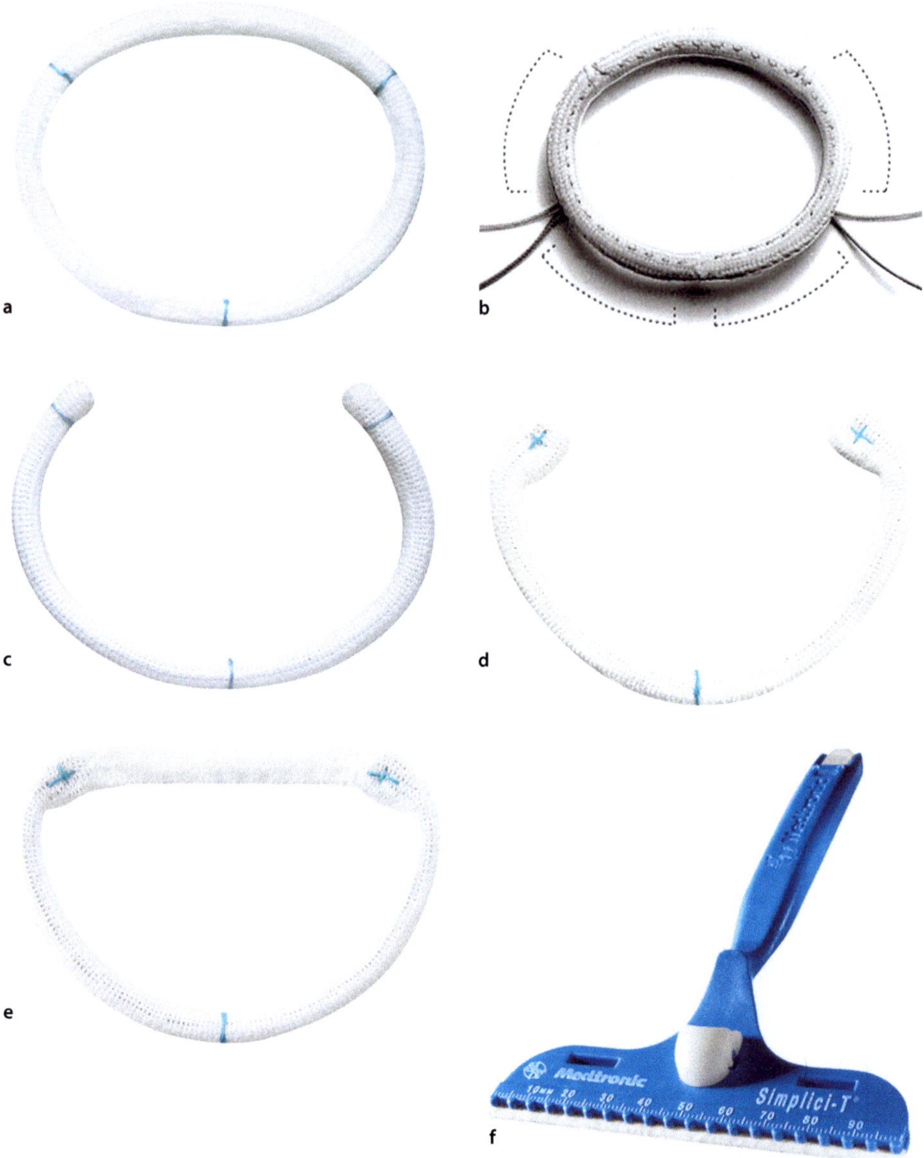

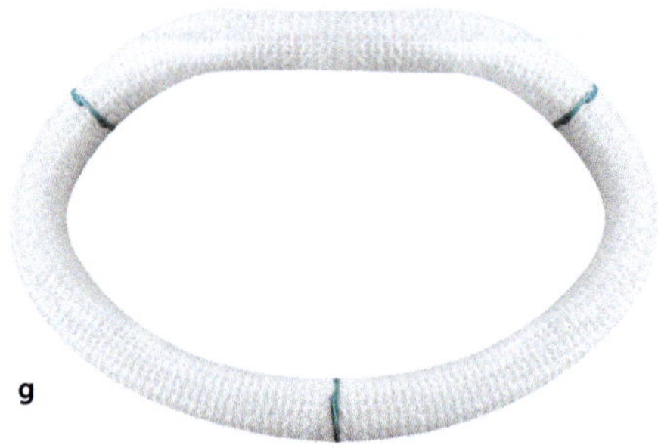

Fig. 21.3. Medtronic mitral annuloplasty rings
a Duran AnCore Ring, flexible – 1975
b Sculptor adjustable D-ring – 1993
c Duran AnCore Band, flexible – 1999
d CG Future Band, semi-rigid – 2001
e CG Future Ring, semi-rigid – 2005
f Simplici-T Band, flexible – 2005
g Profile 3D Ring, rigid – 2008

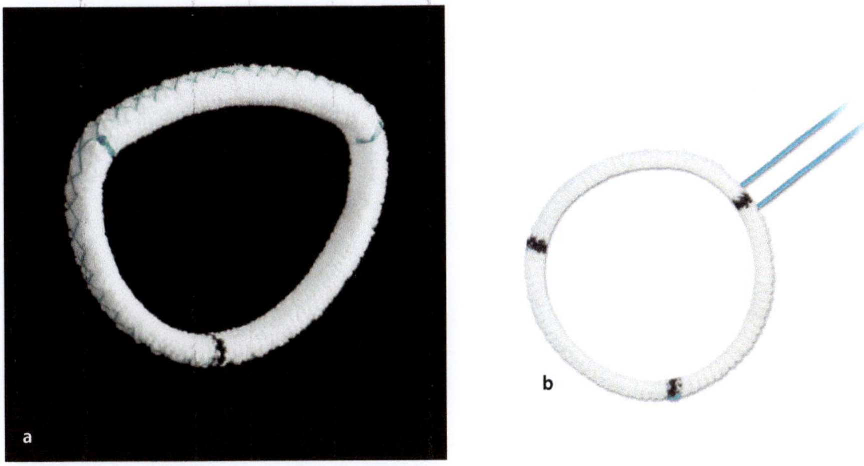

a b

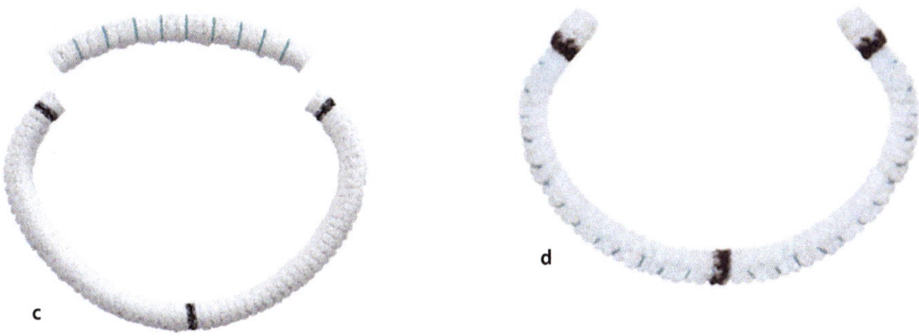

c d

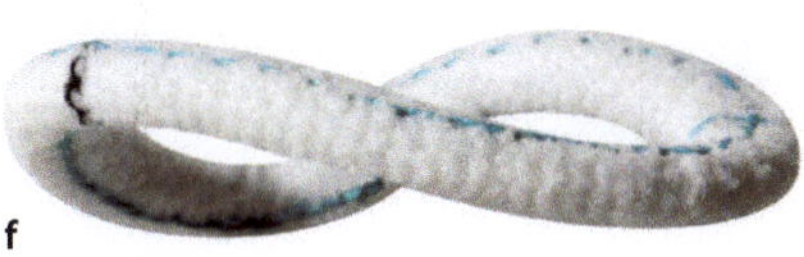

f

Fig. 21.4. St. Jude Medical mitral annuloplasty rings
a Seguin Ring – 1996
b Attune Ring – 2009
c Tailor Ring – 2000
d Tailor Band –2002
e Rigid Saddle Ring – 2005

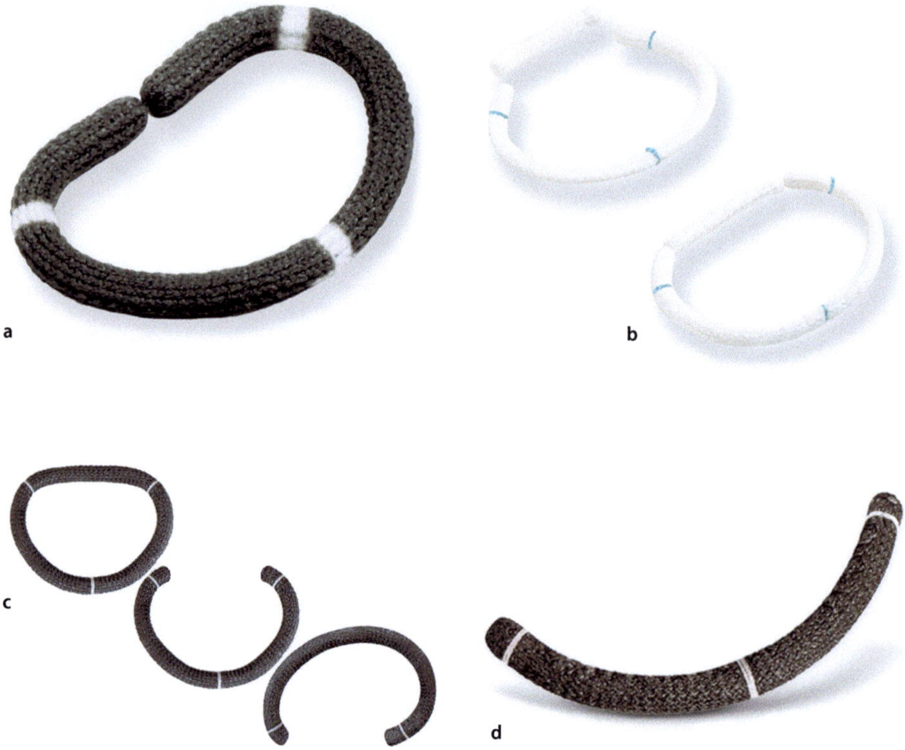

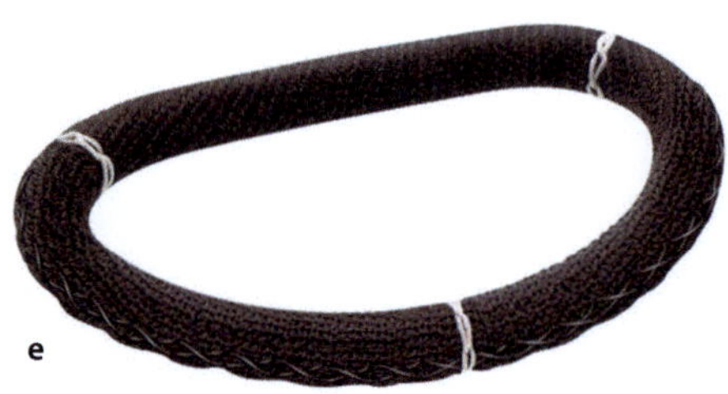

Fig. 21.5. Sorin mitral annuloplasty rings and tricuspid bands
a AnnuloFlo – 1997
b AnnuloFlex – 1999
c Sovering Family – 2001 (Mitral closed ring, Mitral band, Tricuspid band)
d Miniband – 2002
e Memo 3D – 2005

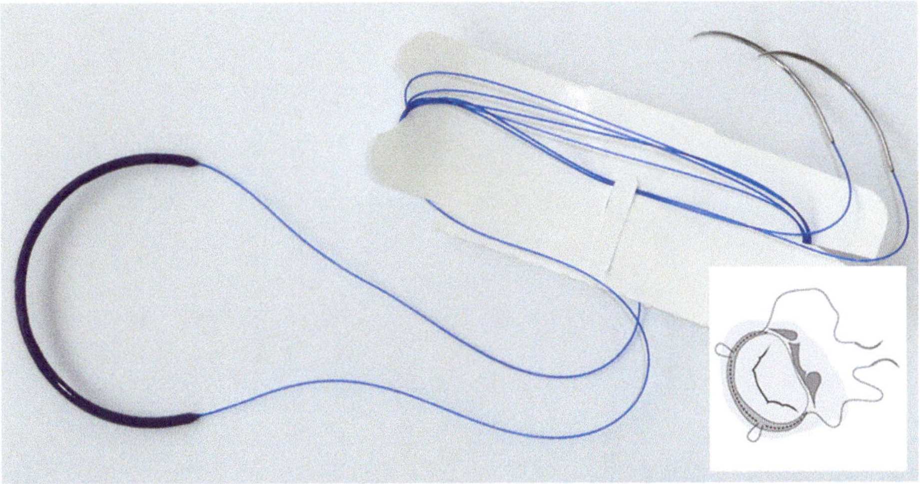

Fig. 21.6. Kalangos Bioring SA biodegradable mitral annuloplasty ring. A re-absorbable polymeric »C« curved segment of poly-1,4-dioxanone polymer which is fixed on the posterior mitral annulus by a 2-0 double-arm monofilament polyvinylidene fluoride (PVDF) suture with a stainless steel needle – 2004

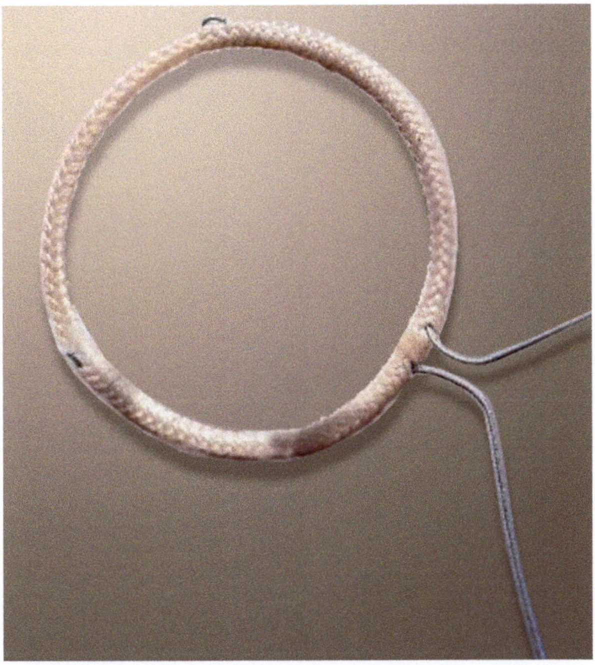

Fig. 21.7. Shiley mitral annuloplasty ring
Puig–Massana–Shiley ring

VII Acknowledgments

Roland Hetzer, J. Scott Rankin, Charles A. Yankah

We are greatly indebted to the authors of the various chapters who are sharing their great knowledge and experience with the readership. To all contributors as well as the manufacturers who provided images for the atlas of the mitral annuloplasty rings, we express our thanks.

In particular, we also thank the Presidents of the Society for Heart Valve Disease, Professor Friedrich W. Mohr, and of the Heart Valve Society of America, Dr. Jeffrey S. Borer, for inviting the Deutsches Herzzentrum Berlin to host the special Mitral Valve Repair session on Monday, June 29, 2009 at the 5th biennial meeting of the Society for Heart Valve Disease from June 27–30, 2009 in Berlin.

Similarly, we are indebted to the Gesellschaft der Freunde des Deutschen Herzzentrums Berlin (President: Professor Peter Fissenewert) for sponsoring the publication of the proceedings of the Mitral Valve Repair session.

We thank not only Ulrike Daechert for the excellent planning and preparation but also all those at Springer publishers in Heidelberg who did their utmost to publish the proceedings on time. We would also like to express our thanks to Anne Gale for editorial assistance, Astrid Benhennour for bibliographic support, and Carla Weber and Helge Haselbach for the graphic design.

VIII Subject Index

A

B

C

D

E

F

G

H

I

L

M

N

O

P

R

S

T

V

MIX
Papier aus verantwortungsvollen Quellen
Paper from responsible sources
FSC® C105338

If you have any concerns about our products,
you can contact us on
ProductSafety@springernature.com

In case Publisher is established outside the EU,
the EU authorized representative is:
Springer Nature Customer Service Center GmbH
Europaplatz 3, 69115 Heidelberg, Germany

Printed by Libri Plureos GmbH
in Hamburg, Germany